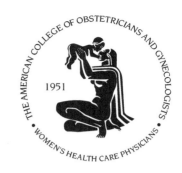

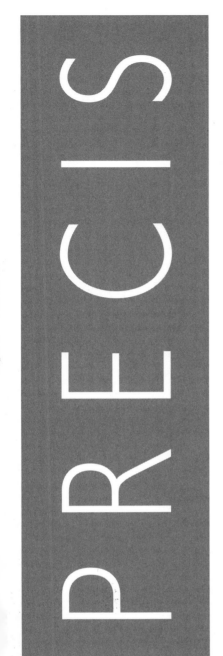

PRECIS

an update in obstetrics and gynecology

Obstetrics

Third Edition

Library of Congress Cataloging-in-Publication Data

Precis : an update in obstetrics and gynecology. Obstetrics.--3rd ed.
     p. ; cm.
Includes bibliographical references and index.
ISBN 1-932328-11-4 (alk. paper)
1. Obstetrics--Outlines, syllabi, etc.
[DNLM: 1. Pregnancy. 2. Delivery, Obstetric. 3. Postpartum Period. 4. Pregnancy Complications. 5. Prenatal Care. 6. Prenatal Diagnosis.]
I. Title: Obstetrics. II.American College of Obstetricians and Gynecologists.

RG533.P74 2005
618.2--dc22

2004029734

The American College of Obstetricians and Gynecologists
409 12th Street, SW
PO Box 96920
Washington, DC 20090-6920

12345/98765

Contents

Contributors

EDITORIAL COMMITTEE

Gary D. V. Hankins, MD, Chair

Radek K. Bukowski, MD

Harold E. Fox, MD

Larry C. Gilstrap III, MD

Charles J. Lockwood, MD

J. Gerald Quirk, MD

Laura E. Riley, MD

David B. Schwartz, MD

Paul B. Tomich, MD

Katharine D. Wenstrom, MD

Isabelle A. Wilkins, MD

ADVISORY COMMITTEE

Donald R. Coustan, MD

Leo J. Dunn, MD

Roger P. Smith, MD

AUTHORS

Pamela Donovan Berens, MD
The Puerperium

Radek K. Bukowski, MD
Intrauterine Growth Restriction

Steven L. Clark, MD
Cardiac Disease

Jane Cleary-Goldman, MD
Multiple Gestation

David S. Cooper, MD
Thyroid Diseases

Donald R. Coustan, MD
Diabetes Mellitus

Donna S. Dizon-Townson, MD
Immunologic Disorders

Leo J. Dunn, MD
Dermatologic Disease

Bruce Flamm, MD
Cesarean Birth, Vaginal Birth After Cesarean
Delivery, Cesarean and Puerperal Hysterectomy,
Perimortem Cesarean

Robert B. Gherman, MD
External Cephalic Version, Shoulder Dystocia,
Fetal and Neonatal Injuries

Larry C. Gilstrap III, MD
Hypertension, Postterm Gestation, Corticosteroid
Therapy, Chronic Hypertension, Fetal Acidemia

Gary D. V. Hankins, MD
Vaginal Breech Delivery

Hassan Harirah, MD
Vaginal Breech Delivery

Joy A. Hawkins, MD
Obstetric Anesthesia and Analgesia

Jay D. Iams, MD
Preterm Labor and Delivery

Donna D. Johnson, MD
Bleeding in the Second Half of Pregnancy

David C. Jones, MD
Renal Disease

Paul W. Ladenson, MD
Thyroid Diseases

Susan M. Lanni, MD
Dermatologic Disease

George A. Little, MD
Neonatal Resuscitation

Charles J. Lockwood, MD
Preconceptional and Routine Antepartum Care,
Endocrinology of Pregnancy, Preterm Labor and
Delivery

Brian Mercer, MD
Premature Rupture of Membranes

Kenneth J. Moise Jr, MD
Fetal Therapy

Thomas E. Nolan, MD
Liver and Alimentary Tract Diseases

Michael Paidas, MD
Hematologic Disorders

Thomas C. Peng, MD
Neurologic Diseases

Charles N. Petty, MD
Acute and Chronic Pain, Headaches

J. Gerald Quirk, MD
Deep Vein Thrombosis and Pulmonary Embolism,
Surgical Complications

Susan M. Ramin, MD
Hypertension, Postterm Gestation, Corticosteroid
Therapy, Chronic Hypertension, Fetal Acidemia

Julian N. Robinson, MD
Multiple Gestation

Andrew J. Satin, MD
Labor Stimulation, Intrapartum Fetal Heart Rate
Monitoring

Megan V. Smith, MPH
Depression During Pregnancy and the Postpartum
Period

David E. Soper, MD
Infection

Catherine Y. Spong, MD
Fetal Death

Paul J. Wendel, MD
Pulmonary Disorders

Katharine D. Wenstrom, MD
Prenatal Diagnosis of Genetic Disorders,
Teratogenic Exposures

Isabelle A. Wilkins, MD
Ultrasonography

Edward R. Yeomans, MD
Forceps Delivery, Vacuum Extraction

Kimberly Yonkers, MD
Depression During Pregnancy and the Postpartum
Period

Staff

Sterling B. Williams, MD
Vice President of Education

Rebecca R. Rinehart
Director of Publications

Joyce Leinberger Mitchell
Senior Editor

Preface

Education is a lifelong process. In no field other than medicine is this process more important. As scientific advances unfold, new techniques and technologies emerge, knowledge expands, and the art and science of medicine undergo dynamic change. Progress in medicine is ongoing, and so too must be the continuing medical education of those in practice.

Precis: An Update in Obstetrics and Gynecology is intended to meet the continuing education needs of obstetricians and gynecologists. It is a broad, yet concise, overview of information relevant to the specialty. As in earlier editions, the emphasis in the third edition is on innovations in clinical practice, presented within the context of traditional approaches that retain their applicability to patient care.

Precis is an educational resource for preparation for the cognitive assessment of clinical knowledge, regardless of the form of the assessment—formal or informal, structured or independent. It is one of the recognized vehicles that are useful in preparing for certification and accreditation processes and is designed to complement those evaluations while serving as a general review of the field.

Each year, 1 volume of this 5-volume set is revised. This process provides continual updates that are critical to the practice of obstetrics and gynecology and that echo the dynamic nature of the field. The focus is on new and emerging techniques, presented from a balanced perspective of clinical value and cost-effectiveness in practice. Hence, discussion of traditional medical practice is limited. The information has been organized to unify the coverage of topics into a single volume so that each volume can stand on its own merit.

This third edition of *Precis: Obstetrics* reflects current thinking on optimal practice. The information is intended to be a useful tool to assist practicing obstetrician–gynecologists in maintaining current knowledge in a rapidly changing field and to better prepare them for the role of primary care provider for women.

Some information from the previous edition continues to be of value and thus has been retained and woven into the new structure. The efforts of authors contributing to previous editions, as well as the work of those authors providing new material, are recognized with gratitude. Collectively, these individuals represent the expertise of the specialty. With such a breadth of representation, differences of opinion are inevitable and have been respected.

Other *Precis* volumes are the second editions of *Gynecology, Reproductive Endocrinology,* and *Oncology* and the third edition of *Primary and Preventive Care.* Each is an educational tool for review, reference, and evaluation. *Precis* establishes a broad scientific basis for the delivery of quality health care for women. Rather than being a statement of ACOG policy, *Precis* serves as an intellectual approach to education. An effort has been made, however, to achieve consistency both within *Precis* and with other ACOG recommendations. Variations in patient care, based on individual needs and resources, are encouraged as an integral part of the practice of medicine.

—THE EDITORS

PRECIS

an update in obstetrics and gynecology

Obstetrics
Third Edition

Introduction

This volume of *Precis* addresses recent advances in technology and provides the reader with concise, updated information in the specialty of obstetrics. New sections have been added on depression and surgical complications. Those knowledgeable in the field of obstetrics provide guidelines for the use of ultrasonography in monitoring the pregnant patient and fetus, fetal heart rate monitoring, and management of premature rupture of membranes. Guidelines are given for the use of fetal fibronectin assessment (as a marker of preterm birth), and new approaches for measurement of intrauterine growth restriction (IUGR) are discussed. Operative obstetric methods are described and compared with other obstetric methods and with cesarean delivery, and strategies and recommendations are provided for optimizing cesarean delivery rates. The section on management of multiple gestations has been expanded, reflecting the increasing numbers of cases seen by obstetrician–gynecologists.

New medications and their use during pregnancy are discussed, including those for women with coexisting medical conditions (eg, immunologic disorders, renal disease, depression) and those for use in labor (eg, misoprostol and prostaglandins for labor stimulation). The use of low-molecular-weight heparin for deep vein thrombosis (DVT) and pulmonary embolism is described. Uses of progesterone have broadened, and limitations have been identified.

Appropriate patient education is key to optimal patient care. Specific areas calling for patient counseling are identified throughout. Such counseling can be enhanced by providing written patient education materials; see Appendix A, "Information Resources," for a list of relevant pamphlets and books available from the American College of Obstetricians and Gynecologists (ACOG). Web sites that may be useful to patients and obstetrician–gynecologists seeking additional information are provided in Appendix A and in resource boxes throughout.

The Editorial Committee, Advisory Board, and other selected individuals have reviewed the content to ensure that the information is accurate, complete, and current. During this review, an effort was made to ensure consistency with other ACOG guidelines as well as to identify emerging areas. As advances unfold, physicians are urged to consult the current version of new documents.

—GARY D. V. HANKINS, MD
Chair, Editorial Committee

Antepartum Care

PRECONCEPTIONAL CARE

Preconceptional health care should include assessment of the reproductive status and plans of all women. Targeting only those women who are actively attempting pregnancy would exclude approximately 50% of women in the United States who have unintended pregnancies, as well as women and teenagers who are unaware of the benefits of preconceptional health care and who seek care only after becoming pregnant.

The critical period of organogenesis—17–56 days after fertilization—occurs before most women are aware that they are pregnant. Therefore, the ideal time for pri-

---

RESOURCES

Antepartum Care

American Association of Clinical Endocrinologists
www.aace.com/clin/guidelines/obesityguide.pdf

American College of Obstetricians and Gynecologists
www.acog.org

American Dietetic Association
www.eatright.org

HealthierUS.gov
www.healthierus.gov

March of Dimes Birth Defects Foundation
www.modimes.org

Maternal Child Health Bureau of HRSA
www.mchb.hrsa.gov

MEDLINEplus
medlineplus.gov

National Center on Birth Defects and Developmental Disabilities
www.cdc.gov/ncbddd

National Institute of Child Health and Human Development
www.nichd.nih.gov

National Women's Health Information Center
www.4woman.gov

Nutrition.gov
www.nutrition.gov

smallstep.gov
www.smallstep.gov

US Department of Agriculture. National Agriculture Library. Food and Nutrition Information Center
www.nal.usda.gov/fnic

---

mary prevention of reproductive health risks is during the preconceptional period. Unfortunately, most women do not seek obstetric care until some weeks after conception. Furthermore, most women are unaware of the health effects of infections, medical conditions, specific drugs and medications, nutrition, genetic risk factors, occupational exposures, and lifestyle behaviors on reproduction. Screening, health maintenance, and continued education in the primary care setting, combined with preconceptional care in obstetric practice, can promote a healthy pregnancy.

Preconceptional health promotion and screening among women of childbearing age should be followed by further assessment of women with identified risk factors. Targeted information and referral services should be provided as appropriate. Patients with unresolved issues (lifestyle habits, medical conditions, and other risk factors) should be provided with contraceptive counseling to reduce the risks associated with unplanned pregnancies.

Preconceptional care should begin with an assessment of a woman's current health. This assessment should include checking on the status of her immunity to certain infections and the need for immunization, the presence and status of any medical conditions, reproductive and family history, nutrition status, and risk of genetic disease. The patient's use of alternative and complementary medicine should be noted, and she should be counseled about the safe use and potential interaction of these therapies with conventional medicine (Box 1). Women contemplating infertility treatments should be encouraged to consider the possibility of multiple gestations and what her options are to minimize this risk.

Infection

Women should be tested for immunity to rubella, and those who are not immune should be vaccinated (Box 2). Women who do not report having chickenpox as a child should be tested and, if not immune, offered vaccination. Women at risk of hepatitis B infection should be offered vaccination. All women should be offered testing for the human immunodeficiency virus (HIV) antibody, with appropriate counseling and consent. In states where it is legally permissible, patients should be informed that HIV testing is part of a recommended battery of tests that enable physicians to better ensure a healthy infant and that they can choose not to be tested. However, even in this setting, counseling should be offered. Screening for sexually transmitted diseases (STDs) may be performed as part of the risk assessment.

BOX 1

Components of Preconceptional Care

- Systematic identification of preconceptional risks through assessment of medical, social, reproductive, and family histories, including genetic risk, drugs, and medication history
- Discussion of possible effects of pregnancy on medical conditions for both the prospective mother and the fetus and introduction of interventions, if appropriate and desired
- Determination of risk of infection and, if indicated, testing and vaccination (if available)
- Nutritional counseling regarding appropriate weight for height, nutrient sources, and importance of folic acid, and avoidance of vitamin oversupplementation (especially vitamin A); referral for in-depth nutrition counseling, if appropriate and desired
- Discussion of social, financial, and psychologic issues in preparation for pregnancy, including lifestyle habits, alcohol use, recreational drugs, and domestic violence screening
- Review of alternative and complementary medicine practices
- Provision of education based on risks
- Discussion of birth spacing and real and perceived barriers to achieving desires, including problems with contraceptive use
- Recommendation to keep menstrual calendar
- Emphasis on importance of early and continuous prenatal care and discussion of how care will be structured based on the woman's risks and concerns

BOX 2

Contents of Preconceptional History

The following information should be obtained during the preconceptional period:

I. Immunization—if serology indicates lack of immunity:
   A. Rubella
   B. Varicella
   C. Hepatitis B
II. Occupational/household risks:
   A. Workplace exposure
   B. Cytomegalovirus
   C. Human immunodeficiency virus
   D. Toxoplasmosis
III. Genetic history risks—carrier status:
   A. Autosomal recessive genes (eg, Tay–Sachs disease, cystic fibrosis, Canavan disease, sickle cell anemia)
   B. X-linked mental retardation (eg, Fragile X syndrome)
   C. Population-specific risk

Medical Conditions

Certain medical conditions may carry risks for both mother and fetus. For example, a pregnant woman with congenital heart disease has an increased risk (usually 2–10%) of having an infant with heart disease in addition to the inherent risk to herself. Some cardiac diseases such as uncorrected coarctation of the aorta, pulmonary hypertension, Eisenmenger's syndrome, and Marfan's syndrome with aortic dilatation greater than 4 cm pose a serious risk to the mother's life, and the risks should be fully explained to the mother. Patients with chronic hypertension and cardiac arrhythmias may continue taking their medications, such as β-adrenergic blocking agents, long-acting calcium channel blockers, and digoxin. Angiotensin-converting enzyme inhibitors should be discontinued. Although exposure to such drugs in early pregnancy is not associated with an increased risk of fetal structural anomalies, continued use can affect the fetal kidney adversely. Patients taking warfarin anticoagulation therapy before pregnancy should be informed of its teratogenic potential if used after 7–8 weeks of gestation and switched to unfractionated or low-molecular-weight heparin with a positive pregnancy test result. Warfarin crosses the placenta and is associated with fetal nasal hypoplasia and central nervous system defects, whereas heparin does not cross the placenta and is safe throughout pregnancy. Possible exceptions to this prohibition include women with mechanical heart valves after the first trimester.

Pregestational diabetes mellitus is a common medical complication encountered during pregnancy. Evidence is strong that preconceptional glucose control is paramount in reducing the risk of serious congenital malformations in offspring. It also may be beneficial to evaluate and treat retinopathy and renal disease before a woman with diabetes becomes pregnant. (For discussion of the complications of diabetes in pregnancy, see "Medical Complications of Pregnancy," "Diabetes Mellitus.")

The risks of microcephaly, mental retardation, congenital heart disease, and IUGR are greater in infants who do not have phenylketonuria but are born to women with classic phenylketonuria or atypical hyperphenylalaninemia with blood phenylalanine levels greater than 10 mg/dL. A protective effect is afforded to the fetus by pre-conceptional reduction of the maternal blood level of phenylalanine to the range of 6 mg/dL and maintenance of the same level throughout pregnancy.

Previously euthyroid women who have known autoimmune thyroiditis, a history of treated hyperthyroidism, or other risk factors for hypothyroidism (eg, family history of thyroid disorders or related autoimmune conditions) should be assessed for the emergence of hypothyroidism in the first trimester.

Maternal epilepsy has been associated with a higher rate of malformations in offspring than in the general population. This teratogenic effect seems to be primarily related to treatment (1). Thus, although anticonvulsant drugs should be continued during pregnancy, if indicated, monotherapy using the lowest possible effective dosage is recommended. If the patient has been free of seizures for 2 years, discontinuation of therapy or a reduction in the number of drugs should be discussed during the prepregnancy period in consultation with the patient's neurologist. Preconceptional folate and predelivery vitamin K supplements should be given.

Treatment planning should begin early for women with bipolar disorder who are considering pregnancy. Stable patients may be able to discontinue taking mood stabilizers before attempting to conceive. If medication is to be discontinued, it should be tapered slowly over at least 2 weeks to avoid the illness recurrence that often follows abrupt discontinuation. For women with severe illness, however, continuation of medication through conception should be considered to reduce morbidity to the mother and fetus. Illness would be deemed severe if the patient's history includes self-harm, protracted recovery time, or impaired insight (2). The risk of Epstein's anomaly following prenatal lithium exposure is 0.1%.

Substance Abuse

Despite public health warnings, alcohol consumption by pregnant women increased 4-fold from 1991 to 1995 (3). Maternal alcohol use is the leading known cause of mental retardation and is the leading preventable cause of birth defects in the western world. Moderate to heavy use of alcohol—7 drinks per week or 5 or more drinks on any occasion—during pregnancy has been associated with cognitive deficits and other neurobehavioral sequelae.

An accurate drinking history taken in a nonthreatening manner is a critical component of a preconceptional inventory. A number of techniques are available for identifying problem drinkers. The TWEAK technique, which has a sensitivity of 87%, appears to be superior. This questionnaire includes the following questions:

- **Tolerance** (2 points): How many drinks can you hold (≥ 6 drinks indicates tolerance), or how many drinks does it take before you begin to feel the first effects of the alcohol (≥ 3 indicates tolerance)?

- **Worried** (2 points): Have close friends or relatives worried or complained about your drinking in the past year?

- **Eye openers** (1 point): Do you sometimes take a drink in the morning when you first get up?

- **Amnesia** (1 point): Has a friend or family member ever told you about things you said or did while you were drinking that you could not remember?

- **"Kut"** down (1 point): Do you sometimes feel the need to cut down on your drinking?

One point indicates reason for concern (moderate-risk drinking); 2 points indicate that a problem is likely (high-risk drinking).

Other techniques for evaluating abuse of drugs and alcohol also have been used. They include the T-ACE, NET, and NIAAA questionnaires (4). Based on further assessment of drinking patterns, appropriate interventions should be afforded to women of childbearing age before pregnancy. (There is no safe level of alcohol consumption during pregnancy.)

The effect of prenatal alcohol exposure is magnified by the abuse of other drugs. Maternal cigarette smoking and cocaine use may augment alcohol's ability to cause IUGR. A complete preconceptional social history should include nonjudgmental, indirect questioning of patients to determine their use of drugs in order to provide education, intervention, contraceptive counseling, and referral for treatment. At every office visit, patients who smoke should be encouraged to stop. Interventions should not only include antismoking advice but also emphasize how to stop smoking and could include prescription of smoking cessation medications. Most of these medications can be used during pregnancy if prior attempts to quit smoking without medications have failed and if the patient is still smoking more than 10–15 cigarettes per day. If the patient smokes at this level, the use of a nicotine replacement system may pose fewer risks than smoking.

Nutrition Status

Nutrition and its importance in reproductive outcome should be emphasized in all preconceptional counseling visits. Appropriateness of the patient's weight for height, special childhood diets (such as that required with phenylketonuria), and nutrition patterns, such as vegetarianism, fasting, pica, bulimia, and vitamin supplementation, need thorough investigation.

In nonpregnant women, the daily folic acid requirement is 50–100 µg/d. Multiple studies have shown the efficacy of preconceptional folic acid supplementation in reducing both the occurrence and recurrence of open neural tube defects (NTDs). Stimulated by these results, the U.S. Public Health Service recommends that all women of reproductive age receive 400 µg per day and those who have had a child with an NTD use folic acid supplements (4.0 mg/d) for 3 months before a planned pregnancy and during the first trimester. Other at-risk patients also may benefit from 4.0 mg folic acid per day: couples with a sibling, niece, or nephew with an NTD have a risk of approximately 0.3–1%; women with type 2 diabetes mellitus have a risk of approximately 1%; and women with seizure disorders who are being treated with valproic acid or carbamazepine have a risk of 1%. Folic acid also can prevent megaloblastic anemia during pregnancy. Although this condition is uncommon, it almost always results from folic acid deficiency. This condition usually is found in women who do not consume fresh, leafy green vegetables or foods with a high content of animal protein. Women with megaloblastic anemia may develop troublesome nausea, vomiting, and anorexia during pregnancy.

Although folate is found naturally in orange juice, in leafy green vegetables such as spinach, asparagus, and broccoli, and in grains, it is difficult to obtain the recommended 0.4 mg daily through diet alone. In January 1998, the U.S. Food and Drug Administration (FDA) ruled that flours, cornmeal, pasta, and rice must be fortified with 100–140 µg of folic acid per serving.

Occasionally obstetricians will encounter patients desiring pregnancy who have undergone obesity surgery, usually either gastric restriction (eg, gastric banding) or gastric bypass procedures. These procedures generally are indicated when a patient's body mass index (BMI) exceeds 40 or their BMI is greater than 35 and they have co-existent serious medical problems (eg, obstructive sleep apnea) that would benefit from weight loss. Although beneficial or even lifesaving, obesity surgery may place a patient at risk for iron deficiency and megaloblastic anemias (B_{12} and folate deficiencies). In addition, decreases in preconceptional folate absorption and concentrations may increase the risk of NTDs. The presence of malabsorption and dumping syndromes may identify patients at increased risk for nutrient deficiencies and inadequate caloric intake. Iron, folate, and B_{12} supplementation should be provided, and consultation with a nutritionist may help assure adequate protein and calorie intake. Serial ultrasound scans for fetal growth may be indicated.

Genetic Assessment

Personal and family histories may reveal risks for genetic diseases such as cystic fibrosis, Tay–Sachs disease, Canavan disease, Fragile X syndrome, or Down syndrome. Screening for carriers is available for some autosomal recessive conditions, such as Tay–Sachs disease, cystic fibrosis, Canavan disease, sickle cell disease, and the thalassemias. Women with significant genetic risks may be referred to specialists for further counseling. With these patients, construction of a genetic pedigree is especially useful in assessing the risk for inheritable disease. All cou-ples of Caucasian ancestry and any with a family history of cystic fibrosis should have their carrier status assessed for cystic fibrosis using a panel that includes 25 of the most common mutations. Couples having Ashkenazi Jewish ancestors should in addition be offered screening for their Tay–Sachs and Canavan disease carrier status and may wish to be screened for other genetic disorders more commonly found in that population (Box 3). Couples of African-American heritage should consider assessment of sickle cell and thalassemia carrier status, those of Mediterranean ancestry should be screened for β-thalassemia, and those of Asian ancestry for α-thalassemia.

Reproductive History

A reproductive history helps in identifying conditions that may have contributed to a previous adverse pregnancy outcome that may be amenable to intervention in a subsequent pregnancy. Adverse pregnancy outcomes should be categorized according to the trimester of their occurrence to provide clues to their etiology and areas for evaluation.

Patients with a prior history of venous thrombosis in a nonpregnant state should be screened for thrombophilias, including deficiencies of protein S, protein C, and antithrombin, antiphospholipid antibody syndrome and the Factor V Leiden, and prothrombin gene mutations, as well as hyperhomocysteinemia. Patients whose prior venous thrombosis did not have an associated nonrecurring risk factor (eg, oral contraceptive use or concurrent surgery) or those with a thrombophilia should have prophylaxis with unfractionated or low-molecular-weight heparin in a subsequent pregnancy. For patients whose venous thrombotic event was associated with a nonrecurring risk factor and who have no thrombophilia, anticoagulation therapy can be reserved for the postpartum period.

Occupational Exposure

As a primary care provider, the obstetrician–gynecologist plays an important role in addressing the concerns of women in the workplace and preventing adverse reproductive and developmental outcomes related to toxic exposures. The preconceptional period is the best time to examine possible exposures; environmental risks can be evaluated and the most current information can be reviewed so that women and their partners can make informed decisions regarding future exposure in the workplace or at home. In some instances, work modification, transfer to another unit, or extra precautions, such as the use of masks or gloves, may be advisable. (See "Routine Care," "Work During Pregnancy.") Radiation exposure should be minimized during pregnancy, although the risks of ionizing radiation less than 0.04 Gy (4 rads) to the developing fetus are considered minimal.

BOX 3

Clinical Features of Autosomal Recessive Genetic Diseases Frequent Among Individuals of Eastern European Jewish Descent

Bloom syndrome is a genetic condition associated with increased chromosome breakage, a predisposition to infections and malignancies, prenatal and postnatal growth deficiency, skin findings (such as facial telangiectasias, abnormal pigmentation), and in some cases learning difficulties and mental retardation. The mean age of death is 27 years and usually is related to cancer. No effective treatment currently is available.

Canavan disease is a disorder of the central nervous system characterized by developmental delay, hypotonia, large head, seizures, blindness, and gastrointestinal reflux. Most children die within the first several years of life. Canavan disease is caused by a deficiency of the aspartoacylase enzyme. No treatment currently is available.

Familial dysautonomia is a neurologic disorder characterized by abnormal suck and feeding difficulties, episodic vomiting, abnormal sweating, pain and temperature insensitivity, labile blood pressure levels, absent tearing, and scoliosis. There currently is no cure for familial dysautonomia, but some treatments are available that can improve the length and quality of a patient's life.

Fanconi anemia group C usually presents with severe anemia that progresses to pancytopenia, developmental delay, and failure to thrive. Congenital anomalies are not uncommon, including limb, cardiac, and genital–urinary defects. Microcephaly and mental retardation may be present. Children are at increased risk for leukemia. Some children have been successfully treated with bone marrow transplantation. Life expectancy is 8–12 years.

Gaucher's disease is a genetic disorder that mainly affects the spleen, liver, and bones; it occasionally affects the lungs, kidneys, and brain. It may develop at any age. Some individuals are chronically ill, some are moderately affected, and others are so mildly affected that they may not know that they have Gaucher's disease. The most common symptom is chronic fatigue caused by anemia. Patients may experience easy bruising, nosebleeds, bleeding gums, and prolonged and heavy bleeding with their menses and after childbirth. Other symptoms include an enlarged liver and spleen, osteoporosis, and bone and joint pain. Gaucher's disease is caused by the deficiency of the β-glucosidase enzyme. Treatment is available through enzyme therapy, which results in a vastly improved quality of life.

Mucolipidosis IV is a neurodegenerative lysosomal storage disorder characterized by growth and psychomotor retardation, corneal clouding, progressive retinal degeneration, and strabismus. Most affected infants never speak, walk, or develop beyond the level of a 1–2 year old. Life expectancy may be normal, and there currently is no effective treatment.

Niemann-Pick disease type A is a lysosomal storage disorder typically diagnosed in infancy and marked by a rapid neurodegenerative course similar to Tay–Sachs disease. Affected children die by age 3–5 years. Niemann-Pick disease type A is caused by a deficiency of the sphingomyelinase enzyme. There currently is no treatment.

Tay–Sachs disease (TSD) is a severe, progressive disorder of the central nervous system leading to death within the first few years of life. Infants with TSD appear normal at birth but by age 5–6 months develop poor muscle tone, delayed development, loss of developmental milestones, and mental retardation. Children with TSD lose their eyesight at age 12–18 months. This condition usually is fatal by age 6 years. Tay–Sachs disease is caused by a deficiency of the hexosaminidase A enzyme. No effective treatment currently is available.

Prenatal and preconceptional carrier screening for genetic diseases in individuals of Eastern European Jewish descent. ACOG Committee Opinion No. 298. American College of Obstetricians and Gynecologists. Obstet Gynecol 2004;104:425–8.

References

1. Holmes LB, Harvey EA, Coull BA, Huntington KB, Khoshbin S, Hayes AM, et al. The teratogenicity of anticonvulsant drugs. N Engl J Med 2001;344:1132–8.

2. Yonkers KA, Wisner KL, Stowe Z, Leibenluft E, Cohen L, Miller L, et al. Management of bipolar disorder during pregnancy and the postpartum period. Am J Psychiatry 2004;161:608–20.

3. At-risk drinking and illicit drug use: ethical issues in obstetric and gynecologic practice. ACOG Committee Opinion No. 294. American College of Obstetricians and Gynecologists. Obstet Gynecol 2004;103:1021–31.

4. National Institute on Alcohol Abuse and Alcoholism. Helping patients with alcohol problems: a health practitioner's guide. Bethesda (MD): NIAAA; 2003. Available at: http://www.niaaa.nih.gov/publications/Practitioner/PractitionersGuideFINAL.pdf. Retrieved January 7, 2004.

ROUTINE CARE

The major goal of prenatal care is to ensure a healthy infant and a healthy mother. Although pregnant women should be aware of this goal, they should be counseled that, with current limitations in medicine and science, its achievement cannot be guaranteed, especially with regard to promising a normal infant. Specific objectives to achieve this goal include the following:

- Evaluation of the health status of mother and fetus
- Estimation of gestational age
- Identification of the patient at risk for complications
- Anticipation of problems before they occur, and prevention if possible
- Patient education and communication

In an attempt to ensure a systematic approach to prenatal care, several standardized prenatal forms have been developed, some of which provide a built-in risk assessment system. The antepartum record produced by ACOG appears in Appendix B.

Diagnosis of Pregnancy

Commercial kits are available for the diagnosis of pregnancy. All of these kits depend on the detection of human chorionic gonadotropin (hCG) by an antibody. The various techniques used to detect hCG include agglutination inhibition, radioimmunoassay, enzyme-linked immunosorbent assay, and immunochromatography. Some tests can detect hCG at levels as low as 25 mIU/mL or as early as 1 week after implantation (1 week before the expected time of the next menstruation).

History and Physical Examination

It is important to identify patients who are at significant risk of having an abnormal fetus or child. This identification may be accomplished by compiling a complete history with the use of a prenatal questionnaire, as described in "Preconceptional Care." Patients at risk of having a infant with a chromosomal or genetic disorder may benefit from genetic counseling. The American College of Obstetricians and Gynecologists currently recommends that screening for cystic fibrosis with a minimal panel of 25 common mutations be offered to all Caucasian patients and patients with a family history of cystic fibrosis.

An important part of the initial physical assessment is the pelvic examination to ascertain uterine size and gestational age and to estimate the expected date of delivery. If there is a discrepancy between uterine size and the last menstrual period or if the latter is unknown, first-trimester or early second-trimester ultrasonography will help establish an expected date of delivery. Ultrasound measurement of the crown–rump length at 6–12 weeks of gestation is the most accurate technique for estimation of gestational age.

Laboratory Tests

The following routine and indicated tests are recommended for individual patients during the initial prenatal visit:

- Blood type
- Rh status
- Antibody screen
- Hemoglobin and hematocrit measurements
- Pap test
- Rubella antibody titer measurement, if indicated
- Venereal Disease Research Laboratory (VDRL) or rapid plasma reagin testing
- Urine culture or screen
- Hepatitis B virus screen (hepatitis B surface antigen)
- Human immunodeficiency virus testing
- Cystic fibrosis carrier testing if of the appropriate ethnicity or when there is a positive family history

Patient Education

Each patient should be given information about the general plan of management for her pregnancy. The plan should include the number and frequency of prenatal visits; plans for diet, nutrition, and weight gain; and signs and symptoms of potential complications. The patient should be counseled about the benefits of exercise and any restrictions that may be needed in her exercise program. Other topics that may be discussed include travel plans and the nature of work outside the home to assess whether there might be environmental hazards. Questions about labor, hospitalization, mode of delivery, and analgesia and anesthesia can be addressed in general terms at the initial visit and discussed in greater detail later in pregnancy.

The initial prenatal visit also can be a good time to discuss the risks of congenital malformations that occur in the general population, as well as specific risks. The patient should be asked if she has ever had chickenpox, and if she has not, she should be counseled on the need for varicella-zoster immune globulin if she is exposed. She also should be counseled about the use of tobacco, alcohol, and other substances that might harm the fetus. Because of the risk of transmission of toxoplasmosis from cats, she should be encouraged to wash her hands after contact with these animals and to avoid changing a cat's litter box. The patient should be counseled about the various methods available to screen for fetal aneuploidy, including first- and second-trimester biochemical screening and, where available, ultrasonographic nuchal translucency measurements at 11–14 weeks. Screening for NTDs with a maternal serum alpha-fetoprotein, either alone or as part of a second-trimester maternal serum aneuploidy screen, also should be offered.

Written information can be helpful. Patients can be referred to patient education materials and web pages for answers to questions. (See Appendix A.)

Nutrition and Weight Gain

All pregnant women should be encouraged to eat a well-balanced diet consisting of the dietary allowances recommended in Table 1. Of particular note, the Centers for Disease Control and Prevention (CDC) has recommended supplemental folic acid in the preconceptional and early prenatal period to prevent NTDs (see "Preconceptional Care").

Recommendations for weight gain during pregnancy are based on prepregnancy BMI, defined as weight (in kilograms) divided by height (in meters squared). Underweight women (those with a BMI of <19.8) should have a weight gain of 12.5–18 kg (28–40 lb), whereas overweight women (BMI ≥26) should have a weight gain of 7–11.5 kg (15–25 lb). The recommended weight gain for women of average weight (BMI = 19.8–26.0) is 11.5–16 kg (25–35 lb). An additional 100–300 kcal per day is recommended.

TABLE 1. Recommended Daily Dietary Allowances for Adolescent and Adult Pregnant and Lactating Women

	Pregnant			Lactating		
	14–18 years	19–30 years	31–50 years	14–18 years	19–30 years	31–50 years
Fat-soluble Vitamins						
Vitamin A	750 µg	770 µg	770 µg	1,200 µg	1,300 µg	1,300 µg
Vitamin D*	5 µg	5 µg	5 µg	5 µg	5 µg	5 µg
Vitamin E	15 mg	15 mg	15 mg	19 mg	19 mg	19 mg
Vitamin K	75 µg	90 µg	90 µg	75 µg	90 µg	90 µg
Water-soluble Vitamins						
Vitamin C	80 mg	85 mg	85 mg	115 mg	120 mg	120 mg
Thiamin	1.4 mg	1.4 mg	1.4 mg	1.4 mg	1.4 mg	1.4 mg
Riboflavin	1.4 mg	1.4 mg	1.4 mg	1.6 mg	1.6 mg	1.6 mg
Niacin	18 mg	18 mg	18 mg	17 mg	17 mg	17 mg
Vitamin B_6	1.9 mg	1.9 mg	1.9 mg	2 mg	2 mg	2 mg
Folate	600 µg	600 µg	600 µg	500 µg	500 µg	500 µg
Vitamin B_{12}	2.6 µg	2.6 µg	2.6 µg	2.8 µg	2.8 µg	2.8 µg
Minerals						
Calcium*	1,300 mg	1,000 mg	1,000 mg	1,300 mg	1,000 mg	1,000 mg
Phosphorus	1,240 mg	700 mg	700 mg	1,250 mg	700 mg	700 mg
Iron	27 mg	27 mg	27 mg	10 mg	9 mg	9 mg
Zinc	13 mg	11 mg	11 mg	14 mg	12 mg	12 mg
Iodine	220 µg	220 µg	220 µg	290 µg	290 µg	290 µg
Selenium	60 µg	60 µg	60 µg	70 µg	70 µg	70 µg

*Recommendations measured as Adequate Intake (AI) instead of Recommended Daily Dietary Allowance (RDA). An AI is set instead of an RDA if insufficient evidence is available to determine an RDA. The AI is based on observed or experimentally determined estimates of average nutrient intake by a group (or groups) of healthy people.

Data from Institute of Medicine. Dietary reference intakes for calcium, phosphorus, magnesium, vitamin D, and fluoride. Washington, DC: National Academy Press; 1997. Institute of Medicine (US). Dietary reference intakes for thiamin, riboflavin, niacin, vitamin B6, folate, vitamin B12, pantothenic acid, biotin, and choline. Washington, DC: National Academy Press; 1998. Institute of Medicine (US). Dietary reference intakes for vitamin C, vitamin E, selenium, and carotenoids. Washington, DC: National Academy Press; 2000. Institute of Medicine (US). Dietary reference intakes for vitamin A, vitamin K, arsenic, boron, chromium, copper, iodine, iron, manganese, molybdenum, nickel, silicon, vanadium, and zinc. Washington, DC: National Academy Press; 2002.

Work During Pregnancy

A woman who has an uncomplicated pregnancy and a normal fetus and whose workplace poses no greater hazards than those encountered in routine daily life in the community may continue to work without interruption until the onset of labor. She may resume working 4–6 weeks after an uncomplicated delivery. Work may be limited or contraindicated during pregnancy in patients with vaginal bleeding, incompetent cervix, uterine malformation associated with perinatal loss, gestational hypertension, IUGR, multiple gestations, a history of preterm birth, or hydramnios. Maternal disorders that warrant special review include renal disease; diabetes mellitus, especially with vasculopathy; heart disease with arrhythmias; pulmonary or arterial hypertension; hemoglobinopathies; a hemoglobin value of less than 8 g/L; seizure disorders; nerve root irritations; back problems; and asthma.

The Pregnancy Discrimination Act requires that employers offering medical disability benefits must treat pregnancy-related disabilities as they do all other disabilities. Pregnant workers must be provided the same insurance benefits, sick leave, seniority credits, and reinstatement privileges that are awarded to workers who are disabled by other causes.

The U.S. Occupational Safety and Health Administration establishes and enforces standards requiring employers to provide a workplace that is free from recognized hazards that are likely to cause serious physical harm. In 1991, the U.S. Supreme Court ruled that a rigid policy banning women of reproductive age from certain jobs discriminated against women on the basis of their sex. Although several toxic substances found in the workplace also could harm men of reproductive age, men were not banned from jobs on that basis. Therefore, the Court reasoned that it is illegal for an employer to ban women from certain jobs because they might become pregnant while they are working there.

Exercise During Pregnancy

A pregnant woman may engage in a moderate level of physical activity if she has no obstetric or medical complications. Exercise helps a woman to maintain cardiorespiratory and muscular fitness throughout her pregnancy. Contraindications to exercise during pregnancy include the following:

- Gestational hypertension
- Preterm premature rupture of membranes
- Preterm labor during a prior or current pregnancy
- Incompetent cervix
- Second- or third-trimester bleeding
- Intrauterine growth restriction

For women who do not have any additional risk factors for adverse maternal or perinatal outcomes, ACOG recommends the following guidelines for exercise during pregnancy:

- Women can continue to exercise and derive health benefits even from mildly to moderately strenuous exercise routines. Regular exercise (at least 3 times per week) is preferable to intermittent activity.

- Women should avoid exercise in the supine position after the first trimester. Such a position is associated with decreased cardiac output in most pregnant women. Because the remaining cardiac output will be preferentially distributed away from the splanchnic beds (including the uterus) during vigorous exercise, such regimens are best avoided during pregnancy. Prolonged periods of motionless standing should also be avoided.

- Women should be aware of the decreased oxygen available for aerobic exercise. They should be encouraged to modify the intensity of their exercise according to their symptoms. Pregnant women should stop exercising when fatigued and not exercise to exhaustion. Weight-bearing exercises may, under some circumstances, be continued throughout pregnancy at intensities similar to those prior to pregnancy. Non–weight-bearing exercises, such as cycling or swimming, will minimize the risk of injury and facilitate the continuation of exercise during pregnancy.

- Morphologic changes in pregnancy should serve as a relative contraindication to types of exercise in which loss of balance could be detrimental to maternal or fetal well-being, especially in the third trimester. Furthermore, any type of exercise involving the potential for even mild abdominal trauma should be avoided.

- Pregnancy requires an additional 300 kcal/d in order to maintain energy balance. Thus, women who exercise during pregnancy should be particularly careful to ensure an adequate diet.

- Pregnant women who exercise in the first trimester should augment heat dissipation by ensuring adequate hydration, appropriate clothing, and optimal environmental surroundings during exercise.

Many of the physiologic and morphologic changes of pregnancy persist for 4–6 weeks postpartum. Thus, prepregnancy exercise routines should be resumed gradually based on a woman's physical capability.

Follow-up Visits

Examinations at each subsequent visit following diagnosis of pregnancy generally should consist of measurement of the uterine fundus, determination of fetal heart tones, measurement of blood pressure and weight, and determination of fetal presentation. Screening of urine for glucose and protein at each visit should be considered.

The interval for subsequent prenatal visits should be individualized according to the patient's needs. In general, women with uncomplicated pregnancies are seen every 4–5 weeks until 28 weeks of gestation, then every 2 weeks until 36 weeks, and then at least weekly until delivery. More frequent visits may be of benefit in monitoring women with diabetes, hypertension, threatened preterm birth, postterm pregnancies, and other complications. Conversely, less frequent visits may be appropriate, depending on the patient's needs and risk factors.

Bibliography

American Academy of Pediatrics, American College of Obstetricians and Gynecologists. Guidelines for perinatal care. 5th ed. Elk Grove Village (IL): AAP; Washington, DC: ACOG; 2002.

Exercise during pregnancy and the postpartum period. ACOG Committee Opinion No. 267. American College of Obstetricians and Gynecologists. Obstet Gynecol 2002; 99: 171–3.

Institute of Medicine, Subcommittee on Nutritional Status and Weight Gain During Pregnancy. Nutrition during pregnancy; part I, weight gain; part IV, nutrient supplements. Washington, DC: National Academy Press; 1990.

TERATOGENIC EXPOSURES

Major congenital anomalies are observed in approximately 3% of all births. Maternal exposure to drugs or environmental chemicals may be responsible for approximately 5% of these anomalies, or approximately 1 in 670 liveborn infants. Only approximately 1% of teratogen-related anomalies can be attributed to pharmaceutical agents; the bulk result from maternal ethanol use.

The most important determinants of the developmental toxicity of an agent are timing, dose, and fetal susceptibility. Many agents have teratogenic effects only if taken while the susceptible fetal organ system is forming. For example, thalidomide produced amelia only if taken between the 27th and 33rd day after conception. Similarly, an agent suspected of causing a cardiac defect would have to be present during the critical period of heart development, from 20 days to 50 days after fertilization. Other agents are teratogenic only at certain doses. Most X-ray exposures (ambient solar radiation, diagnostic X-rays) have no effect on the fetus, but high-dose exposures such as those encountered in cancer radiation therapy might result in fetal abnormalities. Finally, the fetal tissue must be susceptible. Radioiodine ^{131}I can damage the fetal thyroid when the organ is fully formed and functional; ^{131}I given at less than 10 weeks of gestation is unlikely to have an effect.

Susceptibility also is influenced by the genetic makeup of both the fetus and the mother. Genetic variability in susceptibility to developmental toxicity is attributed to differences in the absorption, biotransformation, or elimination of drugs and chemicals. These processes are controlled by enzymes whose activities differ among individuals, a difference called pharmacogenetic variation. For example, variations in the gene encoding epoxide hydrolase, an enzyme required for metabolism of the anticonvulsant phenytoin, may account for major malformations in some exposed babies but not in others.

It is now recognized that some teratogens produce functional rather than structural abnormalities. Although exposure to certain agents during first-trimester organogenesis can result in anatomic anomalies, exposure later in pregnancy may cause functional problems that are less readily identified. For example, first-trimester exposure to alcohol can result in a specific embryopathy, which

---

RESOURCES

Teratogenicity of Agents

American Society of Health-System Pharmacists
www.ashp.org

American Pharmaceutical Association
www.aphanet.org

Center for the Evaluation of Risks to Human Reproduction
cerhr.niehs.nih.gov

Clinical Teratology Web Site
www.depts.washington.edu/~terisweb

U.S. Food and Drug Administration
www.fda.gov

MEDLINEplus Drug Information
www.nlm.nih.gov/medlineplus/druginformation.html

Motherisk
www.motherisk.org

National Center on Birth Defects and Developmental Disabilities
www.cdc.gov/ncbddd

National Institute on Drug Abuse
www.nida.nih.gov

National Institute for Occupational Safety and Health
www.cdc.gov/niosh/homepage.html

Occupational Safety & Health Administration
www.osha.gov

Organization of Teratology Information Services
www.otispregnancy.org

Reprotox
www.reprotox.org

U.S. Pharmacopoeia
www.usp.org

includes distinct facial anomalies, microcephaly, joint contractures, and cardiac defects, whereas exposure during the second and third trimesters can result in learning and behavioral abnormalities that might not be detected before school age. Because infants exposed to potential teratogens are rarely if ever monitored throughout their lives, and exposure-related functional abnormalities are thus unlikely to be detected, the safety of any drug can never be completely assured.

This section covers examples of agents that are believed to be teratogenic and is not intended to be exhaustive. For additional current information sources on these and other agents, see Appendix A.

Drugs and Chemicals

Most drugs commonly used during pregnancy (eg, aspirin, acetaminophen, metronidazole, caffeine) have not been associated with an increased risk of congenital anomalies at ordinary exposure levels. Some agents, however, increase the risk of congenital malformations even under ordinary dosing conditions.

SEDATIVES

Once marketed as a sedative–hypnotic, thalidomide was withdrawn when its use during pregnancy was associated with severe anomalies in 20% of exposed fetuses. The most striking abnormalities were severe upper and lower limb reduction defects known as phocomelia and other abnormalities involving the ears, bowel musculature, kidneys, and heart. This agent has been reintroduced for treatment of the skin manifestations of leprosy. The manufacturer has instituted an elaborate system of controls designed to prevent treatment of pregnant women. The effectiveness of these controls remains to be demonstrated.

ANTIHYPERTENSIVE AGENTS

Angiotensin-converting enzyme inhibitors are used in the treatment of hypertension and other cardiovascular disorders. Their use during pregnancy can cause severe fetal hypotension and, thus, hypoperfusion of the fetal kidney, leading to renal ischemia, renal tubular dysgenesis, and anuria. Use in the first trimester has been associated with fetal limb shortening and with maldevelopment of the calvarium, a structure formed from membranous bone that requires extensive vascularity and high oxygen tension for growth. Exposure during the second or third trimesters can result in oligohydramnios, leading to limb contractures, pulmonary hypoplasia, and sometimes fetal death. Similar problems have been seen with receptor blocker use.

ANTINEOPLASTIC AGENTS

Cyclophosphamide is an alkylating agent that causes cell death and DNA damage in surviving cells; both these mechanisms can adversely affect developing fetal tissues. Fetal anomalies reported after exposure during early pregnancy include missing and hypoplastic digits on hands and feet, cleft palate, single coronary artery, imperforate anus, and IUGR with microcephaly. Suboptimal data suggest that nurses who administer cyclophosphamide may be at increased risk for fetal loss. Alkylating agents should be avoided during early pregnancy, but may be given during the second and third trimester.

Aminopterin and methotrexate are folic acid antagonists that inhibit DNA synthesis and are toxic to rapidly dividing cells. Both have been used to produce abortion, and cases in which the pregnancy was actually intrauterine and the fetus survived have been associated with abnormalities of the cranium, face, and limbs. Methotrexate exposure results in a "clover-leaf" shaped skull, along with low-set ears, prominent eyes, wide nasal bridge, and limb defects (1). Reports of affected fetuses are rare, most likely because a dosage of at least 10 mg per week during weeks 6 through 8 of gestation would likely be required to produce defects.

ANTIINFECTIVES

There are a wide variety of antibiotics that have varying effects in pregnancy. The risk–benefit ratio should be carefully considered on an individual basis. When choosing an antiinfective, the teratogenicity of these drugs should be reviewed.

ANTICOAGULANTS

Warfarin and coumarin inhibit the synthesis of vitamin K-dependent coagulation factors. Their use during pregnancy can produce major and minor congenital anomalies in as many as 25% of exposed fetuses. Fetuses exposed during the first trimester can develop a hypoplastic nose and midface and epiphyseal stippling. Called warfarin embryopathy, these defects occur because warfarin inhibits the posttranslational carboxylation of coagulation proteins called osteocalcins. Exposure during the second and third trimesters can cause hemorrhage that results in scarring of developing tissues, leading to uncoordinated and abnormal tissue growth. The resulting fetopathy is characterized by IUGR and limb defects, along with central nervous system anomalies such as optic atrophy, microcephaly, and hydrocephalus. Heparins, including low-molecular-weight heparins, do not increase the risk of congenital anomalies because they do not cross the placenta.

ANTICONVULSANTS

The older anticonvulsant medications all have been implicated in increasing the incidence of congenital anomalies, including cardiac defects and oro-facial clefts (see "Seizure Disorders"). Phenytoin (diphenylhydantoin) is metabolized to oxidative intermediates called arene oxides or epoxides, which are then detoxified by cytoplasmic epoxide hydrolase. Because fetal epoxide hydrolase activity is weak, oxidative intermediates build up in fetal tissues where they have dose-related mutagenic and toxic effects. As a result, fetal exposure to phenytoin can be associated with abnormal facies, cleft lip or palate, microcephaly, growth deficiency, mild to moderate mental and developmental delay, and hypoplastic nails and distal phalanges. Of exposed offspring, 10% have the full fetal hydantoin syndrome, and 30% have some feature of it; fetuses that inherit a mutation in the gene for epoxide hydrolase that makes it even less functional are at highest risk. Of fetuses exposed to valproic acid, 4–5% have an NTD, usually involving the lumbosacral area. Carbamazepine has been associated with NTDs in some reports. Phenobarbital and lamotrigine reduce folic acid levels, which could increase the risk of NTDs and other malformations associated with decreased folate.

Newer anticonvulsants such as gabapentin and topiramate have not been associated with the same developmental toxicity in animal experiments as have the older medications, and no increase in congenital anomalies has been reported in exposed offspring. However, experience with these medications during pregnancy is not yet as extensive as with the older drugs.

LITHIUM

Although case reports and small series have suggested an association between antenatal lithium use and a rare fetal cardiac malformation called Ebstein's anomaly, these data have been challenged. A Canadian multicenter study of lithium exposure during pregnancy, in which women taking lithium were monitored prospectively and confounding factors were carefully detailed, found no increase in the incidence of birth defects and no association between lithium and any cardiac malformation. Exposure late in pregnancy may produce transplacental lithium intoxication with neonatal cyanosis, hypotonia, bradycardia, goiter with hypothyroidism, diabetes insipidus, and hydramnios.

VITAMIN A AND ITS CONGENERS

The 2 forms of vitamin A found in nature are beta-carotene, a precursor of provitamin A, and preformed vitamin A or retinal. Beta-carotene is found in fruits and vegetables and has never been shown to cause birth defects. Vitamin A is found in many foods, especially animal liver, and also is included in vitamin supplements. Although one report associated intake of more than 10,000 IU of this nutrient per day during pregnancy with a significant risk of fetal renal and craniofacial anomalies, other studies have found no increase in adverse pregnancy outcome in women taking 25,000 to 50,000 IU per day (2, 3). However, given that the American diet is not

deficient in vitamin A, it appears prudent to limit vitamin A supplementation to no more than 5,000 IU per day.

Isotretinoin (the 13-*cis* isomer of retinoic acid), an acne medication, is a vitamin A–like compound. Miscarriage is common after exposure during pregnancy, and serious congenital anomalies occur in approximately 35% of surviving exposed fetuses. The most commonly identified abnormalities are cardiac malformations, thymic agenesis, microphthalmia, hydrocephalus, cleft palate, deafness, and blindness. Because isotretinoin also can cause anotia, a defect that is otherwise exceedingly rare, it was not difficult to identify drug exposure as the cause. Neurobehavioral abnormalities have been described among surviving children.

Etretinate is an oral agent used to treat psoriasis. Case reports link the use of this agent to birth defects similar to those observed after prenatal exposure to isotretinoin. Unlike vitamin A and its congeners, however, etretinate has been detected in the sera of patients for as long as 7 years after cessation of use. Congenital anomalies similar to those observed with isotretinoin have occurred up to 18 months after discontinuing the drug. If possible, this drug should not be used in women who have not completed childbearing.

Tretinoin (all-trans-retinoic acid) is a topical medication. Application of tretinoin to the skin results in little detectable systemic absorption. As a result, it does not increase the incidence of congenital anomalies.

Dietary Additives, Contaminants, and Herbal Remedies

Aspartame is used as an artificial sweetener (Nutrasweet). It is metabolized to aspartic acid, which does not cross the placenta; phenylalanine, which is normally metabolized in individuals who do not have phenylketonuria; and methanol, which is produced at levels lower than those found in an equivalent amount of fruit juice. It is thus not biologically plausible that aspartame is a teratogen, and no adverse effects of aspartame have been reported in human pregnancies. Women with phenylketonuria should be advised to avoid aspartame whether or not they are pregnant.

Mercury, although not a drug, is a known teratogen. The developing nervous system is particularly susceptible. Prenatal exposure to mercury results in a variety of defects ranging from developmental delay and mild neurologic abnormalities to microcephaly and severe brain damage (4). Mercury enters the ecosystem through industrial pollution, gets into surface water, and eventually reaches the ocean where it is absorbed by fish. Several varieties of large fish, including tuna, shark, king mackerel, and tilefish, not only absorb mercury from the water but ingest it when they eat smaller fish and aquatic organisms. Women who eat these large fish ingest mercury as well. Although methyl mercury is metabolized and eventually eliminated from the body, the process is slow; the elimination halftime is 45 to 70 days. The FDA currently recommends that pregnant women refrain from eating these large fish or at least consume no more than 12 ounces per week (6 ounces white tuna or tuna steaks) (5). Albacore has been shown to be more toxic than chunk light tuna.

Because herbal remedies are not regulated as prescription or over-the-counter drugs, the identity and quantity of all ingredients are unknown, and there are virtually no studies of their teratogenic potential. Because it is not possible to assess their safety, pregnant women should be counseled to avoid these substances. Remedies containing substances with pharmaceutical properties that could theoretically have adverse fetal effects include echinacea, which causes fragmentation of hamster sperm at high concentrations; black cohosh, which contains a chemical that acts like estrogen; garlic and willow barks, which have anticoagulant properties; gingko, which can interfere with the effects of monoamine oxydase inhibitors and has anticoagulant properties; real licorice, which has hypertensive and potassium-wasting effects; valerian, which intensifies the effects of prescription sleep aids; and ginseng, which interferes with monoamine oxydase inhibitors. Herbal remedies used as abortifacients also should be avoided; blue and black cohosh and pennyroyal appear to stimulate uterine musculature directly, and pennyroyal also can cause liver damage, renal failure, disseminated intravascular coagulation, and maternal death.

Radiation

Ionizing radiation exposure is universal; most radiation originates from beyond the earth's atmosphere, from the land, and from endogenous radionuclides. The total radiation exposure from these sources is approximately 0.00125 Gy (125 mrad) per year. Although radiation exposure has the potential to cause gene mutations, growth impairment, chromosome damage and malignancy, or even fetal death, large doses are required to produce discernible fetal effects. During the first 2 weeks after fertilization, exposure to 0.10 Gy (10 rads) is required to produce an effect. Because this is the "all or none" period, this level of exposure will either cause death ("all") or have no effect ("none"). In the first trimester, 0.25 Gy (25 rads) are required to produce detectable damage, and 1 Gy (100 rads) are required in later pregnancy. The recommended upper limit of exposure during pregnancy, 0.05 Gy (5 rads), is thus well below the level that could actually produce damage and well below the amount of radiation exposure resulting from diagnostic radiologic studies (Table 2).

The risks of radionuclide exposure during pregnancy depend on the agent used and the amount and kind of particle or wave emitted. Of the radionuclides in common use, only ^{131}I exposes the fetus to dangerous levels of radiation, and only if the exposure occurs after 10 weeks of gestation. Before that, the fetal thyroid is not capable

TABLE 2. Estimated Fetal Exposure From Some Common Radiologic Procedures

Procedure	Fetal Exposure
CT scan of abdomen and lumbar spine	3.5 rad
Barium enema or small bowel series	2–4 rad
Intravenous pyelography	≥1 rad*
CT scan of head or chest	<1 rad
CT pelvimetry	250 mrad
Hip film (single view)	200 mrad
Abdominal film (single view)	100 rad
Mammography	7–20 mrad
Chest X-ray (2 views)	0.02–0.07 mrad
Magnetic resonance imaging	0

CT indicates computed tomography; 1 Gy = 100 rad.
*Amount of exposure depends on the number of films obtained.
Data from Cunningham FG, Gant NF, Leveno KJ, Gilstrap LC 3rd, Hauth JC, Wenstrom KD. General considerations and maternal evaluation. In: Williams obstetrics. 21st ed. New York (NY): McGraw-Hill; 2001. p. 1143–58.
Adapted from Guidelines for diagnostic imaging during pregnancy. ACOG Committee Opinion No. 299. American College of Obstetricians and Gynecologists. Obstet Gynecol 2004;104: 647–51.

of concentrating the iodine; after this time, ^{131}I is concentrated by the fetal thyroid and then ablates the gland.

NONIONIZING ELECTROMAGNETIC RADIATION

Electromagnetic radiation in the nonionizing spectrum includes radiofrequency and microwave radiation as well as visible light. Electronic appliances emit nonionizing radiation, but such exposures have not been shown to affect fetal development adversely. Magnetic resonance imaging results in high-level exposure to radiofrequency radiation, and also appears to have no adverse effect on the fetus (6).

Recreational Drugs

Certain adverse effects can result from the use of recreational drugs during pregnancy. Patient education about the possible deleterious effects of drug use is appropriate during preconceptional and prenatal visits (see "Preconceptional Care").

ALCOHOL

Maternal alcohol ingestion during pregnancy may result in a recognizable pattern of congenital anomalies known as fetal alcohol syndrome. The anatomic features of fetal alcohol syndrome include prenatal and postnatal growth restriction, characteristic facial anomalies (ie, short palpebral fissures, microphthalmia, indistinct or absent philtrum, thin upper lip, midfacial hypoplasia), microcephaly, joint contractures, and cardiac defects. Fetal alcohol syndrome also includes varying degrees of mental retardation, hyperactivity, other behavioral abnormalities, poor coordination, and developmental delays. Alcohol abuse during pregnancy is a leading and completely preventable cause of mental retardation.

Although studies have suggested that as little as 1 drink per day can cause fetal alcohol syndrome, most of the subjects in these studies did not drink 1 drink daily; most drank 6 or more drinks per occasion, which averaged 1 drink per day. It now appears that the fetal effects of alcohol are biphasic, with a linear dose-response effect seen after a threshold of 4–6 drinks per occasion on several occasions per week. Among pregnant women who consume 4 drinks per day during pregnancy, the risk of fetal alcohol syndrome may be as high as 20%; this risk increases to 40% with 6 drinks per day, and goes up to 50% with 8 drinks. One beer, 1 shot of liquor, 1 mixed drink, and 1 glass of wine all contain approximately 14 g (0.5 ounce) of absolute alcohol. Thus, all forms of alcohol are equally hazardous. Although no quantifiable risk has been associated with an occasional alcoholic beverage during pregnancy, it is reasonable to advise pregnant women to avoid alcohol consumption completely.

TOBACCO

Pregnant smokers may be at increased risk of spontaneous abortion, fetal death associated with placental abruption, preterm delivery, and premature preterm rupture of membranes. Smoking approximately doubles the risk of low birth weight, and there is a dose–response relationship between the amount of maternal smoking and the degree of birth weight reduction (7) (see "Preconceptional Care" for discussion of smoking cessation programs). The offspring of women who smoke approximately 20 cigarettes (1 pack) per day during pregnancy have birth weights that are approximately 200 g less than those of infants born to women who do not smoke. If a woman stops smoking during the last 4 months of pregnancy, the risk of giving birth to an infant with lowered birth weight is similar to that of a nonsmoker (8).

The use of smokeless tobacco increases blood nicotine levels to those associated with cigarette smoking and, based on limited data, may result in similarly decreased birth weight. The possible clinical effects of passive smoking during pregnancy have not been clearly established, but a small decrement in birth weight appears possible.

Although cigarette smoking has long been recognized as a cause of lower birth weight and an increased risk of pregnancy complications, an association with congenital anomalies has been identified only recently. Smoking women who carry a certain polymorphism in the gene for transforming growth factor β (TGF-β) appear to have an increased risk of cleft lip and palate in their offspring (9). This polymorphism is not common, and most offspring of women who smoke do not have an increased incidence of birth defects.

COCAINE

Cocaine blocks the presynaptic reuptake of the neurotransmitters norepinephrine and dopamine, causing them to accumulate at postsynaptic receptor sites and resulting in intense vasoconstriction, acute arterial hypertension, and tachycardia. The potentially lethal medical complications associated, directly or indirectly, with cocaine use seem to be attributable to the intense sympathomimetic effects of the drug. These complications include acute myocardial infarction, cardiac arrhythmias, rupture of the ascending aorta, cerebrovascular accidents, seizures, bowel ischemia, and hyperthermia. The effects on pregnancy attributed to the noradrenergic or vasoconstrictive action of cocaine include preterm labor and placental abruption. Cocaine binges can bring on labor, causing some women to binge when they want to bring on labor.

Cocaine also affects fetal vasculature. Vascular disruption caused by the sympathomimetic effects of cocaine can result in skull defects, cutis aplasia, porencephaly, subependymal and periventricular cysts, ileal atresia, visceral infarcts, and cardiac anomalies. Fetuses exposed to cocaine have urinary tract defects 4.4 times more often than unexposed fetuses.

Neonates exposed to cocaine in utero also exhibit neurobehavioral abnormalities, especially irritability and an inability to respond appropriately to stimulation. However, it is difficult to determine whether these problems are caused by cocaine alone. Pregnant cocaine users often seek prenatal care late in pregnancy, if at all, and may have poor nutrition. They also tend to abuse multiple drugs, including tobacco and alcohol. Adverse pregnancy outcomes attributed to cocaine may, therefore, result from the combination of cocaine with other risk factors. When such infants are adopted and raised in nurturing environments, their behaviors appear to normalize. It is, therefore, not clear whether or not these behaviors represent permanent abnormalities of brain development, or whether such children will later manifest permanent neurobehavioral abnormalities.

OTHER ILLICIT DRUGS

Maternal use of heroin, methadone, methamphetamine, or phencyclidine may produce a neonatal withdrawal syndrome characterized by increased muscle tone, tremors, and a high-pitched cry. Lysergic acid diethylamide (LSD) has not been associated with an increase in birth defects, either with use during pregnancy or with use in the past.

References

1. Del Campo M, Kosaki K, Bennett FC, Jones KL. Developmental delay in fetal aminopterin/methotrexate syndrome. Teratology 1999;60:10–2.

2. Miller RK, Hendrickx AG, Mills JL, Hummler H, Wiegand UW. Periconceptional vitamin A use: how much is teratogenic? Reprod Toxicol 1998;12:75–88.

3. Mastroiacovo P, Mazzone T, Addis A, Elephant E, Carlier P, Vial T, et al. High vitamin A intake in early pregnancy and major malformations: a multicenter prospective controlled study. Teratology 1999;59:7–11.

4. Clarkson TW. The three modern faces of mercury. Environ Health Perspect 2002;110:11–23.

5. Center for Food Safety and Applied Nutrition, U.S. Food and Drug Administration. An important message for pregnant women and women of childbearing age who may become pregnant about the risks of mercury in fish. Consumer Advisory. Washington, DC: FDA; 2001.

6. Roberts MD, Lange RC, McCarthy SM. Fetal anatomy with magnetic resonance imaging. Magn Reson Imaging 1995; 13:645–9.

7. Werler MM. Teratogen update: smoking and reproductive outcomes. Teratology 1997;55:382–8.

8. Cliver SP, Goldenberg RL, Cutter R, Hoffman HJ, Davis RO, Nelson KG. The effect of cigarette smoking on neonatal anthropometric measurements. Obstet Gynecol 1995;85: 625–30.

9. Shaw GM, Velie EM, Schaffer D. Risk of neural tube defect-affected pregnancies among obese women. JAMA 1996;275:1093–6.

ULTRASONOGRAPHY

Obstetric ultrasound examination has become an integral part of obstetric practice. Most U.S. women have at least 1 ultrasound examination during their pregnancies.

Types of Examinations

The types of ultrasound examinations are defined by the components. Coding for reimbursement is guided by these components (Table 3). The implications and use of ultrasound examinations have continued to expand.

Brief or limited examinations may be appropriate during emergencies. Depending on the indication, a limited examination should be followed by a basic or comprehensive examination unless the patient previously had such an examination in the second or third trimester. A limited ultrasound examination also may be used to provide guidance during procedures such as amniocentesis, during labor and delivery for quickly assessing fetal position or locating fetal heart tones, and is used during external cephalic version.

Recently, attention has been turned to screening for fetal chromosome anomalies, particularly Down syndrome

in the first trimester (1, 2). It has been found that fetuses with Down syndrome have an increased lucent area behind the head in the nuchal region. The risk of Down syndrome increases with increasing size of the nuchal area. Various authors have used either a cutoff of 3 mm, or more accurately, nomograms that take into account maternal age, gestational age, and crown–rump length, to determine the risk of Down syndrome. Serum screening has been used in conjunction with first-trimester nuchal measurements or subsequently in the second trimester in order to decrease the false-positive rate and increase the detection of Down

TABLE 3. Types of Ultrasound Examinations

Type of Examination	CPT Code	Description
First trimester (<14 weeks)	76801	Fetal and maternal evaluation, transabdominal approach, singleton gestation
Basic (≥14 weeks)	76805	Fetal and maternal evaluation, transabdominal approach; includes anatomy survey, singleton gestation
Detailed fetal	76811	Includes detailed fetal anatomic examination, singleton gestation
Limited	76815	Focused brief examination of fetal heartbeat, placental location, fetal position, and/ or qualitative amniotic fluid volume
Follow-up	76816	Follow-up examination for reevaluation of previously examined fetus, singleton gestation
Transvaginal	76817	Transvaginal examination of pregnant uterus

CPT indicates Current Procedural Terminology.

RESOURCES

Ultrasonography

American College of Obstetricians and Gynecologists
www.acog.org

American Institute of Ultrasound in Medicine
www.aium.org

National Institute of Child Health and Human Development
www.nichd.nih.gov

Society of Diagnostic Medical Sonography
www.sdms.org

syndrome (3). These ultrasound measurements are technically exacting because the areas measured are small and small deviations in methodology may change risk assignment and patient management. Accuracy increases with operator experience (Fig. 1).

Some investigators also noted absence of a nasal bone in fetuses screened in the first trimester with Down syndrome; in the second trimester, this is shortening of the bone, reflecting hypoplasia (4). However, subsequent studies did not show this finding. This presumably corresponds to the mid-face hypoplasia seen in children with Down syndrome (Fig. 2). Fetuses with an increased nuchal lucency and normal chromosomes have an increased risk for congenital heart disease.

Evaluation of Structures

THE PLACENTA

Patients who present with bleeding and do not have placenta previa may well have placental abruption. More than half of patients with significant placental abruption

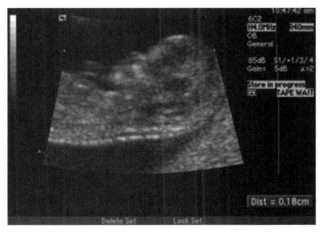

■ **FIG. 1.** Nuchal area. (Courtesy of Isabelle Wilkins, MD)

have ultrasound examination findings that identify an area of separation or a retroplacental hematoma. For many patients, placental abruption remains a diagnosis of exclusion.

Attention has been turned recently to looking for placental abnormalities consistent with placenta accreta. It is unclear how accurate this is as a screening tool, but in patients at risk, for example with placenta previa and a prior cesarean delivery, suspicious areas may be seen by ultrasound examination. In these cases, large vessels can be seen replacing myometrium and often invading or indenting the bladder wall (Fig. 3); color flow Doppler usually is dramatic. Although magnetic resonance imaging has been used as a definitive diagnostic test, ultrasound examination alone may be just as accurate.

THE CERVIX

The cervix may be seen at any time during pregnancy through transabdominal or transvaginal approaches. Reliable, reproducible information about the cervix is best obtained on transvaginal views. The most established use of cervical ultrasonography is to visualize the relationship of a low-lying placenta to the os, thus excluding or making the diagnosis of a placenta previa. The length of the endocervical canal and the contour of the internal os can be seen easily with this approach.

The average length of the cervix at 26–30 weeks is 35–37 mm (Fig. 4). This is longer than is generally described by vaginal examination, no doubt because a portion of the cervix is above the level of the vaginal fornix. Cervical ultrasound examination in this setting has been shown to correlate with eventual preterm delivery (5). Both the shortening of the cervix and the presence of funneling or wedging of the internal os have been correlated with a higher risk of preterm delivery than a normal cervical ultrasound examination result (Figs. 5 and 6).

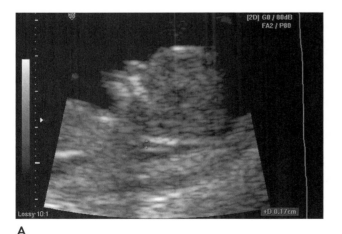

A

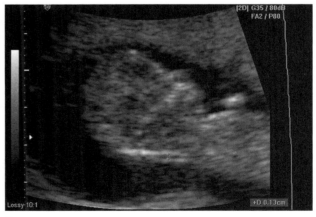

B

■ **FIG. 2. A.** Nasal bone seen. **B.** No nasal bone. (Courtesy of Isabelle Wilkins, MD)

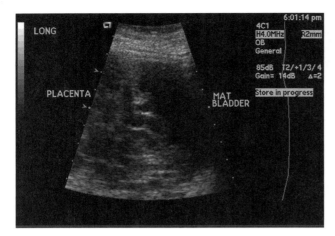

■ **FIG 3.** Placenta accreta. (Courtesy of Isabelle Wilkins, MD)

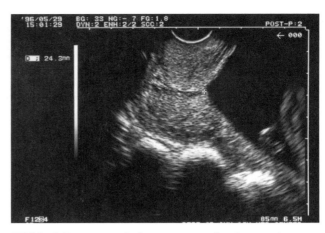

■ **FIG. 5.** Transvaginal ultrasonogram of a shortened cervix. The total length is 24 mm. (Courtesy of Jay Iams, MD)

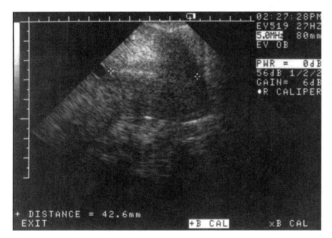

■ **FIG. 4.** Transvaginal ultrasonogram of a normal cervix with a length of 43 mm. (Courtesy of Isabelle Wilkins, MD)

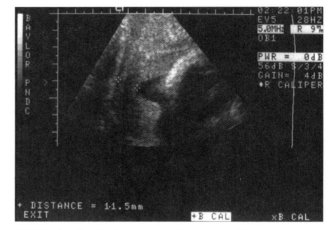

■ **FIG. 6.** Cervix showing beaking or wedging in the area of the internal os; in this case, it is adjacent to the fetal vertex. (Courtesy of Isabelle Wilkins, MD)

When these findings are discovered incidentally during ultrasound examination of low-risk women, such findings do not support a diagnosis of cervical incompetence. In contrast, nonrandomized studies suggest that the findings of progressive shortening and wedging at the internal os in patients at risk for cervical incompetence indicate impending second-trimester loss (Fig. 7) (6).

FETAL ECHOCARDIOGRAM

A specialized adjunct to a comprehensive ultrasound examination is a fetal echocardiogram. Although a thorough evaluation of the fetal heart usually is performed during a comprehensive examination, fetal cardiac anatomy is difficult to visualize completely and remains one area in which the detection rate for anomalies is low (approximately 50–80% in most series). Fetal echocardiograms are more detailed, lengthy examinations performed in specialized centers in which multiple aspects of intracardiac anatomy and function are assessed through the use of 2-dimensional imaging, color flow, and Doppler stud-

ies. Indications for fetal echocardiogram include a suspicion of a cardiac anomaly on a previous examination, a family history of congenital heart disease, maternal diabetes, fetal arrhythmias, and anomalies in other organ systems.

FETAL ARTERY DOPPLER STUDIES

Doppler fetal umbilical artery velocimetry has been used to measure increased placental vascular resistance, which may allow for the recognition of placental dysfunction. However, because of its low positive predictive value, Doppler velocimetry is not a screening test for detecting fetal compromise in the general obstetric population, as was originally proposed. The value of Doppler fetal umbilical artery velocimetry is most established in pregnancies with IUGR (7). In these cases, an abnormal pattern of blood flow is associated with a poor outcome and warrants close surveillance or intervention. After 24 weeks of gestation, measurement of the relationship of peak systolic-to-diastolic flow velocities, with the systolic-diastolic ratio, pulsatility index, or resistance index, is a useful predictor of fetal compromise. Absent or reversed blood flow in diastole reflects extreme placental vascular resistance and is ominous; perinatal mortality in such pregnancies is high. The clinical utility of umbilical artery Doppler velocimetry for antenatal testing in other diagnoses has been less fruitful.

Noninvasive monitoring of the alloimmunized pregnancy is becoming routine. Doppler study of the peak systolic blood velocity in the fetal middle cerebral artery is now becoming the standard for the detection of fetal anemia at many referral centers (9). Serial testing is undertaken every 1–2 weeks starting at 18–20 weeks of gestation once a critical maternal antibody titer has been reached. A value of greater than 1.5 multiples of the median (MoM) indicates a high likelihood for fetal anemia with a false-positive rate of approximately 10%. This

strategy virtually eliminates the need for amniocentesis for ΔOD_{450}.

Three-Dimensional Ultrasound Imaging

Three-dimensional ultrasound imaging is now clinically available in many centers and is frequently sought by patients. In some circumstances, it provides useful adjunctive information to traditional imaging. Most ultrasound machines with 3-dimensional capability employ a transducer that is thicker than that commonly used with 2-dimensional machines. A series of tomograms are obtained over the width of the transducer. After the data are obtained, computer analysis creates a 3-dimensional rendering. The computer also can be used to delete adjacent structures that are not of interest. Fetal movement while these serial tomograms are being captured interferes with resolution.

A number of pilot studies have examined normal and abnormal fetuses with this approach. Many of the initial results have been in areas in which the surface of structures is important and, therefore, 3-dimensional imaging is likely to be superior to 2-dimensional imaging, such as the fetal face (Fig. 8). Three-dimensional imaging also is used for volume calculations. To date, this has been more applicable to gynecologic ultrasonography, but it also has been described to calculate fetal weight or fetal fat stores and to determine more precisely the size of various fetal landmarks.

References

1. American College of Obstetricians and Gynecologists. Prenatal diagnosis of fetal chromosomal abnormalities. ACOG Practice Bulletin 27. Washington, DC: ACOG; 2001.

2. First-trimester screening for fetal aneuploidy. ACOG Committee Opinion No. 296. American College of Obstetricians and Gynecologists. Obstet Gynecol 2004; 104:215–7.

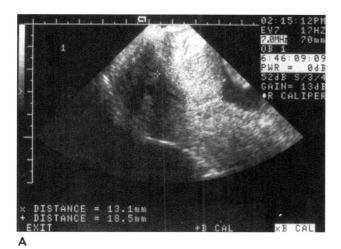

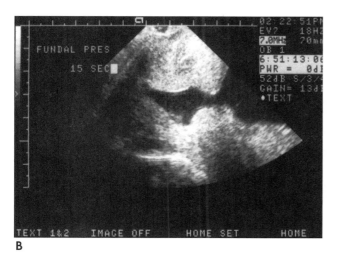

■ FIG. 7. A. Patient at 20 weeks of gestation, with an apparently normal length cervix of 32 mm. **B.** The same patient a few minutes later, after application of fundal pressure, showing prolapsing of the membranes through the cervix. This patient had a normal digital pelvic examination. (Courtesy of Isabelle Wilkins, MD)

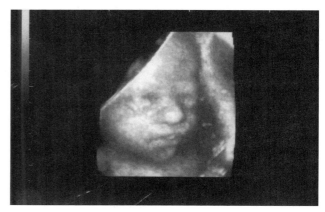

■ FIG. 8. Three-dimensional ultrasonogram of a fetal face, showing normal anatomy, at 20 weeks of gestation. (Courtesy of Christine Comstock, MD)

3. Wapner R, Thom E, Simpson JL, Pergament E, Silver R, Filkins K, et al. First trimester screening for trisomies 21 and 18. First Trimester Maternal Serum Biochemistry and Fetal Nuchal Translucency Screening (BUN) Study Group. N Engl J Med 2003;349:1405–13.

4. Cicero S, Bindra R, Rembouskos G, Spencer K, Nicolaides KH. Integrated ultrasound and biochemical screening for trisomy 21 using fetal nuchal translucency, absent fetal nasal bone, free beta-hCG and PAPP-A at 11 to 14 weeks. Prenat Diagn 2003;23:306–10.

5. Iams JD, Goldenberg RL, Meis PJ, Mercer BM, Moawad A, Das A, et al. The length of the cervix and the risk of spontaneous premature delivery. National Institute of Child Health and Human Development Maternal Fetal Medicine Unit Network. N Engl J Med 1996;334:567–72.

6. Guzman ER, Houlihan C, Vintzileos A, Ivan J, Benito C, Kappy K. The significance of transvaginal ultrasonographic evaluation of the cervix in women treated with emergency cerclage. Am J Obstet Gynecol 1996;175:471–6.

7. American College of Obstetricians and Gynecologists. Utility of antepartum umbilical artery Doppler velocimetry in intrauterine growth restriction. ACOG Committee Opinion 188. Washington, DC: ACOG, 1997.

8. Zimmerman R, Carpenter RJ Jr, Durig P, Mari G. Longitudinal measurement of peak systolic velocity in the fetal middle cerebral artery for monitoring pregnancies complicated by red cell alloimmunisation: a prospective multicentre trial with intention-to-treat. BJOG 2002;109: 746–52.

PRENATAL DIAGNOSIS OF GENETIC DISORDERS

Genetic disorders have a tremendous potential for causing adverse effects for reproductive-aged women and their families. Eight percent (1/13) of conceptuses are chromosomally abnormal, accounting for at least 50% of all first-trimester abortions and 6–11% of all stillbirths and neonatal deaths. By grade school, a major or minor structural birth defect will be recognized in 8% of all children and another 8% will have developmental delays. Additionally, it is estimated that 60% of disease in adults (eg, hypertension, diabetes) has a genetic basis. Specific knowledge of the genetic etiology of these conditions is expanding rapidly. The indications for preconceptional counseling and prenatal diagnosis are expanding as well, as more women request counseling and testing.

Genetic Disorders

CHROMOSOME ABNORMALITIES

Most trisomies result from maternal meiotic nondisjunction, a phenomenon that occurs more frequently as women (and their gametes) age. Numeric sex chromosome abnormalities can result from either maternal or paternal nondisjunction; inversions and translocations may be sporadic or familial.

Autosomal Trisomy

Most fetal trisomies result from an error in maternal meiosis. Although any woman at any age can have a trisomic fetus, the frequency of meiotic errors and resulting fetal aneuploidy increases with each year of age. Traditionally, women who will be aged 35 years or older at the time of delivery are thought to be at sufficient risk to warrant the routine offering of fetal karyotype analysis by chorionic villus sampling (CVS) or genetic amniocentesis. Age 35 years is an arbitrary cutoff chosen because, at that age, the risk of fetal Down syndrome begins to increase sharply with each year of maternal age, and because the midtrimester risk of Down syndrome or the term risk of any aneuploidy roughly equals the risk of pregnancy loss after amniocentesis. Women younger than 35 years also should be offered prenatal genetic testing if their obstetric history, family history, ultrasound examination findings, or maternal serum screening test results suggest an increased risk. Women who have had a previ-

---

RESOURCES

Prenatal Diagnosis of Genetic Disorders

American College of Medical Genetics
www.acmg.net

American College of Obstetricians and Gynecologists
www.acog.org

Genetics Home Reference
ghr.nlm.nih.gov/ghr/page/home

The Human Genome Resources
www.ncbi.nlm.nih.gov/genome/guide/human

March of Dimes Birth Defects Foundation
www.modimes.org

National Center on Birth Defects and Developmental Disabilities
www.cdc.gov/ncbddd

National Human Genome Research Institute
www.genome.gov

National Institute of Child Health and Human Development
www.nichd.nih.gov

National Newborn Screening & Genetics Resource Center
genes-r-us.uthscsa.edu

NINDS Cerebral Palsy Information Page
www.ninds.nih.gov/disorders/cerebral_palsy/cerebral_palsy.htm

ous pregnancy complicated by trisomy 21, 18, or 13 or any other trisomy in which the fetus survived at least to the second trimester should be offered prenatal karyotype analysis. For such women, the risk of having another pregnancy complicated by the same or a different trisomy is estimated to be 1% until the age-related risk exceeds this figure; the risk is then determined by maternal age.

Some younger women may request testing because of anxiety. Testing may be performed in these patients after a full discussion of the risks of the procedure relative to the patient's estimated risk of fetal aneuploidy. Conversely, after an explanation of the risks and benefits of invasive testing, women older than 34 years of age who wish to minimize their risk of pregnancy loss may opt for noninvasive first- or second-trimester aneuploidy screening to further refine their estimated Down syndrome risk before moving to invasive testing.

Sex Chromosome Abnormalities

Sex chromosome abnormalities occur in 1 of every 1,000 births. The most common are 45,X; 47,XXY; 47,XXX; 47,XYY; and mosaicism (the presence of 2 or more cell populations with different karyotypes). A pregnancy complicated by fetal XXX or XXY increases the recurrence risk for another fetal trisomy to 1%; women with this history should be offered prenatal testing in subsequent pregnancies. Although monosomy X (Turner syndrome) and 47,XYY impart no increased risk of recurrence, a woman whose fetus had either of these karyotypes may request genetic testing for reassurance.

Translocations and Inversions

A translocation involves the exchange of genetic material between 2 different (nonhomologous) chromosomes. A break occurs in 1 arm of each chromosome, and all the genetic material distal to each break point is exchanged.

In a balanced translocation, no genetic material is gained or lost, and the individual carrying such a rearrangement usually is phenotypically normal. However, a carrier of a balanced translocation may make unbalanced gametes, resulting in infertility, early pregnancy loss, or structurally or developmentally abnormal offspring. The translocation carrier's risk of having an affected child with an abnormal amount of chromosomal material should be estimated individually, taking into account the chromosomes involved, the amount of genetic material exchanged, the sex of the transmitting parent, and the method of ascertainment. In general, translocation carriers identified after the birth of an abnormal infant are at increased risk (5–30%) of having another abnormal child. Those identified during an infertility workup are at low risk (0–5%) of having an abnormal child but are at increased risk to have continued infertility, most likely because their translocation leads to nonviable gametes or conceptuses.

A robertsonian translocation results from the centromeric fusion of 2 acrocentric chromosomes. Acrocentric chromosomes (chromosomes 13, 14, 15, 21, and 22) have the centromere located very near one end. The carrier of a robertsonian translocation also is at risk of producing unbalanced gametes. Whether the unbalanced gametes will result in abnormal offspring depends on the type of translocation, the chromosomes involved, and the sex of the carrier parent. The most clinically important robertsonian translocations are those involving chromosome 21 and another acrocentric chromosome, most commonly chromosome 14 (t[14;21]). Carriers of these translocations have the potential to have a liveborn child with trisomy 21. The risk of trisomy 21 is 15% if the translocation is maternal and 2% or less if it is paternal.

Inversions arise when 2 breaks occur in the same chromosome and the segment between the break points is inverted before the breaks are repaired. No genetic material is lost, but the gene sequence is altered. Most carriers of inversions are phenotypically normal. However, because inversion carriers usually produce both balanced and unbalanced gametes, fertility may be affected. If both break points occur in the same arm of the chromosome (paracentric inversion), the centromere is not involved. The unbalanced gametes produced contain either no centromere or 2 centromeres, and thus are so abnormal as to preclude fertilization. The carrier of a paracentric inversion, therefore, has virtually no risk of having abnormal offspring. However, if the break points occur in opposite arms of the chromosome (pericentric inversion), the centromere is involved. The unbalanced gametes produced in this case may contain duplications or deletions, but still be capable of fertilization. As a result, the carrier of a pericentric inversion has a 5–10% risk of having abnormal children if the carrier status was ascertained after the birth of an abnormal child and 1–3% if not. All carriers of chromosome rearrangements should be counseled and offered prenatal diagnosis based on their history and estimated risk.

Triploidy

A triploid conception is one in which 3 complete haploid (n = 23) chromosome complements are present, resulting in 69 total chromosomes. This abnormality occurs in 1–2% of recognized pregnancies, accounting for 15% of chromosomally abnormal abortuses. Most commonly, triploidy results from double fertilization of a normal haploid egg (dispermy) or from fertilization with a diploid sperm. Such conceptions usually are partial hydatidiform moles and end spontaneously in the first trimester; the recurrence risk is minimal, and genetic testing in future pregnancies is unnecessary. Rarely, a fetus develops in association with triploidy. Fetuses resulting from the fertilization of a diploid ovum (digenic) are severely growth restricted and have small, noncystic placentas. Fetuses resulting from disperm (diandric) are relatively normal in size but have large, cystic placentas. This form of triploidy often is associated with midtrimester onset of severe preeclampsia. Women who experienced triploidy in association with a fetus surviving past the first trimester have a 1–2% risk of recurrence for any numerical aneuploidy and should be offered genetic testing in subsequent pregnancies.

Spontaneous Pregnancy Loss

At least half of all first-trimester pregnancy losses result from fetal karyotypic abnormalities; the most common abnormalities are monosomy X; polyploidy (triploidy or tetraploidy); and trisomies 13, 16, 18, 21, and 22. Some studies suggest that recurrent pregnancy loss is commonly caused by fetal aneuploidy, whereas others indicate that most recurrent losses are euploid (1). Because the incidence of early pregnancy loss caused by fetal aneuploidy increases with maternal age, failure to account for the maternal age-related risk of aneuploidy may explain these opposite findings. It is controversial as to whether a chromosomally abnormal first-trimester loss increases the risk of having an aneuploid fetus surviving into the second trimester and beyond. It is, therefore,

unclear whether karyotyping products of conception is of value in determining the risk of subsequent viable aneuploid offspring, although it may clarify the etiology of the patient's loss. Because approximately 2% of recurrent abortions occur as the result of a parental translocation, couples with a history of recurrent first-trimester loss in which no genetic studies have been performed should be offered parental karyotype analysis, followed by prenatal genetic testing of the fetus if either parent is a carrier of a chromosome abnormality (2).

Parental Aneuploidy

Women with trisomy 21 or 47,XXX and men with 47,XYY usually are fertile and have a 30% risk of trisomic offspring. Men with trisomy 21 or 47,XXY usually are sterile.

Fetus With Major Structural Defect Identified by Ultrasonography

The discovery of a structural malformation of a major fetal organ or structure (Table 4) or the finding of 2 or more minor malformations (ie, choroid plexus cyst, extra digit, single umbilical artery) increases the risk of aneuploidy sufficiently to warrant genetic testing of the fetus, regardless of maternal age or parental karyotypes. An exception to this dictum is a fetal defect known to be a malformation not associated with aneuploidy (eg, fetal

■ TABLE 4. Aneuploid Risk of Major Anomalies

Structural Defect	Population Incidence	Aneuploidy Risk	Most Common Aneuploidy (Trisomy)
Cystic hygroma	1/120 (EU) – 1/6,000 (B)	60–75%	45X (80%); 21, 18, 13, XXY
Hydrops	1/1,500–1/4,000 B	30–80%*	13, 21 ,18 ,45X
Hydrocephalus	3/10,000–8/10,000 LB	3–8%	13, 18, triploidy
Hydranencephaly	2/1,000 IA	Minimal	–
Holoprosencephaly	1/16,000 LB	40–60%	13, 18, 18p-
Cardiac defects	7/1,000–9/1,000 LB	5–30%	21, 18, 13, 22, 8, 9
Complete AV canal		40–70%	21
Diaphragmatic hernia	1/3,500–1/4,000 LB	20–25%	13, 18, 21, 45X
Omphalocele	1/5,800 LB	30–40%	13,18
Gastroschisis	1/10,000–1/15,000 LB	Minimal	–
Duodenal atresia	1/10,000 LB	20–30%	21
Bowel obstruction	1/2,500–5,000 LB	Minimal	–
Bladder outlet obstruction	1/1,000–2/1,000 LB	20–25%	13, 18
Prune belly syndrome	1/35,000–1/50,000 LB	Low	18, 13, 45X
Facial cleft	1/700 LB	1%	13, 18, deletions
Limb reduction	4/10,000–6/10,000 LB	8%	18
Club foot	1.2 /1,000 LB	20–30%	18, 13, 4p-,18q-
Single umbilical artery	1%	Minimal	–

B indicates birth; EU, early ultrasound; IA, infant autopsy; LB, live birth; SAB, spontaneous abortion.

*30% if diagnosed ≥24 weeks; 80% if diagnosed ≤17 weeks.

cleft lip discovered during an ultrasound examination ordered because the mother has a cleft lip).

SINGLE-GENE DISORDERS

Patient or Family History

Single-gene disorders generally are transmitted in autosomal dominant, autosomal recessive, or X-linked recessive fashion. An exception is any new single-gene disorder that results in death before reproduction or infertility; these occur as the result of a spontaneous new mutation. For example, deletions of genes on the Y chromosome are frequently not transmissible because they result in infertility.

The number of single-gene disorders that can be diagnosed prenatally is increasing rapidly. The list of diagnosable diseases currently includes autosomal dominant diseases, such as neurofibromatosis, myotonic dystrophy, adult polycystic kidney disease, Huntington's disease, and osteogenesis imperfecta; autosomal recessive conditions, such as cystic fibrosis, phenylketonuria, congenital adrenal hyperplasia, and Tay–Sachs and other enzyme deficiency diseases; and X-linked diseases, including hemophilia A, Duchenne's muscular dystrophy, and Fragile X syndrome. Any patient with a personal or family history of a monogenic disorder should be referred before conception or early in pregnancy for genetic counseling and consideration of carrier testing or prenatal diagnosis.

Ethnic Groups at High Risk

Although single-gene disorders generally are rare, some ethnic groups are at higher risk of having certain diseases than the general population and should be counseled and offered genetic screening accordingly (Table 5). If only one person in a couple is a member of the high-risk group, that person can be tested first; if he or she is determined not to be a carrier, the partner may not need to be screened.

African Americans are at increased risk of having sickle cell disease, the most common hemoglobin disorder in the United States. Hemoglobin is a tetrameric protein composed of 2 α and 2 β polypeptide chains. Hemoglobin S results from the alteration of a single peptide in the β chain—the substitution of valine for glutamic acid at the sixth position of the polypeptide.

Approximately 8% of African Americans carry the sickle hemoglobin gene, which also is found with increased frequency in those of Mediterranean, Caribbean, Latin American, or Middle Eastern descent. Southeast Asians are at increased risk for carrying hemoglobin E, the second most common abnormal hemoglobin in the world. The homozygous state results in microcytosis but not marked anemia, whereas individuals with hemoglobin E β-thalassemia can have severe hemolytic anemia requiring transfusion during pregnancy. Women whose ancestors came from high-risk areas should be offered hemoglobinopathy screening. Hemoglobin electrophoresis is the test of choice because it will identify all abnormal hemoglobins, not just hemoglobin S. If the patient is a hemoglobinopathy carrier, the partner should be screened as well so that the couple's risk of having an affected child can be determined.

Individuals of Mediterranean or Asian origin are at increased risk of having α-thalassemia or β-thalassemia. The thalassemias occur as the result of a functional deletion of 1 or more of the 2 β genes or 2 or more of the 4 α genes (Table 6). The loss of these genes leads to decreased production of the hemoglobin chain in question, reduced production of the intact hemoglobin molecule, hemolysis, and anemia, which can be severe. Carrier testing begins with determination of red blood cell indices; a mean corpuscular volume (MCV) of less than 79 m^3 indicates increased risk. Because the most common explanation for a reduced MCV is iron deficiency, the patient with a low MCV first should be evaluated with iron studies or begin iron therapy presumptively. If iron studies are normal or there is no response to therapy, hemoglobin electrophoresis should be performed.

If the patient has a functional deletion of a β gene and makes reduced quantities of the β chain, the excess α chains will combine with δ chains instead to make hemoglobin A$_2$. A hemoglobin A$_2$ level of at least 3.5% (determined by hemoglobin electrophoresis) confirms the diagnosis.

In α-thalassemia, 2 or more α chain genes must be deleted before the MCV is decreased. In contrast to β-thalassemia, α-thalassemia does not result in the production of an alternate hemoglobin molecule because there is no protein that can substitute for the α chain. The loss of 2 or more genes encoding the α chain thus results only in reduced production of normal hemoglobin A. As a result, α-thalassemia cannot be diagnosed by hemoglobin electrophoresis, but approximately 20% of α-thalassemia cases can be identified by molecular genetic testing. Patients with 2 or more deleted α chain genes will have normal iron studies as well as normal levels of hemoglobin A$_2$. The patient with a low MCV, normal iron studies, and normal hemoglobin electrophoresis should, therefore, be referred for genetic counseling and molecular genetic testing. Prenatal diagnosis by molecular testing can identify all forms of β-thalassemia.

Individuals of Jewish descent are at increased risk for Tay–Sachs disease, Canavan disease, and Gaucher's disease, each of which is caused by a different enzyme deficiency (hexosaminidase A, aspartoacylase, and glucocerebrosidase, respectively), and other less common enzyme deficiency diseases such as Niemann–Pick, Bloom syndrome, and Fanconi anemia type C. Individuals with these autosomal recessive disorders all have in common the inability to degrade certain byproducts of normal catabolism, leading to a neurovisceral storage abnormality and a rapidly progressive neurodegenerative course. The carrier rate among individuals

■ **TABLE 5.** Ethnic Groups at Risk for Single-Gene Disorders

Ethnic Group	Disease	Heterozygote (Carrier) Rate	Incidence of Disease
African American	Hemoglobin SS (sickle cell disease)	1/12	1/576
	Hemoglobin CC	1/40	1/4,790
	Hemoglobin SC	Variable	1/757
	Hemoglobin S/ β-thalassemia	1/22	1/1,672
Mediterranean (also Asian)	β-thalassemia	1/10–1/20	1/10–1/20* (β-thal minor)
Asian (also Mediterranean)	α-thalassemia	1/5	1/50 (α-thal minor)†
Jewish	Tay–Sachs disease	1/30	1/3,600
	Canavan disease	1/40	1/6,400
	Gaucher's disease	1/12–1/25	1/576–1/2,500
	Cystic fibrosis	1/24–1/90	1/2,304–1/32,400
North European Caucasian	Cystic fibrosis	1/20–1/25	1/2,500
Native American	Cystic fibrosis	1/20–1/31	1/1,580–1/3,970
Southeast Asian	Hemoglobin EE	1/10–1/400	
	Hemoglobin E/ β-thalassemia	Variable	1/400–1/800
	Hemoglobin E/ α-thalassemia	Variable	1/200

*Deletion of both chain genes results in Cooley anemia and usually is lethal.

†Deletion of 3 chain genes results in hemoglobin H, which is transfusion dependent and often lethal; deletion of 4 chain genes results in hemoglobin Barts and hydrops fetalis and is lethal.

■ **TABLE 6.** Hemoglobinopathies

Clinical Class	Genotype	Hemoglobin Electrophoresis
Silent carrier		
α+ Thalassemia silent	$-\alpha/\alpha\alpha$	Normal
Thalassemia minor		
β-Thalassemia trait	β/β^0	
α^0 Thalassemia trait	$.../\alpha\alpha$	
Hgb Constant Spring	$\alpha^{CS}/\alpha\alpha^{CS}$	Decreased A_2
α+ Thalassemia trait	$-\alpha/-\alpha$	
Lepore trait	$\beta/(\delta\beta)^{+Lepore}$	
δβ-Thalassemia trait	$\beta/(\delta\beta)^{0\ or\ +}$	Increased A_2
Thalassemia intermedia		
$\beta^{+Africa}$ –Thalassemia trait		
α^+ and β^0 –Thalassemia	$\beta^{+Africa}/\beta^{+Africa}\ -\alpha/\ -\alpha\beta/\beta^0$	
Double heterozygote trait		
β^0 –Thalassemia major with high Hgb F	β/β^0 with incr F production	
$(\delta\beta)$ 0 or $^{+/Lepore}$ homozygotes	(δ/β) 0 or $^{+/Lepore}/(\delta\beta)$ 0 or $^{+/Lepore}$	Increased A_2
Thalassemia major		
β^0–Thalassemia	β^0/β^0	
β^0/Hemoglobin E disease	β^0/β^E	Increased Hgb F

Data from Poole JH. Thalassemia and pregnancy. J Perinat Neonat Nurs 2003;17:196–208.

of Jewish heritage is 1 in 30 for Tay–Sachs disease, 1 in 40 for Canavan disease, and 1 in 12 to 1 in 25 for Gaucher's disease. Counseling and carrier screening for Tay–Sachs and Canavan diseases should be offered to all patients of Jewish heritage because prenatal diagnosis of both diseases is possible. Tay–Sachs carriers are identified by measuring their hexosaminidase A levels, which are reduced to 50% of normal. Carriers of Canavan disease are identified by molecular testing, but given that virtually all cases in individuals of Ashkenazi Jewish heritage are caused by only 2 mutations, this is not difficult.

For Gaucher's disease, however, screening and diagnosis is frustrating for at least 2 reasons. First, carriers cannot be identified by measuring enzyme levels, so they must be identified by molecular genetic testing to determine whether they carry any of the many known Gaucher's mutations. Second, prediction of the homozygous fetus's phenotype is difficult if there are no other affected family members (eg, if the parents underwent genetic testing only because of their ethnic origin). The difficulty arises from the fact that there are 3 clinical forms of Gaucher's disease, representing different degrees of enzyme deficiency, and 1 of these 3 forms is characterized by mild symptoms with adult onset. It is not currently possible to determine prenatally whether a fetus inheriting 2 Gaucher's mutations will have the mild or the severe form. For these reasons, prenatal screening for Gaucher's disease remains controversial.

Some centers offer screening for a battery of diseases that affect the Jewish population. The screening profile typically includes Tay–Sachs disease, Canavan disease, and Gaucher's disease, possibly along with Niemann–Pick disease, Bloom's syndrome, and Fanconi anemia type C. The low carrier rate and disease incidence for these disorders have led to controversy regarding screening.

Caucasians of Northern European descent are at increased risk of cystic fibrosis. A chronic pulmonary and exocrine pancreatic disease, cystic fibrosis is the most common monogenic disorder in this population. It is transmitted in autosomal recessive fashion and has a carrier frequency of 1 in 22 in Caucasians of Northern European heritage. Native Americans also are at increased risk, as are individuals of Jewish heritage. Hispanic individuals are at lower risk, with a carrier frequency of 1 in 49. More than 900 different gene mutations are known to cause cystic fibrosis. The most common cystic fibrosis mutation in Caucasians, ΔF508, accounts for 75% of cases of the disease.

If a specific gene mutation has been identified in an affected family, individuals at risk can be tested for that particular mutation. In a family with no history of cystic fibrosis, the laboratory receives no specific guidance regarding the gene deletions for which it should screen. Because it is not possible to screen for all 900 known mutations during carrier testing, most laboratories screen for a panel of 25 mutations that each have a frequency of at least 0.1% in American cystic fibrosis patients, and 1 or more of 7 second-tier mutations if certain specific mutations are identified in the first mutation panel (3).

An individual who has a negative cystic fibrosis screening test cannot be told that she does not carry the cystic fibrosis gene. However, she can be informed that the negative test result significantly reduces her risk of carrying the gene. For example, if the test result indicates that the patient does not carry any of the 25 most common mutations causing cystic fibrosis, her risk is reduced by 90%— from 1 in 22 (the a priori risk based solely on ethnic origin) to 1 in 246. If both members of the couple test negative, their risk of having a child with cystic fibrosis is reduced to 1 in 242,100.

The National Institutes of Health (NIH) and ACOG have recommended that cystic fibrosis screening be *offered* to all pregnant Caucasians of Northern European descent, and *made available* to pregnant women of other ethnic groups.

Nonmendelian Inheritance

Certain single-gene disorders are transmitted in nonclassical (nonmendelian) ways. For example, some inherited diseases occur as a result of a mutation in mitochondrial DNA (ie, Leber's hereditary optic atrophy, Kearns–Sayre syndrome, and myoclonic epilepsy with ragged red fibers). Because mitochondria are passed to the ovum exclusively by the mother, mitochondrial disorders are characterized by maternal inheritance.

Another nonclassical inheritance pattern involves germline mosaicism. Although it was previously believed that conditions caused by new autosomal dominant mutations (ie, osteogenesis imperfecta type II, tuberous sclerosis, or achondroplasia) occurred sporadically and had no recurrence risk, it is now believed that some individuals carry 2 or more populations of germ cells, 1 of which contains the new mutation. The risk of having another child with the same condition caused by a new autosomal dominant mutation is, therefore, not zero, but somewhere between 1% and 7%.

Genomic imprinting results in gene expression that differs according to the parent of origin. The differential expression is related to sex-specific differences in DNA methylation patterns. The methylation patterns are not permanent, but are altered with each generation to reflect the sex of the transmitting parent. The function of the gene and thus the course of certain diseases is altered by genomic imprinting. For example, when the gene for Huntington's disease is transmitted by the father, the symptoms have a much earlier onset than when the gene is transmitted by the mother.

Uniparental disomy occurs when both copies of 1 chromosome are transmitted by the same parent. A person with uniparental disomy, therefore, has 2 copies of certain genes from one parent and no copies of the same genes from the other parent. Because of genomic imprinting and resulting differential gene expression, this situation may cause phenotypic abnormalities. If the 2 copies inherited from one parent are abnormal, the individual may express features of an autosomal recessive disease even though only one parent carries the abnormal gene.

MULTIFACTORIAL DISORDERS

Multifactorial disorders are caused by a combination of factors, some genetic and some nongenetic (ie, environmental). Multifactorial disorders recur in families but are not transmitted in any distinctive pattern. Many congenital, single-organ system structural abnormalities are multifactorial, having an incidence in the general population of approximately 1 per 1,000. Examples of multifactorial traits include the following:

- Cleft lip, with or without cleft palate
- Congenital cardiac defects
- Diaphragmatic hernia
- Hydrocephalus
- Müllerian fusion defects
- Neural tube defects
- Omphalocele
- Posterior urethral valves
- Pyloric stenosis
- Renal agenesis
- Talipes equinovarus

Because most of the defects on this list also may occur as the result of a genetic syndrome, a single-gene disorder, or a chromosome abnormality, a thorough evaluation by a geneticist or fetal pathologist (in the case of pregnancy loss) may be necessary before multifactorial inheritance can be assumed. When multifactorial inheritance has been ascertained, the patient can be counseled regarding the following points:

- The risk to first-degree relatives of the affected individual (mother, father, brother, sister) is higher than in the general population. The most commonly quoted risk is an empiric risk based on experience with similar families (1–5% in most cases).
- The risk is sharply lower (<1%) for second-degree and more distant relatives.
- The recurrence risk is higher when more than 1 family member is affected and when the defect is more severe (indicating the presence of more abnormal genes or environmental influences).
- If the trait is more common in one sex than in the other, the risk is higher if the affected individual is of the less susceptible sex (again, indicating the presence of more abnormal genes).

Techniques

MATERNAL SERUM SCREENING FOR DOWN SYNDROME

Genetic amniocentesis to identify fetal aneuploidy in women at high risk for trisomy 21 (Down syndrome) has been available for 40 years. The definition of "high risk" in a singleton pregnancy has traditionally included being 35 years or older at the time of delivery. Although age 35 years was chosen somewhat arbitrarily as a cutoff, it roughly corresponds to the time when the incidence of trisomy related to maternal age starts to increase dramatically. In addition, the midtrimester risk of having a singleton fetus with Down syndrome or the term risk of any aneuploidy is roughly equivalent to the most commonly quoted risk of a procedure-related fetal loss (1/200). However, most Down syndrome pregnancies (80%) occur in women younger than 35 years. Younger women at risk for having a child with Down syndrome can be identified by the multiple-marker screening test. The second-trimester triple screen, consisting of maternal serum alpha-fetoprotein, unconjugated estriol, and β-hCG, identifies approximately 60% of all Down syndrome cases in women younger than 35 years and 75–90% in women aged 35 years and older. In addition, a unique pattern of analyte levels (low levels of all 3 serum analytes) identifies 60–75% of all cases of fetal trisomy 18. Dimeric inhibin A improves the detection of Down syndrome when added to the 3 traditional markers. Many laboratories now report that this second-trimester "quad screen" detects 70% of Down syndrome cases in women younger than 35 years and 80–90% in women aged 35 years and older (4).

In many centers across the country, first-trimester Down syndrome screening is offered using maternal serum analytes either alone or in combination with ultrasonographic markers. The most discriminatory first-trimester maternal serum analytes are either free β-hCG or intact hCG and pregnancy-associated plasma protein A (PAPP-A) (4, 5). The most predictive ultrasonographic marker is measurement of the nuchal translucency, an echolucent area seen in longitudinal midsagittal views of the back of the fetal neck between 10 and 14 weeks of gestation. Because the nuchal translucency naturally increases in size as the fetus grows, using a specific size cutoff to define an abnormal result leads to decreased test sensitivity. Expressing the nuchal translucency as a multiple of the median accounts for gestational age–associated size changes and also allows it to be combined with serum analytes to calculate a composite risk (6).

Two large trials of combined first-trimester ultrasonographic and serum screening have now been completed. One trial enrolled more than 8,000 women who underwent screening between 10 weeks 4 days and 13 weeks 6 days of gestation (7). The risks of Down syndrome and trisomy 18 were calculated based on maternal age, free β-hCG, PAPP-A, and nuchal translucency measurement.

A screen positive cutoff of 1 in 270 resulted in a Down syndrome detection rate of 85% and a false-positive rate of 9.4%. If the screen positive cutoff was set so that the screen positive rate was only 5%, the detection rate was 79%. In addition, 91% of the trisomy 18 cases were identified at a false-positive rate of 2%.

The FASTER (First and Second Trimester Evaluation of Risk) trial included more than 38,000 women who underwent both first-trimester screening (free β-hCG, PAPP-A, nuchal translucency measurement, and maternal age) *and* second-trimester screening (hCG, alpha-fetoprotein, estriol, and inhibin and maternal age). When women completed *both* first- and second-trimester screening tests and then underwent definitive testing if either test result was positive, the Down syndrome detection rate was 94% at a screen positive rate of 10.8%; the detection rate was 90% when the screen positive rate was set at 5.4% (8).

Nuchal translucency measurements are difficult to do accurately and reproducibly. The accuracy of the measurement depends on a number of factors, including the operator, the ultrasound equipment, proper magnification and contrast, fetal position, correct caliper placement, and body habitus (9). In the FASTER trial, the nuchal translucency medians varied from center to center as well as from operator to operator, and the medians obtained by a single operator varied over time (10). Nuchal translucency measurement should be performed only by operators with specific training, and each operator's medians should be monitored carefully and adjusted as necessary.

Development of the first-trimester and second-trimester quad (alpha-fetoprotein, hCG, unconjugated estriol, and inhibin-A) screening tests allows tailoring of the test to patient needs. Combined first-trimester screening (nuchal translucency, pregnancy-associated plasma protein A, and free β-hCG) for many patients has the important advantage of the opportunity for early diagnosis using chorionic villus sampling. For patients who miss the testing window for first-trimester screening at 11–14 weeks of gestation, the second-trimester quad test provides similar detection rates. In practices that do not have access to high-quality first-trimester ultrasonography, or appropriate quality assurance, another option is serum integrated screening, using PAPP-A in the first trimester and the quad screen in the second trimester. This test has Down syndrome detection and false-positive rates similar to its performance as a combined first-trimester screen, but does not require an ultrasound examination. For patients who desire the lowest false-positive rate, as many infertility patients or patients with prior adverse outcomes do, the optimal approach is a fully integrated screening that additionally incorporates nuchal translucency measurement in the first trimester. This test's reported detection rate is 88% with a false-positive rate of 1% (8).

Current ACOG guidelines regarding screening for fetal Down syndrome recommend that all women younger than 35 years be offered some form of maternal serum screening. Women aged 35 years and older should be offered definitive fetal testing (genetic amniocentesis or CVS); genetic counseling may include the relative risks and benefits of maternal serum screening as an alternative.

MATERNAL SERUM SCREENING FOR NEURAL TUBE DEFECTS

All variations of the second-trimester multiple marker screening test include maternal serum alpha-fetoprotein because this marker also screens for fetal NTDs. Because 95% of all NTDs occur in families with no previous history, all women should be offered NTD screening regardless of their family history. Maternal serum alpha-fetoprotein screening identifies 80–90% of fetuses with open spina bifida or anencephaly, and at least half of all fetuses with a ventral wall defect.

All pregnancies characterized by confirmed elevated maternal serum alpha-fetoprotein should be evaluated by ultrasonography. In the second-trimester fetus, 90–99% of open spinal defects are diagnosed by ultrasound examination. As the resolution of ultrasound imaging has improved, controversy has increased concerning the value of amniocentesis to measure alpha-fetoprotein levels in amniotic fluid when the ultrasound evaluation is reassuring (11). Although some highly skilled ultrasonographers report nearly 100% diagnostic accuracy with ultrasonography alone, this figure is strongly influenced by the skill and experience of the person evaluating the images, the quality of the ultrasound equipment, and individual factors affecting neural tube imaging, such as fetal position, maternal BMI, or abdominal wall scarring. Amniotic fluid alpha-fetoprotein analysis identifies all NTDs except the 3–5% of fetuses whose spinal defect is covered by skin. The decision of whether to perform amniocentesis should be individualized, considering both the quality of the ultrasound evaluation and the patient's desires.

ULTRASOUND SCREENING

Ultrasonographic Findings Indicating High Risk of Aneuploidy: Major Structural Defects

Most structural abnormalities involving a major organ or structure or the finding of 2 or more minor structural abnormalities in the same fetus indicate a high risk for fetal aneuploidy. The presence of a major anomaly increases the risk enough that invasive testing is justified regardless of the patient's age, family history, or maternal serum screening results. The specific risk associated with each of several major anomalies is listed in Table 4.

Major structural fetal anomalies in otherwise low-risk pregnancies usually are discovered during an ultrasound examination performed for pregnancy dating, evaluation of size and growth, or as part of a workup of complications such as vaginal bleeding. It is a matter of controversy whether to perform early second-trimester ultrasound examinations routinely to look for structural fetal abnormalities in women believed to be at low risk for such abnormalities. Before this issue can be resolved, the detection and false-negative rates for such examinations need to be improved; data from several large studies indicate that only 16–50% of major structural defects typically are identified during a second-trimester ultrasound examination.

Second-Trimester Ultrasonographic Findings Indicating Increased Risk of Aneuploidy: Dysmorphic Features

Minor dysmorphisms, by definition, are not major structural abnormalities and are commonly found in many normal individuals. Such dysmorphisms arouse interest because they are found with greater frequency in aneuploid fetuses. The dysmorphisms associated with Down syndrome are listed in Table 7. It is controversial as to whether an ultrasound evaluation for such dysmorphisms should be offered as the sole Down syndrome screening test to low-risk women. Much of the research concerning ultrasound evaluation of fetal dysmorphisms as a screening test for fetal chromosome abnormalities has been performed on high-risk women, primarily women aged 35 years and older who are already scheduled to undergo invasive genetic testing. Because the predictive value of a screening test is determined not only by the sensitivity and specificity of the test but also by the prevalence of the abnormality in the population studied, it is unknown whether this type of data can or should be extrapolated to younger, low-risk women. Other concerns include the

TABLE 7. Down Syndrome Risk of Dysmorphism

Ultrasound Marker	No. of Studies	DR (%)	FPR (%)
Nuchal fold = 6 mm	16	38	1.3
Femur length (O/E)^X	10	34	5.9
Femur length (BPD/FL)	4	22	5.9
Humerus length (O/E)^X	6	37	5.3
Femur plus humerus (O/E)^X	3	36	3.7
Pyelectasis	4	19	2.4
Hyperechogenic bowel	3	11	0.7
Cerebral ventricular dilatation	1	6	0
Choroid plexus cyst	1	0	1.8
Ear length	1	78	8.0
Fifth-digit mid-phalanx hypoplasia	1	75	18.0
Increased iliac length	1	50	2.0
Short frontal lobe	1	21	4.8

DR indicates Down syndrome detection rate; FPR, false-positive rate; (O/E)^X, observed compared to expected; BPD, biparietal diameter; FL, femur length.

transient nature of many dysmorphisms (eg, choroid plexus cysts), the difficulty in clearly visualizing all dysmorphisms (eg, absence of the middle phalanx of the little finger), and variations in both measurement technique and the methods used to classify the size of a structure as abnormal (eg, nuchal fold). The utility of ultrasound screening for both major structural malformations and dysmorphisms in low-risk women, therefore, remains unresolved.

Current Strategies for Fetal Aneuploidy Detection

AMNIOCENTESIS

Amniocentesis for prenatal diagnosis of aneuploidy or genetic disease usually is offered between 15 and 20 weeks of gestation. Early amniocentesis, performed between 11 and 14 weeks, results in significantly higher rates of pregnancy loss and procedural complications than does traditional amniocentesis. In a recent multicenter randomized trial, the rate of spontaneous pregnancy loss after early amniocentesis was 2.5%, whereas this rate was only 0.7% after traditional amniocentesis. Early amniocentesis also was associated with significantly more cases of talipes than was traditional amniocentesis. There were significantly more failures of amniotic fluid cultures after the early procedure, necessitating an additional invasive diagnostic procedure. For all these reasons, many centers no longer offer amniocentesis before 14 weeks of gestation.

CHORIONIC VILLUS SAMPLING

The primary advantage of CVS is that results are available earlier in pregnancy. There have been reports of an association between CVS and limb reduction and oromandibular defects. Cavernous hemangiomas also have been reported. Although a few reports have caused concern, several large studies indicate that CVS does not increase the risk of these anomalies above the background risk. Patients can be counseled that a CVS procedure performed at or beyond 10 weeks of gestation is believed to be as safe as second-trimester amniocentesis; in some reports, the transabdominal approach is even safer than the transvaginal method.

PERCUTANEOUS UMBILICAL CORD BLOOD SAMPLING

Percutaneous umbilical cord blood sampling, also known as cordocentesis, has been used to obtain fetal blood cells for prenatal diagnosis when a rapid diagnosis is needed. The overall rate of procedure-related pregnancy loss is 1.4%. However, the loss rate probably varies with the indication for the procedure, from much less than 1.4% for evaluation of isoimmunization with a nonanemic fetus to more than 1.4% for evaluation of severe IUGR. The fetal blood sample may be sent for cytogenetic or molecular DNA analysis, complete blood count, metabolic and hematologic studies, acid–base analysis, virus cultures, and immunologic studies.

New Horizons

One disadvantage of amniocentesis is the need to culture cells for several days before karyotype analysis. Fluorescent in situ hybridization (FISH) for the rapid detection of chromosomal aneuploidies in uncultured amniocytes is now offered by many centers. In this technique, fluorescently tagged, specific DNA probes for chromosomes 13, 18, 21, X, and Y are used to rapidly detect the ploidy status of these particular chromosomes. Fluorescent in situ hybridization may not detect mosaicism and does not detect structural chromosomal abnormalities or aneuploidies in other chromosomes. It typically is used as an adjunct to traditional cytogenetic analysis with high-resolution chromosome banding. The benefit of FISH is rapid availability of preliminary results.

Experience with preimplantation diagnosis (embryo biopsy) also has been reported. After in vitro fertilization, a blastomere (at the 8-cell stage) or polar body biopsy is performed, followed by intrauterine transfer of the embryo once it is confirmed that the embryo is unaffected. The benefits of preimplantation diagnosis are obvious, as are the drawbacks of having to conceive by using reproductive technology.

Trisomy 21 has been diagnosed in fetal cells isolated from maternal blood obtained during the first trimester. Fetal cell sorting techniques currently are being developed for the noninvasive diagnosis of fetal aneuploidy, with recovered fetal cells analyzed using FISH.

Patient Counseling

Screening for carriers of genetic diseases is voluntary. For some patients, it can be difficult to decide whether to have a specific test. There are many factors patients may consider, including the prevalence of the disease, the carrier risk, the disease severity, and treatment options, cost, and reproductive choices. Counseling by a genetic counselor, geneticist, or physician with expertise in these diseases may assist patients in making an informed decision about carrier testing.

References

1. Stern JJ, Dorfmann AD, Gutierrez-Najar A, Cerrillo M, Coulam CB. Frequency of abnormal karyotypes among abortuses from women with and without a history of recurrent spontaneous abortion. Fertil Steril 1996;65:250–3.

2. American College of Obstetricians and Gynecologists. Management of recurrent early pregnancy loss. ACOG Practice Bulletin 24. Washington, DC: ACOG; 2001.

3. American College of Obstetricians and Gynecologists, American College of Medical Genetics. Preconception and prenatal carrier screening for cystic fibrosis. Clinical and laboratory guidelines. Washington, DC: ACOG; 2001.

4. Wald NJ, George L, Smith D, Densem JW, Petterson K. Serum screening for Down's syndrome between 8 and 14 weeks of pregnancy. International Prenatal Screening Research Group. Br J Obstet Gynaecol 1996;103:407–12.

5. Haddow JE, Palomaki GE, Knight GJ, Williams J, Miller WA, Johnson A. Screening of maternal serum for fetal Down's syndrome in the first trimester. N Engl J Med 1998;338:955–61.

6. Snijders RJ, Noble P, Sebire N, Souka A, Nicolaides KH. UK multicentre project on assessment of risk of trisomy 21 by maternal age and fetal nuchal-translucency thickness at 10-14 weeks of gestation. Fetal Medicine Foundation First Trimester Screening Group. Lancet 1998;352:343–6.

7. Wapner R, Thom E, Simpson JL, Pergament E, Silver R, Filkins K, et al. First-trimester screening for trisomies 21 and 18. First Trimester Maternal Serum Biochemistry and Fetal Nuchal Translucency Screening (BUN) Study Group. N Engl J Med 2003;349:1405–13.

8. Malone FD, Wald NJ, Canick JA, Ball RH, Nyberg DA, Comstock C, et al. First- and second-trimester evaluation of risk (FASTER) trial: principal results of the NICHD multicenter Down syndrome screening study [abstract]. Am J Obstet Gynecol 2003;189:S56.

9. First trimester screening for fetal aneuploidy. ACOG Committee Opinion No. 296. American College of Obstetricians and Gynecologists. Obstet Gynecol 2004;104: 215–7.

10. D'Alton ME, Malone FD, Lambert-Messerlian G, Ball RH, Nyberg DA, Comstock CH, et al. Maintaining quality assurance for nuchal translucency sonography in a prospective multicenter study: results from the FASTER trial [abstract]. Am J Obstet Gynecol 2003;189:S79.

11. Sepulveda W, Donaldson A, Johnson RD, Davies G, Fisk NM. Are routine alpha-fetoprotein and acetylcholinesterase determinations still necessary at second-trimester amniocentesis? Impact of high-resolution ultrasonography. Obstet Gynecol 1995;85:107–12.

FETAL THERAPY

The advent of fetal therapy occurred in the early 1960s with reports of successful intrauterine transfusion for severe hemolytic disease of the newborn. Later efforts at open maternal–fetal surgery were complicated by excessive perinatal morbidity related to premature labor. Minimally invasive surgical techniques and gene therapy hold real promise to advance fetal therapy.

Conditions Treated Noninvasively

CONGENITAL ADRENAL HYPERPLASIA

Neonates with congenital adrenal hyperplasia typically have ambiguous genitalia or cardiovascular collapse from the salt-wasting form of the disease. A genetic defect in

1 of 2 enzymes (21-hydroxylase or 11-hydroxylase) involved in the production of adrenal steroids creates a block in these metabolic pathways, with a resulting increase in adrenal androgens. Virilization of a female fetus can then occur. Because the disease is inherited in an autosomal recessive fashion, 1 of 4 subsequent offspring will be affected. In such cases, maternal dexamethasone therapy is initiated after biochemical confirmation of pregnancy. Early suppression of the fetal adrenal axis is important because development of the external genitalia is complete by 7–12 weeks of gestation. A chorionic villus biopsy is then undertaken at 10–12 weeks of gestation. Steroids are discontinued if a male fetus or an unaffected female fetus is identified through karyotype and DNA analysis. A tapering steroid regimen should be used. If an affected female fetus is identified, maternal dexamethasone is continued until delivery. Stress doses of steroids are indicated to prevent maternal addisonian crisis in labor. Mixed results in the neonate have been reported with this approach: one third of fetuses are still completely virilized, and an additional one third exhibit partial virilization. This may result from inadequate dosing or late entry into therapy (1).

Fetal Arrhythmias

Tachyarrhythmias

Supraventricular tachycardia usually is diagnosed in an uncomplicated pregnancy when fetal heart rate evaluation indicates a rate in excess of 200 beats per minute. If this arrhythmia is sustained, hydrops fetalis can result. Fetal echocardiography rarely reveals structural abnormalities. In gestations of 35 or more weeks, delivery with subsequent cardioversion in the nursery would appear prudent. In a preterm gestation, in utero therapy is aimed at decreasing the conduction time of the fetal atrioventricular node to allow adequate time for ventricular filling. This usually is accomplished by administration of digoxin to the mother. In most cases, hospitalization with monitoring of maternal digoxin levels is indicated. In addition, larger doses of digoxin than are typically used in the nonpregnant patient are needed secondary to increased maternal glomerular filtration. If fetal supraventricular tachycardia persists, oral flecainide or sotalol is added as second-line therapy (2). Because many of these agents increase digoxin levels, the maternal digoxin dose should be reduced appropriately. In cases of recalcitrant fetal tachycardia or severe fetal hydrops, medications can be administered directly to the fetus through intramuscular injection performed under ultrasound guidance. Maternal administration of oral sotalol appears to be the therapy of choice in cases of fetal atrial fibrillation. A reversal of hydrops can be expected once the fetal supraventricular tachycardia resolves. Maternal medications should be continued until delivery.

Bradyarrhythmias

More than 50% of cases of congenital heart block result from structural cardiac abnormalities. The remaining cases are secondary to immune destruction of the fetal cardiac conduction system in response to maternal autoantibodies (anti-Ro/SSA and anti-La/SSB).

Maternal administration of steroids (dexamethasone) that cross the placenta has been attempted in an effort to ameliorate the inflammatory action on fetal conduction. Steroid therapy after the detection of fetal bradycardia has not proved beneficial. The disease tends to recur in subsequent offspring because of the persistence of maternal antibodies. Steroid therapy before 14 weeks of gestation may prevent recurrence.

Fetal Thyroid Disorders

Small amounts of maternal thyroxine (T_4) cross the human placenta. By 12 weeks of gestation, however, the fetal thyroid begins to produce T_4, and by 20 weeks of gestation the fetal pituitary–thyroid axis is functionally mature and independent of the maternal endocrine system. Fetal thyroid disorders usually are unrecognized until after birth, when they are detected through mandated neonatal screening programs. Fetal goiter on routine antenatal ultrasonography is sometimes detected; however, this finding can be associated with both hypothyroidism and hyperthyroidism in the fetus, as well as a euthyroid state. It is often associated with polyhydramnios due to external compression of the fetal esophagus. Intrauterine growth restriction has been reported in fetal hypothyroidism and hyperthyroidism. Congenital heart block and cardiac failure are noted in some cases of fetal hypothyroidism; tachycardia, hydrops fetalis, and craniosynostosis can be seen in hyperthyroid cases.

Hypothyroidism

Although neonatal supplementation will avert most cases of delayed neurologic development when the fetus is hypothyroid, language, motor, and spatial visual development still may be impaired. Most cases of fetal goiter and hypothyroidism are related to overzealous use of maternal propylthiouracil or methimazole, which readily enter the fetal compartment. Direct fetal causes include dysgenesis of the thyroid gland or enzymatic defects in the formation of thyroid hormones.

In cases of maternal thyrotoxicosis, antithyroid medications should be adjusted to maintain serum thyroid hormone levels in the upper limits of the normal range. If a fetal goiter is noted in the euthyroid pregnant patient or in the hyperthyroid patient receiving appropriate doses of antithyroid medications, cordocentesis should be undertaken to determine the fetal free T_4 and TSH levels (3). Amniotic fluid levels of these hormones are not indicative of the fetal status. If hypothyroidism is detected, the fetus can be treated with weekly intraamniotic injections of thyroxine. Fetal blood sampling should be repeated 4–6 weeks later to confirm the fetal response.

Hyperthyroidism

Maternal Graves' disease is associated with fetal hyperthyroidism in 2–10% of cases. High levels of maternal thyroid-stimulating antibody (TSAb) can stimulate the fetal thyroid gland after transplacental passage. Maternal TSAb levels should be measured in women who are euthyroid but previously have been treated with ^{131}I ablation. Cordocentesis at 20–24 weeks of gestation is undertaken to measure fetal thyroid function in the pregnant patient with previous or current Graves' disease and with any of the following:

- History of a previously affected infant
- Elevated TSAb level (>160% of normal)
- Ultrasound findings suggestive of fetal hyperthyroidism—goiter, tachycardia, growth restriction, hydrops, or cardiomegaly (4)

Maternal treatment with propylthiouracil (with thyroxine supplementation if necessary) can be implemented if the fetus is found to be hyperthyroid. Repeat cordocentesis should be undertaken in 4–6 weeks to confirm fetal response. Close supervision of the neonate by pediatricians is warranted in cases of fetal hypothyroidism or hyperthyroidism requiring in utero treatment.

Management of Fetal Anemia and Thrombocytopenia

RED CELL ALLOIMMUNIZATION

Maternal sensitization or alloimmunization to erythrocyte antigens produces hemolytic disease of the fetus and newborn. More than 40 erythrocyte antigens can cause the disorder; however, the 3 major antigens that often lead to the need for in utero therapy include Rh D, Rh C, and Kell (K1). The following established protocols for therapy can ensure optimal outcomes.

Prevention of Rh D Alloimmunization

Most cases of spontaneous fetomaternal hemorrhage occur late in pregnancy. In the United States, the use of 300 µg of intramuscular anti-D immune globulin (formerly referred to as Rho[D] immune globulin) at 28 weeks of gestation has produced a 10-fold reduction in cases of antepartum sensitization to the Rh D antigen. Whether a maternal antibody screen is needed before administering antenatal anti-D immune globulin is controversial, and it may not be cost-effective. At delivery, approximately 15–20% of patients are found to have a positive indirect Coombs' test for Rh D antibody secondary to the persistence of antenatal anti-D immune

globulin. Titers in this situation are 4 or less and should not prevent the use of postpartum prophylaxis. However, in situations where a high titer is noted at delivery, indicating maternal sensitization, anti-D immune globulin has not been shown to be advantageous (5).

Anti-D immune globulin should be administered in a dose of 300 µg within 72 hours of delivery if cord blood indicates that the neonate of an Rh D-negative, nonsensitized patient is Rh D positive. Because some protective effects have been reported with the use of anti-D immune globulin for up to 28 days after delivery, inadvertent omission of anti-D immune globulin within 72 hours of delivery should not preclude the use of anti-D immune globulin after this time. All patients should be screened for excessive fetomaternal hemorrhage in the immediate postpartum period. Testing requires quantification of the amount of fetomaternal hemorrhage and appropriate dose administration of anti-D immune globulin. The amount of fetal–maternal transfer must be quantified to determine the appropriate dosage. Negative results warrant the administration of 1 vial of anti-D immune globulin (300 µg). The volume is then divided by 30 to determine the number of vials of anti-D immune globulin needed. Although anti-D immune globulin products manufactured in the United States can be given only intramuscularly, an intravenous preparation made in Canada is now available. Dosing of the Canadian product is equivalent to intramuscular preparations (15,000 IU in 2.5 mL = 300 µg). The product may be beneficial in patients with thrombocytopenia when intramuscular injections are contraindicated.

Patients with a weak D-positive type (once termed D^u positive) are not candidates for anti-D immune globulin. In these patients, Rh D antigens are expressed on the surface of the erythrocytes in a weaker concentration than in most Rh D-positive individuals. Patients with a weak D-positive type are therefore not at risk for sensitization. However, an error can occur when a weak D-positive type patient undergoes her first blood typing at delivery. If a significant fetomaternal hemorrhage occurred after delivery, a mixed field agglutination reaction will result from the Rh D-positive fetal cells in the maternal circulation, yielding an erroneous weak D-positive type. Such confusing cases can be prevented by routine screening for fetomaternal hemorrhage at delivery.

If delivery occurs within 3 weeks of antenatal anti-D immune globulin administration, the dose need not be repeated if there is no evidence of excessive fetomaternal hemorrhage. This recommendation would apply also to the use of anti-D immune globulin after late third-trimester amniocentesis or external cephalic version. Controversy remains as to whether an antenatal dose of anti-D immune globulin should be repeated after 40 completed weeks of gestation; some experts recommend a repeat dose.

Intrauterine Transfusion

Values of ΔOD_{450} that reach the upper 80th percentile of the Liley curve or an MCA Doppler finding of more than 1.5 MoM warrant fetal blood sampling to determine the fetal hematocrit. Typically, the umbilical cord is targeted at its insertion into the placenta using continuous ultrasound guidance. On some occasions, the intrahepatic portion of the umbilical vein can be used. An initial fetal hematocrit value is obtained; a value of less than 30% warrants transfusion. Standardized formulas based on fetal weight estimated by ultrasonography are then employed to calculate the volume of erythrocytes to be given. In many instances, neuromuscular blocking agents, such as pancuronium or vecuronium, are administered into the umbilical cord to prevent fetal movement. Maternal packed erythrocytes can be used as the source of red cells after extensive washing to remove the antibody-containing plasma. Leukoreduction and irradiation with 25 Gy are performed to prevent graft-versus-host reaction. If donor red cells are used, a fresh source that tests negative for cytomegalovirus (CMV) should be identified. These cells also should be leukoreduced and irradiated. Intrauterine transfusions are continued at 1–3-week intervals until approximately 35 weeks of gestation, when delivery of the fetus probably represents a safer alternative than continued in utero therapy. Induction of labor is undertaken 2–3 weeks later. An overall survival rate of 85% can be expected, with slightly lower rates of survival if the fetus is hydropic at the first procedure.

Although the need for neonatal exchange transfusion has become less frequent with aggressive in utero therapy, many of these infants require simple transfusions in the first few months of life because of persistent bone marrow suppression. These children, therefore, should be monitored with weekly hematocrit determinations and reticulocyte counts. Data to date have indicated normal developmental outcomes in infants who survive intrauterine transfusion.

Kell Alloimmunization

In cases of Kell alloimmunization, the use of amniocentesis to monitor ΔOD_{450} values has been questioned. Recent clinical and basic laboratory data suggest that unlike Rh disease, the Kell antibody causes both hemolysis and suppression of erythropoiesis (6). Bilirubin levels in serum and amniotic fluid are lower in Kell-positive fetuses than in newborns with Rh D hemolytic disease. One compromise is to suggest a lower threshold for fetal blood sampling, such as the 50th percentile of zone 2 of the Liley curve. Other centers have abandoned the use of amniocentesis in cases of Kell alloimmunization and use serial fetal blood sampling or Doppler measurements of peak velocity in the middle cerebral artery or a combination of the two.

FETOMATERNAL HEMORRHAGE

A limited number of cases of fetal hydrops secondary to fetomaternal hemorrhage have been reported in which the intrauterine transfusion of erythrocytes resulted in a successful outcome. In these cases, a presentation of decreased fetal movement led to ultrasound detection of the hydrops. Kleihauer–Betke testing of maternal blood can confirm the diagnosis of fetomaternal hemorrhage. Although intrauterine transfusion prolongs most pregnancies, some may benefit from premature delivery secondary to continued fetomaternal hemorrhage.

ALLOIMMUNE THROMBOCYTOPENIA

Alloimmune thrombocytopenia (AIT) affects approximately 1 in 1,200 pregnancies. Similar to red cell alloimmunization, maternal antibodies to platelet-specific antigens are actively transported across the placenta, resulting in profound fetal thrombocytopenia. Platelet function also appears to be affected as spontaneous intracranial bleeding can occur in 10–20% of cases, with 25–50% of these occurring in utero (7). Important differences between AIT and hemolytic disease of the newborn include the possibility of an affected fetus or infant in the patient's first pregnancy (50% of cases) and the inability of the maternal anti-platelet antibody titer to predict perinatal disease. The HPA-la (PLA[1]) platelet antigen is involved in more than 80% of cases in Caucasians. The HPA-3a (Bak[a]) and HPA-5b (Br[a]) antigens comprise most of the remaining cases. In Asians, antibodies to the HPA-4 (Pen, Yuk) antigen system are the most common etiology.

Typically, AIT is first diagnosed after the birth of an affected infant who exhibits clinical manifestations of severe thrombocytopenia. Platelet typing of the parents will reveal an antigen incompatibility with evidence of maternal antibodies against both neonatal and paternal platelets. Once there is an antecedent history, subsequent offspring are equally or more severely affected. A history of a previous fetus with intracranial bleeding or a sibling with a platelet count of less than $20 \ K \times 10^9/L$ represents a high-risk factor for recurrent severe perinatal disease. Without treatment, recurrence of intracranial bleeding occurs in up to 70% of cases. In a subsequent pregnancy, paternal testing should be reviewed to determine if there is a heterozygous state (25% of cases of HPA-1a). If this is the case, amniocentesis can be performed in the second trimester for fetal platelet typing of the involved antigen through DNA analysis.

Prevention and treatment strategies vary between North America and Europe. The most widely accepted prevention strategy in the United States is antenatal administration of intravenous immunoglobulin (IVIG) weekly, typically initiated around 20 weeks of gestation (8). Other treatment options include daily antenatal oral steroid administration or a combination of IVIG and steroid administration. Treatment options in AIT treatment protocols have been based on the degree of thrombocytopenia found at cordocentesis in the index pregnancy and the presence of intracranial hemorrhage detected antenatally (the earlier the diagnosis, the more severe the disease). Studies have demonstrated that IVIG is effective in reducing the risk of intracranial hemorrhage when compared with outcomes of prior affected siblings (9). Intravenous gamma globulin (1g/kg/wk) resulted in a higher platelet count in 78% of cases. The remaining cases were treated additionally with prednisone; 50% of these had a higher platelet count. However, cases of failure of IVIG have been reported in the literature (8). In the most refractory cases, weekly in utero platelet transfusions have been performed (preferably with maternal-derived platelets), but this carries a risk of fetal loss associated with cordocentesis.

Potential risks of prednisone administration include osteoporosis, glucose intolerance and gestational diabetes, depressed immunity, mood swings, and gastrointestinal irritation. These potential risks are reversible. The risks of administering IVIG, a blood product, include local reaction at the administration site, fever, rash, altered immunity, and transmission of infectious agents.

Fetal blood sampling could be performed to establish thrombocytopenia and monitor progress in pregnancy. This should be performed as rarely as possible to minimize risks to the pregnancy. Risks for exsanguination at cordocentesis are related to the degree of thrombocytopenia and the presence of intracranial hemorrhage in a prior affected sibling detected antenatally. Although knowing the platelet count at the beginning of therapy has the advantage of aiding the interpretation of platelet counts later on, it does present an added risk of pregnancy loss. In general, cordocentesis is associated with an approximate 1–2% risk of fetal loss, and this risk can be substantially higher in high-risk cases, such as AIT. Because IVIG has been shown to be effective in most cases, a current protocol (8) for the treatment of AIT offers fetal blood sampling later in pregnancy (mid-third trimester) at a time when the fetus would survive with less prematurity risk but still with enough time left in the pregnancy to change therapy if needed. Fetal blood sampling should be performed by experienced maternal–fetal medicine specialists and with the availability of direct infusion of maternal-derived platelets. In utero transfusion of maternal-derived platelets should occur if the fetal platelet count is less than 50×10^9/L to prevent exsanguination from the needle site of cordocentesis. Liberal use of cesarean delivery is recommended; vaginal delivery should be considered only if the fetal platelet count is greater than 50×10^9/L at cordocentesis prior to delivery.

Fetal Surgery

Since the first reported case of open fetal surgery in 1983, such surgery has been restricted to fetal conditions such as diaphragmatic hernia that were considered likely to be lethal in neonatal life (10). More recently, spina bifida, a fetal condition associated with life-long morbidity, has become the most common indication for this procedure. Proposed requirements to consider invasive intervention for fetal conditions include the following:

- The morbidity (both maternal and fetal) of the antenatal intervention is acceptable.
- The diagnosis of the condition can be made accurately.
- The condition can be differentiated from other nonsurgical anomalies.
- The natural evolution of the disease, if left untreated, should be predictable and the condition should be lethal or severely debilitating.
- Adequate postnatal treatment should not exist.
- The proposed in utero intervention should be technically feasible.

MINIMALLY INVASIVE TECHNIQUES

Percutaneous Shunting

Ultrasound-guided placement of a double-pigtail, polymeric silicone shunt has been successfully employed to drain excessive collections of intracavitary fluid that might compromise fetal renal or pulmonary function. The most common indication for this technique is the treatment of severe oligohydramnios in cases of bladder outlet obstruction (urethral atresia or posterior urethral valves). Serial bladder aspirations are undertaken initially to evaluate the fetal karyotype and urinary electrolytes. An abnormal karyotype or evidence of poor renal reserve based on elevated electrolytes and β_2 microglobulin precludes placement of the shunt. Percutaneous shunts also have been employed to drain large collections of thoracic fluid associated with fetal hydrops secondary to lateral displacement of the fetal heart. Such cases include unilateral pleural effusions and type I cystic adenomatoid malformations of the lung.

Laser Therapy

Twin–twin transfusion is a major contributor to perinatal morbidity and mortality in monochorionic gestations. Although initially thought to be caused by simple transfusion of excessive blood volume from one fetus to another, recent insight suggests that the pathophysiology is more complex. The severity of the disease is graded using a staging system of ultrasound criteria:

Stage 1: There is polyhydramnios in association with the "recipient" twin and severe oligohydramnios associated with the "donor" or "stuck" twin. The bladder of the donor twin is still seen; Doppler studies are normal.

Stage 2: The bladder of the donor twin is absent; Doppler studies are normal.

Stage 3: Abnormal Doppler studies, such as absent or reversed end-diastolic flow in the umbilical artery or reversed diastolic flow in the ductus venosus or pulsatile venous flow in the umbilical vein, are noted in one or both twins.

Stage 4: Ascites, pleural effusions, scalp edema, or overt hydrops is present in one or both twins.

Stage 5: One or both twins are dead (11).

Stages 1 and 2 probably can be treated by serial amniocenteses to reduce the excess amniotic fluid volume in the recipient twin's sac (amnioreduction). The intentional perforation of the intervening twin membrane (septostomy) with a small-gauge needle is equally effective in early stage disease and may require fewer total procedures for treatment. The yttrium–aluminum–garnet laser is now being used at select centers worldwide to coagulate anastomotic vessels that are shared between the twin circulations. The fiber used to deliver the laser energy is introduced into the amniotic cavity through a fetoscope (a small-diameter, laparoscopelike device). Prospective data would suggest enhanced overall survival and intact neurologic survival in twin–twin transfusion syndrome at stages more advanced than stage 2 (12).

OPEN MATERNAL–FETAL SURGERY

The ultrasound finding of right-sided displacement of the fetal heart should lead to a suspicion of a fetal diaphragmatic hernia. When a hernia is present, lesions are predominantly left-sided, and the stomach or liver often can be herniated into the thoracic cavity. Direct compression of the ipsilateral lung and deviation of the heart with compression of the contralateral lung can lead to pulmonary hypoplasia. Kinking of the gastroesophageal junction produces polyhydramnios. Initial efforts to correct this lesion with open maternal–fetal surgery met with poor success because of preterm premature rupture of membranes and preterm labor after maternal hysterotomy. In addition, high rates of fetal loss were noted when hepatic herniation into the chest was present. Such outcomes have led to the abandonment of open maternal–fetal surgery for the direct repair of diaphragmatic hernia.

Investigations into animal models for diaphragmatic hernia revealed that occlusion of the fetal trachea prevented the egress of pulmonary fluid, leading to enlargement of the fetal lungs and displacement of the abdominal viscera from the thorax. Clinical trials in humans were initiated with surgical clips placed on the trachea first by open hysterotomy and later by fetoscopy. Subsequently, the procedure was modified to use a detachable balloon placed inside the trachea through a fetoscope. Results to date have been disappointing, with survival rates equal to aggressive neonatal management.

Large and predominantly solid fetal sacrococcygeal teratomas can cause the development of nonimmune hydrops because of high-output cardiac failure. Open maternal–fetal surgery has been employed in such cases with mixed success. In many cases, the pregnant patient develops mirror syndrome, consisting of maternal fluid retention and respiratory compromise secondary to adult respiratory distress syndrome, and the fetus must be delivered. Minimally invasive techniques for the in utero treatment of sacrococcygeal teratomas have been of limited success to date.

A cystic adenomatoid malformation can present as a solid or cystic hamartomatous growth in the fetal lung. A progressive increase in size can lead to hydrops fetalis or pulmonary hypoplasia. Approximately 20% of lesions can regress. Cystic adenomatoid malformation must be distinguished from pulmonary sequestration, which is universally associated with a good neonatal prognosis. Cystic adenomatoid malformation is the fetal condition in which fetal surgery has yielded the highest rate of successful outcomes. Unfortunately, deciding which fetus with cystic adenomatoid malformation is a candidate for such surgery remains problematic.

Maternal–fetal surgery for meningomyelocele was originally attempted laparoscopically through the use of maternal skin grafts; success was limited. Centers turned to open hysterotomy for definitive repair of the lesion. To date, more than 250 procedures have been performed. Outcomes of these infants have revealed a decrease in the incidence of neonatal ventriculoperitoneal shunting by 30–50% for lumbosacral lesions. The greatest effect was associated with lesions below L2, moderate ventriculomegaly, and repair before 25 weeks of gestation. The Chiari II malformation associated with meningomyelocele has been noted to reverse in utero in virtually all cases of fetal repair. Neonatal urodynamic follow-up has not revealed clear improvement in function. Developmental studies regarding lower extremity function have revealed conflicting results. In 2000, the NIH held a consensus conference that called for a randomized clinical trial to study open hysterotomy for the correction of meningomyelocele. The MOMS study (www.spinabifidamoms.com) was initiated in January 2003. Entry criteria include:

- Myelomeningocele defect between T1 and S1, inclusive
- Hindbrain herniation (Chiari II malformation) identified by fetal magnetic resonance imaging
- Maternal age of 18 years or older
- Normal fetal karyotype
- Gestational age of 19^0 to 25^3 weeks at randomization

A moratorium on open maternal–fetal surgery for spina bifida has been called until the trial is completed.

STEM CELL TRANSPLANTATION

The human fetus is thought to be immunologically tolerant in early gestation. This has led several investigators to attempt stem cell transfusions early in gestation for conditions such as Krabbe disease and severe combined immunodeficiency syndrome. Both paternal bone marrow and frozen banked cells from abortuses have been used as sources. The cells are typically placed into the fetal peritoneal cavity. Thus far, the only successful cases of engraftment have involved cases of severe combined immunodeficiency syndrome.

References

1. Garner PR. Congenital adrenal hyperplasia in pregnancy. Semin Perinatol 1998;22:446–56.

2. Oudijk MA, Ruskamp JM, Ambachtsheer BE, Ververs TF, Stoutenbeek P, Visser GH, et al. Drug treatment of fetal tachycardia. Pediatr Drugs 2002;4:49–63.

3. Abuhamad AZ, Fisher DA, Warsof SL, Slotnick RN, Pyle PG, Wu SY, Evans AT. Antenatal diagnosis and treatment of fetal goitrous hypothyroidism: case report and review of the literature. Ultrasound Obstet Gynecol 1995;6:368–71.

4. Kilpatrick S. Umbilical blood sampling in women with thyroid disease in pregnancy: is it necessary? Am J Obstet Gynecol 2003;189:1–2.

5. American College of Obstetricians and Gynecologists. Prevention of Rh D alloimmunization. ACOG Practice Bulletin 4. Washington, DC: ACOG; 1999.

6. Vaughan JI, Manning M, Warwick RM, Letsky EA, Murray NA, Roberts IA. Inhibition of erythroid progenitor cells by anti-Kell antibodies in fetal alloimmune anemia. N Engl J Med 1998;338:798–803.

7. Bussell JB. Alloimmune thrombocytopenia in the fetus and newborn. Semin Thromb Hemost 2001;27:245–51.

8. Birchall JE, Murphy MF, Kaplan C, Kroll H, European Fetomaternal Alloimmune Thrombocytopenia Study Group. European collaborative study of the antenatal management of feto-maternal alloimmune thrombocytopenia. Br J Haematol 2003;122:275–88.

9. Bussel JB, Berkowitz RL, Lynch L, Lesser ML, Paidas MJ, Huang CL, et al. Antenatal management of alloimmune thrombocytopenia with intravenous gamma-globulin: a randomized trial of the addition of low-dose steroid to intravenous gamma-globulin. Am J Obstet Gynecol 1996;174:1414–23.

10. Albanese CT, Harrison MR. Surgical treatment for fetal disease. The state of the art. Ann N Y Acad Sci 1998;847:74–85.

11. Quintero ROA, Morales WJ, Allen MH, Bornick PW, Johnson PK, Kruger M. Staging of twin-twin transfusion syndrome. J Perinatol 1999;19:550–5.

12. Senat MV, Deprest J, Boulvain M, Paupe A, Winter N, Ville Y. Endoscopic laser surgery versus serial amnioreduction for severe twin-to-twin transfusion syndrome. N Engl J Med 2004;351:136–44.

Endocrinology of Pregnancy

Pregnancy is characterized by an extraordinary interplay among maternal, placental, and fetal endocrine systems. These systems facilitate 1) implantation and maintenance of pregnancy, 2) maternal homeostasis to maximize nutritional support for the developing fetus, and 3) parturition and preparation for lactation.

IMPLANTATION

After ovulation and fertilization, the zygote and blastocyst migrate from the ampullary portion of the fallopian tube to the uterine cavity, where implantation takes place 5–7 days after fertilization. Before implantation, the blastocyst secretes specific proteins and hormones that may enhance endometrial receptivity. Successful implantation requires precise synchronization between blastocyst development and endometrial maturation. At the time of implantation, the embryo is actively secreting human chorionic gonadotropin (hCG), which can be detected in maternal serum as early as the 8th day after ovulation. The primary role of hCG is to prolong the biosynthetic activity of the corpus luteum, which allows continued progesterone production to maintain the decidualized endometrium.

Progesterone inhibits endometrial stromal cell expression of plasminogen activator and matrix metalloproteinase and stimulates production of the following factors:

- The hormones prolactin and type 1 insulinlike growth factor–binding protein
- The hemostatic proteins, tissue factor, and type 1 plasminogen activator inhibitor
- The basement membranelike extracellular matrix components (eg, fibronectin, laminin, type III collagen, and glycosaminoglycans).

Thus, the decidua modulates trophoblast invasion to permit controlled endovascular invasion and the establishment of the uteroplacental circulation without causing potentially life-threatening hemorrhage or unrestrained trophoblast invasion.

Between 6 and 7 weeks of gestation, corpus luteum function begins to decline. During this luteal–placental transition period, the production of progesterone shifts to the developing placenta. This transition is marked by a decline in circulating 17α-hydroxyprogesterone caused by the minimal expression of 17α-hydroxylase in the placenta. Thus, removal of the corpus luteum before 6 weeks of gestation increases the risk of abortion. Patients who have corpus luteum dysfunction or who are undergoing in vitro fertilization with donor oocytes after ovarian failure or removal should be given supplemental exogenous progesterone until approximately 10 weeks of gestation.

ENDOCRINE SYSTEMS AND MATERNAL–FETAL HOMEOSTASIS

Placental Compartment

The placenta delivers nutrients to and removes toxic metabolites from the fetus. It also produces numerous steroid and protein hormones and growth factors.

PROGESTERONE

The placenta is the main source of progesterone during pregnancy. From the luteal phase to term, maternal progesterone levels increase 6-fold to 8-fold (Fig. 9). Although the placenta produces large amounts of progesterone, it has a limited capacity to synthesize cholesterol de novo. Thus, maternally derived low-density lipoprotein cholesterol is the principal precursor (>97%) for biosynthesis of progesterone during pregnancy. Progesterone produced by the placenta maintains endometrial decidualization and serves as a substrate for the fetal adrenal gland to produce glucocorticoid and mineralocorticoid. The latter of these functions is necessary

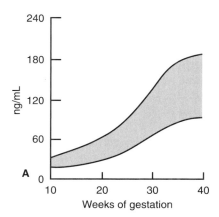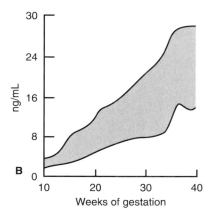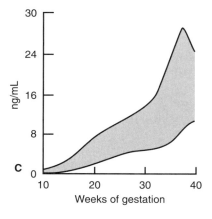

■ FIG. 9. Progesterone **(A)**, estradiol-17β **(B)**, and estriol **(C)** in plasma of normal pregnant women as a function of weeks of gestation (mean ± standard deviation). (Parker CR Jr, Illingsworth DR, Bissonnette J, Carr BR. Endocrine changes during pregnancy in a patient with homozygous familial hypobetalipoproteinemia. N Engl J Med 1986;314:557–60. Copyright © 1986 Massachusetts Medical Society. All rights reserved.)

because the fetal adrenal gland is unable to synthesize these steroids from cholesterol de novo, owing to a relative deficiency of 3β-hydroxysteroid dehydrogenase. Progesterone also inhibits the contractility of myometrial smooth muscle, decreases the formation of decidual and fetal membrane prostaglandin, and inhibits T lymphocyte–mediated responses involved in graft rejection.

ESTROGEN

The rate of estrogen production and the concentration of estrogens in plasma increase markedly during pregnancy (Fig. 9). The corpus luteum is the principal source of estrogen during early pregnancy, after which time nearly all the estrogen comes from the placenta, which is rich in aromatase (P450arom). The placenta is unable to convert the 21-carbon precursors progesterone and pregnenolone into estrogen because it lacks the 17α-hydroxylase /17-20 desmolase (P450c17) enzyme. Thus, the placenta relies on 19-carbon androgen precursors produced by the maternal and fetal adrenal glands. These precursors are readily available from the fetus due to the aforementioned deficiency in 3β-hydroxysteroid dehydrogenase activity in the fetal intermediate zone of the adrenal gland. Fetal adrenal dehydroepiandrosterone sulfate (DHEAS) is readily hydrolyzed to free dehydroepiandrosterone by sulfatase in the placenta and converted to estradiol (E_2) and estrone (E_1). In addition, almost half of the E_2 and E_1 formed in the placenta is derived from dehydroepiandrosterone sulfate secreted from the maternal adrenal. Whereas almost all (>90%) of the estriol (E_3) synthesized by the placenta is from fetal adrenal DHEAS that has been 16α-hydroxylated to 16α-dehydroisoandrosterone sulfate in the fetal liver. The sources of estrogen biosynthesis by the maternal–fetal–placental unit are shown in Figure 10. The major substrate for fetal adrenal DHEAS synthesis is

cholesterol derived from low-density lipoprotein and circulating in fetal blood. A minor source of fetal adrenal DHEAS is pregnenolone secreted by the placenta.

HUMAN CHORIONIC GONADOTROPIN

Human chorionic gonadotropin is secreted by the syncytiotrophoblast of the placenta into both the fetal and the maternal circulation. It is a glycoprotein consisting of 2 noncovalently linked α and β subunits and is similar in structure and action to luteinizing hormone. Indeed, these 2 hormones appear to exert their actions through a single receptor. Plasma levels of hCG double in concentration every 2–3 days between 60 and 90 days of gestation. Thereafter, the concentration of hCG in maternal plasma decreases, reaching a plateau at about 120 days after conception. The half-life of circulating hCG is 24 hours. The most widely accepted theory about the function of hCG is support of the early corpus luteum of pregnancy to ensure continued progesterone secretion until this function is taken over by the placenta. Another function of hCG is the regulation of sexual differentiation in males by the stimulation of testosterone secretion in the fetal testes.

HUMAN PLACENTAL LACTOGEN

Human placental lactogen (hPL), a single-chain polypeptide consisting of 191 amino acid residues with 2 disulfide bonds, has primarily lactogenic activity but exhibits some growth-hormone-like activity. The structures of hPL, prolactin, and growth hormone are quite similar. Human placental lactogen is secreted by syncytiotrophoblasts. Unlike hCG levels, hPL levels continue to increase with advancing gestational age and appear to reach a plateau at term. Although the level of hPL in serum at term is the highest of all the protein hormones

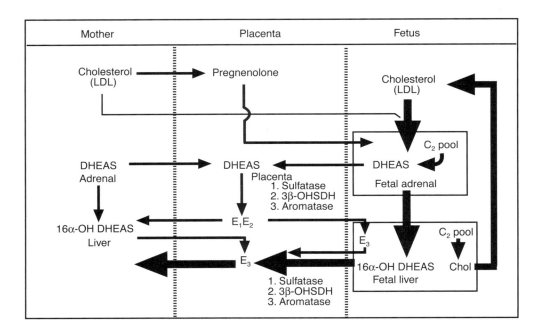

■ **FIG. 10.** Sources of estrogen biosynthesis in the maternal–fetal–placental unit. LDL indicates low-density lipoprotein; C_2 pool, carbon–carbon unit; DHEAS, dehydroepiandrosterone sulfate; 3β-OHSDH = 3β-hydroxysteroid dehydrogenase; 16α-OH DHEAS = 16α-hydroxylase DHEAS; E_1, estrone; E_2, estradiol-17β; E_3, estriol; Chol, cholesterol. (Modified from Carr BR, Gant NF. The endocrinology of pregnancy-induced hypertension. Clin Perinatol 1983;10:737–61.)

secreted by the placenta, its clearance rate is so rapid (half-life is 10 minutes) that it cannot be detected after the first postpartum day.

Because hPL is secreted primarily into the maternal circulation, most of its proposed functions have focused on its sites of action in maternal tissues. Human placental lactogen stimulates type 1 insulinlike growth factor to induce insulin resistance, which then stimulates lipolysis to increase circulating ketones and free fatty acids and stimulate gluconeogenesis. These metabolic effects favor the transportation of glucose, amino acids, and fatty acids to the fetus to provide nutrition. Hypoglycemia stimulates hPL release. Thus, in the fasting state, hPL enhances lipolysis and antagonizes insulin to make free fatty acids and ketones available to the mother while continuing to provide the fetus with glucose. Conversely, hyperglycemia inhibits hPL release. Thus, in the fed state, glucose is available for both mother and fetus, increasing the ability of maternal insulin to augment fat storage. The powerful antiinsulin effects of hPL are responsible, at least in part, for the development of gestational diabetes in some women.

Fetal Compartment

The regulation of the fetal endocrine system is not completely independent but relies to some extent on precursor hormones secreted by the placenta or maternal tissues. As the fetus develops, its endocrine system matures and becomes more independent, preparing the fetus for extrauterine existence.

FETAL HYPOTHALAMIC–PITUITARY AXIS

The fetal hypothalamus begins to differentiate from the forebrain during the first few weeks of fetal life; by 12 weeks, hypothalamic development is well advanced. Most of the hypothalamic-releasing hormones, including gonadotropin-releasing hormone, thyrotropin-releasing hormone, corticotropin-releasing hormone (CRH), dopamine, norepinephrine, and somatostatin, are present by 6–8 weeks of fetal life. The anterior pituitary cells that develop from the cells lining the Rathke pouch are capable of secreting growth hormone, prolactin, follicle-stimulating hormone, luteinizing hormone, and corticotropin in vivo at as early as 7 weeks of fetal life (Fig. 11). The portal system that delivers releasing hormones to the anterior pituitary is fully developed by 18 weeks of gestation.

FETAL THYROID GLAND

The fetal hypothalamic–pituitary–thyroid axis appears to develop and function independently of the mother, although it depends on an adequate supply of iodine from the maternal circulation. The levels of thyroid-stimulating hormone (TSH) and thyroid hormones are relatively low in fetal blood until midgestation. At 24–28 weeks of gestation, serum thyroxine (T_4) and reverse triiodothyronine (rT_3) concentrations begin to increase progressively until term, while the T_3 concentration remains low. At birth there is an abrupt release of TSH, T_4, and T_3. The relative hyperthyroid state of the newborn is believed to facilitate thermoregulatory adjustments for extrauterine life.

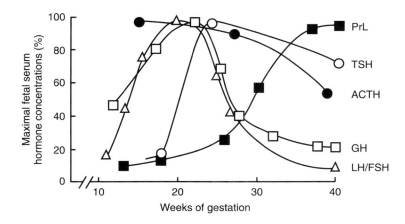

■ FIG. 11. Ontogeny of pituitary hormone levels in human fetal sera. PrL indicates prolactin; TSH, thyroid-stimulating hormone; ACTH, corticotropin; GH, growth hormone; LH/FSH, luteinizing hormone/follicle-stimulating hormone. (Parker CR Jr. The endocrinology of pregnancy. In: Carr BR, Blackwell RE, editors. Textbook of reproductive medicine. Norwalk [CT]: Appleton & Lange; 1993. p. 28. Copyright The McGraw-Hill Companies, Inc.)

FETAL GONADS

The pattern of luteinizing hormone expression in fetal plasma parallels that of follicle-stimulating hormone, and the decrease in gonadotropin pituitary content and plasma concentration of gonadotropins after midgestation is believed to result from the maturation of the hypothalamus. The hypothalamus also becomes progressively more sensitive to sex steroids circulating in fetal blood and those originating from the placenta. In the male, fetal testosterone secretion begins soon after differentiation of the gonad into a testis and formation of Leydig cells, which occurs at 7 weeks of life. Maximum levels of fetal testosterone are observed at about 15 weeks and decrease thereafter. The early secretion of testosterone is important in initiating sexual differentiation in the male. It is believed that the primary stimulus to the early development and growth of Leydig cells and the subsequent peak of testosterone is hCG, supplemented by fetal luteinizing hormone. In the female, the fetal ovary is involved primarily in the formation of follicles and germ cells and less in hormone secretion.

FETAL ADRENAL GLAND

At term, the fetal adrenal gland secretes up to 200 mg of steroid daily. This rate of steroidogenesis is 5 times that observed in the adrenal glands of adults at rest. The principal steroids secreted are C-19 steroids (mainly DHEAS), which, as noted, serve as a precursor substrate for the biosynthesis of estrogen by the placenta. The fetal adrenal gland contains a unique fetal (intermediate) zone that accounts for the rapid growth of the adrenal gland; this zone regresses during the first few weeks after birth. In addition to the fetal zone, an outer layer of cells forms the neocortex (definitive zone). The fetal zone differs histologically and biochemically from the neocortex. It is deficient in 3β-hydroxysteroid dehydrogenase and secretes excess C-19 steroids. In contrast, the neocortex of the fetal adrenal gland secretes primarily cortisol.

Studies of the fetal adrenal gland have attempted to determine what factors stimulate and regulate its growth and steroidogenesis and why the fetal zone undergoes atrophy after delivery. All investigations have shown that corticotropin stimulates steroidogenesis in vitro. Furthermore, there is clinical evidence that corticotropin is the major trophic hormone of the fetal adrenal gland in vivo. In anencephalic fetuses, for example, the plasma levels of corticotropin are very low and the fetal zone is markedly atrophic. Maternal corticosteroid therapy effectively suppresses fetal adrenal steroidogenesis by suppressing fetal corticotropin secretion. Conversely, the progressive increase in placenta-derived CRH synthesis and secretion during the second half of pregnancy may directly stimulate fetal adrenal DHEAS synthesis and drive fetal pituitary corticotropin release to overcome the inhibitory effects of increasing fetal cortisol levels, thus maintaining the fetal zone and its C-19 steroid biosynthetic activity. Interestingly, after birth, the adrenal gland shrinks by more than 50% because of regression of fetal zone cells. After regression of the fetal zone, the neocortex zone increases to develop into the adult cortex, which secretes primarily cortisol.

FETAL PARATHYROID GLAND AND CALCIUM HOMEOSTASIS

The transplacental transfer of calcium from the maternal compartment regulates the level of calcium in the fetus. During pregnancy there is an increase in calcium and D3 absorption from the maternal gastrointestinal tract. In addition, maternal parathyroid hormone levels are elevated. These changes in the maternal compartment allow for a net transfer of sufficient calcium to the fetus to sustain fetal bone growth. Although levels of total calcium and phosphorus decline in the maternal serum, ionized calcium levels remain unchanged. The "placental calcium pump" allows for the maintenance of a positive gradient of calcium and phosphorus to the fetus. Circulating fetal calcium and phosphorus levels increase steadily throughout gestation. Fetal levels of total and ionized calcium, as well as phosphorus, exceed maternal levels at term.

The fetal parathyroid gland secretes parathyroid hormone by 10–12 weeks of gestation. Fetal plasma levels of parathyroid hormone are low but increase after delivery. The neural crest-derived ultimobranchial cells embedded in the fetal thyroid gland produce calcitonin. In contrast to the lack of changes in calcitonin levels in the mother, those in the fetus are elevated. Because there is no transfer of parathyroid hormone or calcitonin across the placenta, the effects of the observed changes in these hormones on fetal calcium are consistent with an adaptation to conserve and stimulate fetal bone growth. After birth, serum calcium and phosphorus levels decrease in the neonate. Parathyroid hormone levels begin to increase 48 hours after birth, and calcium and phosphorus levels gradually increase over the following several days, depending on dietary intake of milk.

FETAL ENDOCRINE PANCREAS

The fetal pancreas appears during the fourth week of fetal life. The cells containing glucagon and the cells containing somatostatin develop before cell differentiation, although insulin can be recognized in the developing pancreas before apparent cell differentiation. Total human pancreatic insulin and glucagon levels increase with fetal age and are higher than concentrations in the adult human pancreas. Studies of fetal blood samples show that fetal insulin secretion is low and relatively unresponsive to acute changes in glucose. In poorly controlled maternal diabetes mellitus, fetal islet cells undergo hypertrophy and secrete increased levels of insulin.

Maternal Compartment

A variety of maternal homeostatic adaptations occur during pregnancy. For example, to provide effective exchange and transport of nutrients between mother and fetus, the maternal vascular system undergoes a significant increase in capacity. This is reflected by increases in uterine and renal blood flow, maternal plasma and erythrocyte volume, and cardiac output. To accommodate the increase in blood volume without a concomitant increase in blood pressure, there is a corresponding decrease in peripheral vascular resistance, owing in part to progesterone-mediated relaxation of arteriolar smooth muscle and development of a low-resistance uteroplacental circulation. The latter may be mediated in part by increased endothelial prostacyclin and nitric oxide production.

HYPOTHALAMUS AND PITUITARY GLAND

The anterior pituitary enlarges 2-fold to 3-fold during pregnancy, primarily because of hyperplasia and hypertrophy of the lactotrophs secondary to estrogen stimulation. This accounts for the progressive increase in plasma prolactin levels throughout gestation. In contrast to lactotrophs, other pituitary cells decrease in size or remain unaltered during pregnancy. Thus, maternal levels of growth hormone are low and the level of TSH remains relatively unchanged. Corticotropin and endorphin levels appear to increase with advancing gestation, likely driven by increasing placental CRH synthesis and secretion. However, excess CRH action is inhibited by the action of CRH-binding protein until term. Maternal plasma levels of arginine vasopressin remain low throughout gestation and are not believed to play a role in human parturition. Maternal oxytocin levels are reported to be low and do not vary throughout pregnancy but increase during the later stages of labor.

THYROID GLAND

The thyroid gland increases slightly in size during pregnancy due to increased vascularity and glandular hyperplasia. There is a modest increase in the basal metabolic rate secondary to fetal requirements. During pregnancy, the mother generally is in a euthyroid state. However, circulating TSH levels may be below normal during the first trimester as a result of the thyrotropic effects of hCG. Conversely, because renal clearance of iodine virtually doubles across gestation, impairing the iodination of tyrosine residues in thyroglobulin, TSH levels may be elevated in the third trimester to maintain a euthyroid state. Total T_4 and T_3 levels increase but do not result in hyperthyroidism because of estrogen-induced increases in T_4-binding globulin. There is reduced transfer of T_4 and T_3 and virtually no transfer of TSH across the placenta.

ADRENAL GLAND

The maternal adrenal gland does not change morphologically during pregnancy. Plasma adrenal steroid hormones increase with advancing gestation. The increase in total plasma cortisol results principally from a concomitant increase in cortisol-binding globulin. There is a slight increase in plasma free cortisol (from 1% to 2%) and urinary free cortisol, but pregnant women do not exhibit any overt signs of hypercortisolism. As in the fetus, this increase in the second half of pregnancy may be driven by progressive increases in placental CRH production. Cortisol-driven placental CRH production blunts the negative feedback effects of cortisol on hypothalamic CRH and pituitary corticotropin release. Levels of renin and angiotensinogen increase during pregnancy. This leads to elevated angiotensin II levels and markedly elevated levels of aldosterone, which in turn contribute to pregnancy-associated increases in plasma volume.

ENDOCRINE PANCREAS

A key metabolic adaptation to pregnancy is the sparing of maternal glucose for the fetus. In response to a glucose load, there is a greater release of insulin from pancreatic cells, as well as a greater suppression of glucagon release from the cells than in the nonpregnant state. Pregnancy is not associated with a change in insulin clearance. In association with the increased release of insulin, the maternal pancreas undergoes cell hyperplasia and islet cell hypertrophy, accompanied by an increase in blood flow to the endocrine pancreas. During pregnancy, the effects of hPL and the increasing utilization of glucose by the fetoplacental unit result in decreasing fasting blood glucose levels and increasing postprandial glucose values. Glucagon levels are suppressed in response to a glucose load, with the greatest suppression occurring near term.

PARTURITION

The initiation of labor in many mammals results from an abrupt decrease in progesterone levels. This decrease is mediated by increasing fetal cortisol levels that activate placental 17α-hydroxylase to shunt steroid precursors away from the progesterone to the estrogen synthetic pathway. Although parturition in humans and higher primates is not associated with plasma progesterone withdrawal, activation of the fetal hypothalamic–pituitary–adrenal axis and functional progesterone withdrawal at the receptor level appears to play a crucial role in the onset of human parturition.

Corticotropin-releasing hormone is a 41–amino acid peptide initially localized to the hypothalamus, where its release into the portal circulation mediates pituitary corticotropin secretion. The latter enhances adrenal cortisol secretion that, in turn, inhibits hypothalamic CRH release. Besides its expression in the central nervous system, CRH is expressed by trophoblasts in the placenta and the chorion and by amnion and decidual cells. Plasma CRH levels increase dramatically during the second half of pregnancy, peak during labor, and rapidly decrease in the postpartum period.

Although glucocorticoids inhibit the hypothalamic release of CRH, they increase the expression of CRH by cultured trophoblasts and amnion, chorion, and decidual cells. As noted, fetal and maternal cortisol levels increase steadily during the second half of gestation. However, fetal cortisol levels most strongly correlate with placental CRH secretion. One explanation for this paradoxical cortisol stimulation of placental CRH expression may rest with the absence of progesterone receptor expression in trophoblasts. Thus, progesterone and cortisol compete for trophoblast glucocorticoid receptor binding sites. In the

first half of gestation, progesterone dominates, inhibiting glucocorticoid receptor–mediated gene expression. However, in the third trimester, as maternal and fetal cortisol levels increase, the tonic inhibition of cortisol/glucocorticoid receptor–mediated CRH expression by progesterone is functionally overcome, and a "feed-forward" loop between cortisol and placental CRH expression ensues. Increasing placental CRH production in turn drives increasing fetal pituitary corticotropin release, stimulating adrenal cortisol production to further enhance placental CRH production. This creates a potent positive-feedback circuit. This preparturition increase in CRH also is accompanied by a fall in CRH-binding protein, leading to increases in circulating bioactive CRH at term (Fig. 12).

Corticotropin-releasing hormone enhances prostanoid production by isolated amnion, chorion, and decidual cells. Prostaglandins act as direct uterotonins but also enhance myometrial receptivity by increasing oxytocin receptors and the formation of gap junctions. Prostaglandins also elicit cervical change by enhancing cellular degradation. Conversely, prostanoids stimulate CRH release in isolated placental tissue, fetal membrane, and decidual cells, establishing a second positive-feedback loop to potentiate the parturition process. Multiple investigators have now reported that elevated maternal plasma levels of CRH precede preterm, term, and postterm labor and have designated CRH as a potential "placental

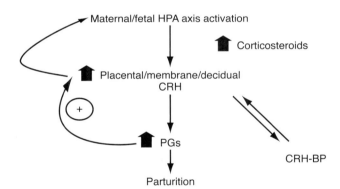

■ **FIG. 12.** Role of activation of the maternal or fetal hypothalamic–pituitary–adrenal (HPA) axis (or both) in the genesis of parturition. CRH indicates corticotropin-releasing hormone; PG, prostaglandin; BP, binding protein. Activation of the maternal or fetal (or both) HPA axis will lead to enhanced fetal adrenal glucocorticoid production. Cortisol in turn stimulates placental, fetal membrane, and decidual CRH expression. Reproductive tract–derived CRH in turn further activates the maternal or the fetal HPA axis or both. Increasing levels of CRH in serum reduce concentrations of CRH-BP to increase CRH bioavailability. Moreover, CRH can stimulate PG production in the placenta, fetal membranes, and decidua, which can induce parturition. Finally, PGs further stimulate reproductive tract CRH expression, establishing yet another proparturition positive-feedback loop.

clock" regulating the onset of parturition. In addition to the direct effects of CRH on prostanoid biosynthesis, cortisol appears to directly enhance amnion cyclooxygenase expression, the key step in prostaglandin synthesis, while inhibiting chorionic prostaglandin dehydrogenase expression, the primary mediator of prostaglandin metabolism.

Activation of the fetal hypothalamic–pituitary–adrenal axis also is associated with enhanced corticotropin (ACTH) hormone-mediated fetal adrenal synthesis of DHEAS, which can be 16-hydroxylated in the fetal liver. Corticotropin-releasing hormone also may exert direct stimulatory effects on adrenal DHEAS synthesis. Upon transfer to the placenta, DHEAS is converted to E_2 and E_1, whereas 16-hydroxy-DHEAS is converted to E_3. These estrogens interact with the myometrium to enhance gap junction (connexin 43) formation and oxytocin receptor mRNA levels, as well as prostaglandin $F_{2\alpha}$ synthase, myosin light chain kinase, and calmodulin expression. This proparturition cycle may be further enhanced by estrogen stimulation of placental 11 α-hydroxysteroid dehydrogenase activity. The latter enzyme converts cortisol to cortisone, reducing the transplacental passage of maternal cortisol to further stimulate fetal corticotropin release. It has long been proposed that estrogens regulate the events leading to parturition because pregnancies are often prolonged when estrogen levels in maternal blood and urine are low, as in placental sulfatase deficiency, or when associated with inadequate fetal adrenal function, as with anencephaly. Near term, there appears to be a shift in myometrial progesterone receptor subtypes from the "proprogestational" PR-B form to the "antiprogestational" PR-A form. Although the precise mediators of this isoform shift are yet to be elucidated, the net effect could be localized "progestational withdrawal." Finally, in labor, increasing concentrations of maternal plasma oxytocin enhance contractile activity. These proparturition mechanisms are delineated in Figure 13.

Bibliography

Becker KL, Bilezikian JP, Bremner WJ, Hung W, Kahn CR, Loriaux DL, et al., editors. Principles and practice of endocrinology and metabolism. 3rd ed. Philadelphia (PA): Lippincott Williams & Wilkins; 2001.

Lockwood CJ, Schatz F. A biological model for the regulation of peri-implantational hemostasis and menstruation. J Soc Gynecol Investig 1996;3:159–65.

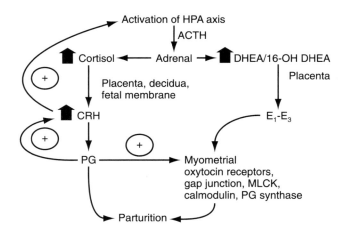

■ FIG. 13. Role of estrogens (E_1, estrone; E_2, estradiol-17β; E_3, estriol) and corticotropin-releasing hormone (CRH) in the initiation of parturition. HPA indicates hypothalamic–pituitary–adrenal; ACTH, corticotropin; DHEA, dehydroepiandrosterone; DHEAS, dehydroepiandrosterone sulfate; PG, prostaglandin; MLCK, myosin light chain kinase. Activation of the fetal HPA axis leads to increasing fetal adrenal synthesis and release of cortisol and DHEAS, which can be 16-hydroxylated in the fetal liver to 16-OH DHEA. Increasing fetal cortisol levels stimulate fetal membrane, decidual, and placental production of CRH, which in turn stimulates PG production in these tissues (as described in Fig. 10). Fetal adrenal-derived DHEA is converted by the placenta to E_1 and E_2 while 16-hydroxy-DHEA is converted into E_3. These estrogens activate the myometrium by enhancing gap junction (connexin 43) formation, increasing oxytocin receptor density, and increasing expression of uterine $PGF_{2\alpha}$ synthetase, MLCK, and calmodulin.

Loke YW, King A. Human implantation: cell biology and immunology. Cambridge: Cambridge University Press; 1995.

Norwitz ER, Schust DJ, Fisher SJ. Implantation and the survival of early pregnancy. N Engl J Med 2001;345:1400–8.

Speroff L, Glass RH, Kase NG. The endocrinology of pregnancy. In: Clinical gynecologic endocrinology and infertility. 6th ed. Baltimore (MD): Lippincott Williams & Wilkins; 1999. p. 275–335.

Tulchinsky D, Little AB, editors. Maternal-fetal endocrinology. 2nd ed. Philadelphia (PA): WB Saunders; 1994.

Yanagimachi R. Mammalian fertilization. In: Knobil E, Neill JD, editors. The physiology of reproduction. 2nd ed. New York (NY): Raven Press; 1994. p. 189–318.

Complications of Pregnancy

HYPERTENSION

Hypertension is the most common medical risk factor among women who give birth to live babies. It affects as many as 8% of all pregnant women and remains a significant cause of maternal and neonatal morbidity and mortality (1).

Terminology and Clinical Manifestations

The report of the National High Blood Pressure Education Program Working Group on High Blood Pressure in Pregnancy (2) has classified hypertensive disorders in pregnancy as follows:

- Chronic hypertension
- Preeclampsia/eclampsia
- Gestational hypertension
- Chronic hypertension with superimposed preeclampsia

This classification also has been adopted by ACOG (3). Both the Working Group and ACOG have provided criteria and definitions for diagnosing the various hypertensive disorders during pregnancy.

Chronic hypertension is preexisting hypertension that is present before 20 weeks of gestation (see "Chronic Hypertension").

Gestational hypertension is presumed after 20 weeks of gestation in the absence of proteinuria or other signs and symptoms of preeclampsia and when the blood pressure returns to normal by 12 weeks postpartum. Many of these women will develop actual preeclampsia as pregnancy progresses. If not, they are given the designation of "transient hypertension." The term *gestational hypertension* has replaced the older term, *pregnancy-induced hypertension.*

Preeclampsia is a pregnancy-specific syndrome that occurs after 20 weeks of gestation and is characterized by systolic pressure of 140 mm Hg or higher or diastolic pressure of 90 mm Hg or higher occurring with proteinuria (≥300 mg of protein over 24 hours or a random dipstick urine determination of ≥1+ protein or ≥30 mg/dL). Blood pressure should be elevated on at least 2 occasions 6 hours apart. From a clinical standpoint, it is not necessary to wait for repeat elevation of blood pressure to confirm the diagnosis of preeclampsia (especially near term) when the patient has severe hypertension in the 180/120 mm Hg range. Preeclampsia can be subdivided further into 2 categories: mild and severe (Box 4).

Edema is no longer used as a diagnostic criterion for preeclampsia. Moreover, the incremental increase of 30 mm Hg systolic or 15 mm Hg diastolic above the baseline blood pressure is not used as a diagnostic criterion. However, although not diagnostic, such changes in blood pressure should not be ignored and warrant close observation (2). In a recent longitudinal study, such changes in blood pressure ("30 and 15") were not risk factors for adverse outcomes (4).

Superimposed preeclampsia in women with chronic hypertension often is difficult to diagnose but includes new-onset proteinuria, a sudden increase in proteinuria, a sudden sustained increase in hypertension, or the development of any component of HELLP syndrome (hemolysis, elevated liver enzymes, and low platelet count), or symptoms of severe preeclampsia (2, 3).

Eclampsia is defined as new-onset grand mal seizures in women with preeclampsia or gestational hypertension. Other etiologies such as arteriovenous malformations, ruptured aneurysm, or idiopathic seizures should be considered when seizures occur after 48–72 hours postpartum (2, 3). However, eclamptic seizures may occur up to 2 weeks postpartum.

BOX 4

Preeclampsia: Severe Versus Mild

Criteria for Diagnosis of Preeclampsia:

- Blood pressure of 140 mm Hg systolic or higher or 90 mm Hg diastolic or higher that occurs after 20 weeks of gestation in a woman with previously normal blood pressure
- Proteinuria, defined as urinary excretion of 0.3 g protein or higher in a 24-hour urine specimen

Diagnosis of Severe Preeclampsia:

Women with any one of the following additional findings are categorized as having severe preeclampsia:

- Systolic blood pressure of 160 mm Hg or higher or diastolic blood pressure of 110 mm Hg or higher on 2 occasions 6 hours apart*
- Proteinuria of more than 5 g in 24 hours (normal <300 mg/24 h) or ≥3+ on 2 random urine samples collected 4 hours apart
- Elevated serum creatinine (>1.2 mg/dL)
- Grand mal seizures (eclampsia)
- Pulmonary edema
- Oliguria of less than 500 mL in 24 hours
- Microangiopathic hemolysis (fragmented red blood cells, schizocytosis, spherocytosis, reticulocytosis, anemia, elevated lactate dehydrogenase level).
- Thrombocytopenia (platelet count <100,000/µL, for overt severe disease)
- Hepatocellular dysfunction (elevated alanine aminotransferase, aspartase)
- Intrauterine growth restriction or oligohydramnios
- Symptoms suggesting significant end organ involvement: headache, visual disturbances, epigastric pain, or pain in the right upper quadrant

Diagnosis of Mild Preeclampsia:

Women with none of these additional findings are categorized as having mild preeclampsia.

*The diastolic blood pressure is the pressure at which the cardiac cycle sounds disappear (Korotkoff phase V). Moreover, blood pressure should be taken with the woman in a sitting or left lateral recumbent position with her arm at the level of the heart. (Report of the National High Blood Pressure Education Program Working Group on High Blood Pressure in Pregnancy. Am J Obstet Gynecol 2000;183:S1–22.)

Modified from Diagnosis and management of preeclampsia and eclampsia. ACOG Practice Bulletin No. 33. American College of Obstetricians and Gynecologists. Obstet Gynecol 2002;99: 159–67.

A subclassification of preeclampsia—early-onset (<34 weeks of gestation) and late-onset (≥34 weeks of gestation)—has been proposed (5). This subclassification makes sense from both a clinical standpoint and a research standpoint and is of paramount importance in trying to establish evidence-based protocols for the management of women with preeclampsia remote from term.

Epidemiology and Risk Factors

Numerous risk factors are associated with preeclampsia and gestational hypertension (6). These include first pregnancies, multifetal gestations, the presence of certain vascular disorders such as those seen with insulin-dependent diabetes (types 1 and 2), lupus erythematosus, renal disease, antiphospholipid antibody syndrome, obesity, advanced maternal age, African-American race, and chronic hypertension (2, 3). Other less common conditions associated with preeclampsia include fetal hydrops and gestational trophoblastic disease.

Pathophysiology

The major pathophysiologic derangements are focal vasospasm and a transfer of fluid from the intravascular space to extravascular spaces (a "porous" vascular tree). The exact cause of vasospasm is unclear, but research has focused on an interaction of various vasodilators and vasoconstrictors, such as prostacyclin, nitric oxide, endothelin 1, angiotensin II, and thromboxane. The literature regarding etiology and pathophysiology of preeclampsia has focused on the role played by angiogenic factors and their inhibitors (eg, soluble FLT-1) as well as the degree of endovascular trophoblastic invasion, which appears to be incomplete (2, 3). Oxidative stress and an intense inflammatory response appear to play a role (1, 2).

The physiologic maternal consequences of preeclampsia include cardiovascular and hematologic effects (eg, hemolysis and thrombocytopenia) and regional perfusion abnormalities. The porous vascular tree is related primarily to an increase in vascular permeability and a decrease in colloid osmotic pressure, which usually is decreased in pregnant women with normal blood pressure but is decreased further in women with preeclampsia. The most frequently cited hemodynamic consequence of preeclampsia is constriction of plasma volume and focal vasospasm, which results in decreased perfusion of certain specific organs. Women with preeclampsia are volume constricted but not hypovolemic in the usual sense of the word (2, 3). Peripheral resistance and cardiac output are increased in women with preeclampsia. In fact, before hydration, cardiac output actually is in a hyperdynamic state in women with preeclampsia.

Thrombocytopenia is the most frequently observed coagulation abnormality in women with preeclampsia, and disseminated intravascular coagulation rarely develops. Microangiopathic hemolytic anemia probably is the consequence of endothelial damage resulting from the arteriolar spasm that accompanies preeclampsia. Abnormalities of hepatic function tests often are found and are elevated in association with thrombocytopenia in HELLP syndrome. The serum uric acid level has not proved to be a clinically useful aid in diagnosing preeclampsia (2, 3, 7).

Women with early-onset (<34 weeks) severe preeclampsia may be candidates for testing for lupus erythematosus and antiphospholipid antibodies. There is considerable controversy about the role of maternal inherited thrombophilia in the genesis of early-onset, severe preeclampsia. The clinical utility and cost-effectiveness of testing for these factors are unclear and await further study.

Clinical Management

There is no known cure for preeclampsia other than fetal delivery. With rare exceptions, delivery is appropriate regardless of gestational age in a woman with eclampsia, renal failure, or rapidly worsening maternal manifestations such as HELLP syndrome. The urgency for delivery can be evaluated on the basis of the severity of maternal manifestations and an assessment of fetal status.

For women with severe preeclampsia before viability, pregnancy termination, preferably performed at a tertiary-care center, is recommended because fetal survival is very unlikely, and the likelihood of maternal complications is great. Testing for antiphospholipid antibody syndrome may help explain this occurrence and lead to therapy for subsequent pregnancies. Women should be counseled that they are at increased risk for repeat preterm preeclampsia, insulin resistance, and chronic hypertension.

Women with severe preeclampsia at 23–34 weeks should be admitted for intensive assessment of maternal and fetal disease status at a tertiary-care center. Initial therapy includes administration of corticosteroids (24–34 weeks of gestation) and magnesium sulfate and control of blood pressure during the first 24–48 hours of hospitalization. Under optimal conditions, the pregnancy can be continued under intensive daily surveillance unless there is evidence of HELLP syndrome, maternal disease progression, or nonreassuring fetal status. As long as blood pressure is neither excessive nor trending upward, maternal laboratory values are stable, oliguria and symptoms of worsening disease (headache, scotomata, epigastric pain) are absent, and fetal monitoring and assessments remain reassuring, delivery can be postponed to maximize the chance for fetal survival.

Women with mild preeclampsia or worsening chronic hypertension but without criteria for severe disease may benefit from brief hospitalization to evaluate maternal–fetal status thoroughly and develop a management plan. Some form of regular antepartum fetal surveillance, such as a weekly biophysical profile, should begin between 32 and 34 weeks of gestation for pregnant women with a hypertensive disorder or earlier if there are concerns about reduced fetal growth or amniotic fluid volume. Blood pressure, urinary protein levels, and laboratory values should be monitored.

At term (≥37 weeks), delivery should be strongly considered for all women with hypertensive disorders of pregnancy. Once gestational age reaches 32–34 weeks of gestation, depending on the capability of the nursery, the neonatal unit, or both, delivery is indicated for any woman with severe preeclampsia and is an option for women with mild preeclampsia because disease progression is likely. The rationale is that risks posed to the fetus by increasing placental compromise or sudden abruption may exceed those posed to the neonate by prematurity. When the diagnosis of preeclampsia is questionable, outpatient management may be appropriate if frequent maternal–fetal assessments are continued. When prompt delivery is not clearly mandated by severe disease but is chosen as a preference, documentation of fetal lung maturity by amniocentesis should be considered.

Management of Labor

Induction of labor (preceded by cervical ripening, if necessary) is preferred to elective cesarean delivery for women with hypertensive disorders unless there are obstetric indications such as malpresentation or there is clear evidence of nonreassuring fetal status. The type of anesthesia used depends on the clinical circumstances, the expertise of the anesthesiologist, and the patient's preference, after informed consent has been obtained.

It is now well established that magnesium sulfate is the anticonvulsant of choice for the prevention or treatment of eclamptic seizures (2, 3, 8). When induction of labor is indicated for a woman with preeclampsia, magnesium sulfate to prevent seizures generally is given intravenously as a 4–6-g loading bolus over 15–20 minutes, followed by a controlled infusion at 1.5–2.0 g/h. Discontinuation of therapy and determination of serum magnesium levels are indicated whenever there is a loss of deep tendon reflexes, the respiratory rate is less than 12 respirations per minute, diplopia is present, or urinary output is less than 25 mL/h. The therapeutic range for serum magnesium is 4.8–8.4 mg/dL. The effects of an overdose of magnesium can be reversed by administering calcium, such as 1 g intravenous calcium gluconate given slowly. If necessary, respiration should be supported mechanically until recovery occurs. In rare cases when a woman is not a candidate for magnesium sulfate administration (such as someone with myasthenia gravis), phenytoin sodium is an alternative drug for seizure prophylaxis. If creatinine is elevated, or urine output is low, the dosage may need to be adjusted. Phenytoin is not used routinely because it is less effective than magnesium in this situation.

Antihypertensive agents are used to maintain systolic blood pressures below 170–180 mm Hg. Hydralazine hydrochloride or labetalol or both are the preferred antihypertensive agents. The goal is to maintain diastolic pressure at less than 110 mm Hg (target range, 90–99 mm Hg).

Invasive hemodynamic monitoring rarely is indicated in women with preeclampsia and may be associated with serious complications. However, it may help guide therapy in rare cases of persistent severe oliguria unresponsive to a fluid challenge. Although dexamethasone administered intravenously (10 mg every 12 hours) to the woman with worsening HELLP syndrome has been shown to improve some of the laboratory abnormalities, the question of whether it affects the actual disease process awaits further study.

Postpartum

Although delivery is recognized as the most definitive event in the cure of preeclampsia, the manifestations of this disorder may continue well into the postpartum period but not longer than 12 weeks. Hypertension persisting beyond 12 weeks is consistent with chronic hypertension. Most patients are free of clinical manifestations within the first postpartum week. Occasionally, hypertensive disease may not become evident until after delivery. Postpartum eclampsia occurs most often in the first 72 hours postpartum but has been reported up to several weeks after delivery. Magnesium sulfate usually is indicated for up to 24 hours after delivery.

Prevention

Use of low-dose aspirin and calcium supplements has not been found to reduce the incidence of preeclampsia (2, 3, 9, 10). Current evidence suggests that women at high risk for preeclampsia because of antiphospholipid antibodies may benefit from therapy with heparin and low-dose aspirin (60–80 mg/d) (11). Research focusing on the use of antioxidant therapy for the prevention of preeclampsia is underway in the National Institute of Child Health and Human Development Network of Maternal–Fetal Medicine Units (NICHD MFMU).

References

1. Roberts JM, Pearson GD, Cutler JA, Lindheimer MD; National Heart, Lung and Blood Institute. Summary of the NHLBI Working Group on Research on Hypertension During Pregnancy. Hypertens Pregnancy 2003;22:109–27.

2. Report of the National High Blood Pressure Education Program Working Group on High Blood Pressure in Pregnancy. Am J Obstet Gynecol 2000;183:S1–22.

3. Diagnosis and management of preeclampsia and eclampsia. ACOG Practice Bulletin No. 33. American College of Obstetricians and Gynecologists. Obstet Gynecol 2002;99:159–67.

4. Ohkuchi A, Iwasaki R, Ojima T, Matsubara S, Sato I, Suzuki M, Minakami H. Increase in systolic blood pressure of > or = 30 mm Hg and/or diastolic blood pressure of > or = 15 mm Hg during pregnancy: is it pathologic? Hypertens Pregnancy 2003;22:275–85.

5. von Dadelszen P, Ornstein MP, Bull SB, Logan AG, Koren G, Magee LA. Fall in mean arterial pressure and fetal growth restriction in pregnancy hypertension: a meta-analysis. Lancet 2000;355:87–92.

6. Dekker GA, Sibai BM. Etiology and pathogenesis of preeclampsia: current concepts. Am J Obstet Gynecol 1998;179:1359–75.

7. Lim KH, Friedman SA, Ecker JL, Kao L, Kilpatrick SJ. The clinical utility of serum uric acid measurements in hypertensive diseases of pregnancy. Am J Obstet Gynecol 1998;178:1067–71.

8. Which anticonvulsant for women with eclampsia? Evidence from the Collaborative Eclampsia Trial [published erratum appears in Lancet 1995;346:258]. Lancet 1995;345:1455–63.

9. Levine RJ, Hauth JC, Curet LB, Sibai BM, Catalano PM, Morris CD, et al. Trial of calcium to prevent preeclampsia. N Engl J Med 1997;337:69–76.

10. Sibai BM, Ewell M, Levine RJ, Klebanoff MA, Esterlitz J, Catalano PM, et al. Risk factors associated with preeclampsia in healthy nulliparous women. The Calcium for Preeclampsia Prevention (CPEP) Study Group. Am J Obstet Gynecol 1997;177:1003–10.

11. Caritis S, Sibai B, Hauth J, Lindheimer MD, Klebanoff M, Thom E, et al. Low-dose aspirin to prevent preeclampsia in women at high risk. National Institute of Child Health and Human Development Network of Maternal Fetal Medicine Units. N Engl J Med 1998;338:701–5.

BLEEDING IN THE SECOND HALF OF PREGNANCY

Because the uterus of a pregnant woman receives 20% of maternal cardiac output, obstetric hemorrhage in the second half of pregnancy can be catastrophic for mother and fetus. To avoid untoward outcomes, the physician must respond quickly to ensure maternal cardiovascular stability, develop a differential diagnosis, and institute definitive therapy.

Initial maternal stabilization includes supplemental maternal oxygen and adequate venous access. Although crystalloid and colloid therapies provide initial volume expansion, neither improves oxygen-carrying capacity. Blood component therapy often is necessary for resuscitation. If cross-matched blood is unavailable, type-specific blood can be administered to a patient with a negative antibody screen. Clinical experience has shown that type-specific therapy carries approximately the same low risk of a major transfusion reaction as cross-matched blood. Platelets and fresh frozen plasma should be administered only with clinical or laboratory evidence of a coagulopathy (1).

Only after maternal stabilization should the physician focus on fetal well-being. Otherwise, a cesarean delivery may be performed for transient fetal jeopardy. In this case, not only is the fetus delivered unnecessarily, but maternal health is further jeopardized by surgery in the face of hemodynamic instability. Often, fetal status becomes reassuring after the maternal condition has improved.

Initial laboratory work includes blood type and cross-match, complete blood count, platelet count, prothrombin time, partial thromboplastin time, fibrinogen, and arterial blood gas. Metabolic acidosis often indicates shock and the need for aggressive fluid and blood replacement. To assess quickly whether the patient has a coagulopathy, a red-topped tube of blood should clot firmly within 7 minutes. If it does not, a coagulopathy should be suspected and a transfusion of platelets and fresh frozen plasma should be considered (1).

The 2 most common causes of significant bleeding in the second trimester are placental abruption and placenta previa. After initial assessment and before pelvic examination, the location of the placenta should be determined with ultrasonography. If the relationship between the placental edge and the internal cervical os cannot be defined transabdominally, gentle transvaginal ultrasonography may be used. The improved resolution of modern equipment has made the double set-up virtually obsolete when placenta previa is suspected. In contrast, visualization of a placental abruption is more difficult by ultrasonography because the acoustic characteristics of a fresh retroplacental clot often are indistinguishable from the placenta (2).

A careful history usually can differentiate previa from abruption. Placenta previa generally is associated with painless vaginal bleeding in the third trimester. Its overall incidence is 1 in 200 pregnancies and decreases with gestational age. Risk factors for placenta previa include prior uterine surgery, multiparity, and advanced maternal age. Although cesarean birth is the preferred mode of delivery, its timing depends on gestational age, amount of bleeding, maternal stability, and fetal well-being (3). If the bleeding stops and the fetus is premature, conservative management should be considered and may include outpatient management (2).

The physician should be particularly aware of the risk of placenta accreta in a patient who has had a cesarean delivery and now has an anterior placenta previa. This risk approaches 25% with 1 prior cesarean delivery and increases exponentially with the number of prior cesarean deliveries (4). Either ultrasonography or magnetic resonance imaging may be used antenatally to detect placenta accreta (5); however, both lack precision. When imaging studies firmly suggest placental invasion of the myometrium, the clinician should make different preparations for delivery; preoperative cross-matching for 4 units of packed red blood cells and the availability of additional surgical expertise are prudent. In cases where the patient does not wish to preserve fertility, an elective cesarean hysterectomy should be considered. In these circumstances, the fetus can be delivered through a transfundal uterine incision and the placenta left in situ. The uterine incision can then be closed or the edges clamped to control bleeding from the uterine incision while a hysterectomy is performed. This method may reduce blood loss and improve visualization compared with traditional cesarean delivery followed by hysterectomy, in which uncontrollable bleeding may be encountered while manually extracting the placenta.

Other reported techniques for controlling massive intraoperative hemorrhage associated with placenta previa complicated by accreta include aortic compression, a Penrose tourniquet at the uterocervical junction, and preoperative placement of intraarterial hypogastric balloons (6). Others have reported interrupted 2–3-cm circular sutures placed 1 cm apart on the serosal surface of the uterus, transvaginal pressure packing, and medical management with methotrexate chemotherapy (7). No large studies exist to support the efficacy, risk, or benefit of each approach, but the clinician may consider these options on a case-by-case basis.

Acute placental abruption usually has a more dramatic presentation that may include vaginal bleeding, a hypertonic uterus, maternal coagulopathy, fetal distress, or even fetal death. The magnitude of these signs and symptoms depends on the degree of placental separation. Some of the most dramatic presentations may be seen with a massive concealed abruption with very little vaginal bleeding. Recognized risk factors include maternal hypertension, prior abruption, cigarette smoking, abdominal trauma, and cocaine or amphetamine abuse (8). As with placenta previa, the timing of delivery depends on gestational age, volume of hemorrhage, maternal hemodynamic stability, degree of coagulopathy, and fetal well-being. In many cases, volume replacement, component blood product therapy, and treatment of any coagulopathy allow a vaginal delivery. A cesarean delivery should be reserved for traditional obstetric indications, such as labor dystocia and nonreassuring fetal status (3, 9).

In some cases, a pregnant woman presents with a small chronic abruption that stabilizes or bleeds intermittently. If the woman's pregnancy is remote from term and without evidence of coagulopathy or fetal jeopardy, tocolysis and betamethasone therapy may be considered. Magnesium sulfate is the tocolytic of choice in this situation because β-mimetics may mimic the cardiovascular effects of acute blood loss (9), and indomethacin may contribute to bleeding problems.

When confronted with bleeding in the second half of pregnancy, the clinician should always treat and stabilize the mother before directing attention to the fetus. A logical, chronological, and aggressive treatment algorithm usually results in a good outcome for mother and fetus.

References

1. Hippala S. Replacement of massive blood loss. Vox Sang 1998;74(suppl 2):399–407.

2. Baron F, Hill WC. Placenta previa, placenta abruptio. Clin Obstet Gynecol 1998;41:527–32.

3. Neilson JP. Interventions for suspected placenta praevia. The Cochrane Database of Systematic Reviews 2003, Issue 1. Art. No.: CD001998. DOI: 10.1002/14651858. CD001998.

4. Clark SL, Koonings PP, Phelan JP. Placenta previa/accreta and prior cesarean section. Obstet Gynecol 1985;66:89–92.

5. Levine D, Hulka CA, Ludmir J, Li W, Edelman RR. Placenta accreta: evaluation with color Doppler US, power Doppler US, and MR imaging. Radiology 1997;205:773–6.

6. Dubois J, Garel L, Grignon A, Lemay M, Leduc L. Placenta percreta: balloon occlusion and embolization of internal iliac arteries to reduce intraoperative blood losses. Am J Obstet Gynecol 1997;176:723–6.

7. Buckshee K, Dadhwal V. Medical management of placenta accreta. Int J Gynaecol Obstet 1997;59:47–8.

8. Zaki ZM, Bahar AM, Ali ME, Albar HA, Gerais MA. Risk factors and morbidity in patients with placenta previa accreta compared to placenta previa non-accreta. Acta Obstet Gynecol Scand 1998;77:391–4.

9. Hladky K, Yankowitz J, Hansen WF. Placental abruption. Obstet Gynecol Surv 2002;57:299–305.

MULTIPLE GESTATION

Epidemiology

According to the National Vital Statistics Reports for 2001, the twinning rate has increased 33% since 1990 and 59% since 1980 (1). Furthermore, triplets and high-order multiple gestations have increased more than 400% since 1980. Multiple pregnancy accounts for a disproportionate share of adverse obstetric and neonatal outcomes. In 2001, 1.6% of singletons, 11.8% of twins, 36.7% of triplets, 64.5% of quadruplets, and 78.6% of quintuplets were delivered prior to 32 completed weeks of gestation (1). Even more noteworthy, the incidence of extreme prematurity (delivery before 28 weeks of gestation) for both triplets and quadruplets may be as high as 14% (2).

Zygosity and Chorionicity

Multiple pregnancy presents increased risk for perinatal morbidity and mortality. Monochorionic twins, which are approximately 20% of all twin pregnancies, have a worse prognosis than their dichorionic counterparts (3). In patients at risk for multiple gestations (based on clinical examination, family history, and use of artificial reproductive technology), an early ultrasound examination to determine chorionicity and amnionicity may be offered. The effect of zygosity on outcomes is less clear. The out-come of dichorionic monozygotic pregnancies seems to be more similar to those of dizygotic pregnancies than to monochorionic pregnancies (4).

Zygosity refers to the genetic makeup of the pregnancy. Twins are either monozygotic or dizygotic, whereas high-order multiple gestations are monozygotic, dizygotic, or a combination of the two. Dizygotic pregnancies result from the fertilization of multiple ova. These fetuses have different genotypes and phenotypes. Monozygotic twins result from the division of 1 zygote arising from the fertilization of 1 ovum by 1 sperm. These offspring have similar genotypes and phenotypes. The incidence of dizygous twins is influenced by various factors, including race, ethnicity, maternal age, and use of assisted reproductive technology. In the past, it was taught that the rate of monozygous twinning was constant (1/250) (5). It is now known that assisted reproductive technology increases the incidence of monozygosity. The mechanism is currently unclear but may be secondary to trauma during the procedure or may be associated with increased gonadotropins (6, 7).

Chorionicity indicates the membrane composition of the pregnancy—the chorion and amnion. Although early determination of chorionicity is a primary objective in the management of multifetal pregnancies, extenuating circumstances, such as late diagnosis of a multiple gestation or inconclusive early ultrasound examination results, may make this goal unattainable. Optimal management of certain obstetric situations, such as discordant anatomic and genetic anomalies, requires knowledge of chorionicity. DNA zygosity studies on amniocytes have been used successfully to help with the management of complex cases requiring definitive diagnosis of chorionicity (8).

Complications

The risk for maternal complications and for perinatal morbidity and mortality increases in direct proportion to the number of fetuses in the gestation (Table 8). Multifetal pregnancies appear to be at increased risk for a number of conditions (Box 5).

PRETERM LABOR

Preterm labor and delivery is the most common complication of multiple pregnancy. Gestational age and fetal weight at the time of delivery may affect long-term out-

TABLE 8. Complications of Multiple Gestation

Complication	Twins	Triplets
Preterm delivery (<32 weeks)	12%	37%
Gestational hypertension	10–20%	25–60%
Acute fatty liver	17%	7%
Intrauterine fetal demise of 1 twin	0.5–7%	4–17%

BOX 5

Multifetal Pregnancy Risks

Multifetal pregnancies appear to be at increased risk of the following conditions:

- Acute fatty liver
- Anemia
- Abnormal placentation
- Amniotic fluid volume abnormalities
- Congenital malformation
- Preeclampsia
- Growth abnormalities
- Intrauterine fetal demise of 1 twin
- Operative vaginal delivery
- Premature rupture of membranes
- Preterm labor and delivery
- Postpartum hemorrhage
- Umbilical cord prolapse

comes. The prophylactic use of cerclage, bed rest, tocolytics, and home uterine activity monitoring has not been shown to prolong pregnancies (9, 10). Patient education regarding the signs and symptoms of preterm labor is important. Cervical surveillance may help predict preterm labor. A score based on digital examination (length minus internal os dilation in centimeters) has been suggested. When the score was greater than 0, preterm labor occurred in 3% of patients in the following week. When the score was less than 0, there was a 75% positive predictive value for preterm labor.

Ultrasound evaluation of cervical length and cervicovaginal assays for fetal fibronectin may help predict preterm labor. In twins, a cervical length of no more than 2.5 cm at 24 weeks of gestation was associated with a 6.9-fold increased risk of preterm delivery before 32 weeks of gestation. Of note, at 28 weeks of gestation, a cervical length of 2.5 cm or less was not associated with spontaneous preterm birth. At 28 and 30 weeks of gestation, a positive cervicovaginal fetal fibronectin assay was also significantly associated with preterm delivery before 32 weeks of gestation (odds ratio of 9.4 and 46.1 respectively). Patients whose fetal fibronectin test result was positive and whose cervix was 2.5 cm or less in length at either 24 or 28 weeks of gestation were at increased risk of preterm delivery before 32 weeks of gestation (11).

Twins discordant for fetal anatomic abnormalities also may be at increased risk for preterm labor and delivery (12). If preterm labor is diagnosed, aggressive tocolysis may be warranted to achieve antenatal corticosteroid benefit. It is important to remember that the physiologic

adaptations to multiple gestation may predispose these women to pulmonary edema when they are treated with these therapies (9, 10).

INTRAUTERINE GROWTH RESTRICTION AND DISCORDANT GROWTH

Serial ultrasonography is ideal for evaluating fetal growth in multiple pregnancies. Although twin and triplet growth curves exist, singleton fetal weight standards are commonly used to assess fetal growth in multiple gestations and are clinically acceptable. Until 30–32 weeks of gestation, when the abdominal circumference begins to lag, growth in twins is similar to that of singletons.

Intrauterine growth restriction seems to be more common in twins and high-order multiple gestations than in singletons. Although there is no concrete definition of IUGR in multiple gestations, it usually is diagnosed when the estimated fetal weight is less than the 10th percentile for singleton gestations or when there is discordance (difference in estimated fetal weight of greater than 20% or 25% between twin A and twin B divided by the larger twin's weight and expressed as a percentage). Once intrauterine growth discordance is diagnosed or IUGR is thought likely, serial ultrasonography (every 2–3 weeks) to check fetal growth is suggested. Antenatal testing is indicated, and early delivery may be considered (9).

FETAL WASTAGE

In patients with twin gestations scanned in the first trimester, rates of demise ranged from 13% to 78%. This phenomenon has been termed the *vanishing twin*.

During the second and third trimester, intrauterine fetal death of 1 fetus in a multiple gestation is uncommon, complicating approximately 2–5% of twin pregnancies. Studies have indicated single intrauterine fetal death rates up to 17% in triplet pregnancies (3). Intrauterine fetal death of 1 twin in the second and third trimesters can adversely affect the surviving fetus or fetuses in 2 ways: 1) risk for multicystic encephalomalacia and multiorgan damage in monochorionic pregnancies; and 2) preterm labor and delivery in both dichorionic and monochorionic twins, resulting in prematurity.

In the period immediately following fetal death, the surviving twin often develops hypotension of a degree that may cause fetal injury. It is thought that blood from the surviving twin may rapidly "back-bleed" into the dead twin through placental anastomosis (a capacitance effect). The shunting of blood from the surviving to the dead twin results in hypotension and hyperperfusion in the live twin. The dead twin may become congested while the surviving twin may become anemic. If the hypotension is grave, the surviving twin is at risk for ischemic damage to vital organs. As a result, immediate delivery of the co-twin following single intrauterine fetal death in a monochorionic pregnancy does not improve outcomes but can increase risk due to prematurity. Normal fetal heart rate patterns and biophysical profile scores should be used to monitor the surviving twin. If tests are not reassuring, delivery should be performed. Even if the results are reassuring, multicystic encephalomalacia cannot be ruled out. Normal fetal magnetic resonance imaging results may be reassuring, but the technique is still investigational (13). In addition to multiorgan ischemic damage in monochorionic pregnancies, studies have demonstrated that intrauterine fetal death of one twin can result in preterm delivery.

It has been established that retention of a dead fetus for 4–5 weeks in a singleton pregnancy results in an increased risk of maternal consumptive coagulopathy (3). Patients with a multiple gestation complicated by intrauterine fetal death also seem to be at a 25% risk of coagulation disorder. Disseminated intravascular coagulation following intrauterine fetal death of one twin in a multiple gestation also has been reported. Other studies have suggested that women with intrauterine fetal death in a multiple gestation are not at the same risk as women with singleton gestations. Transient fibrin-split products and hypofibrinogenemia have been reported; medical therapy was not required. Because there have been few cases of maternal coagulopathy in patients with single intrauterine fetal death in multiple gestation, the 25% risk seems to represent an overestimation (3). Cases of clinically significant coagulopathy have not been reported in multifetal pregnancy reduction and selective reduction (14).

When intrauterine fetal death occurs in a multiple pregnancy, baseline maternal hematologic laboratory tests, including a preoperative prothrombin, partial thromboplastin, fibrinogen level, and platelet count, are suggested. If these values are within normal limits, further surveillance is not indicated. Of note, mothers with intrauterine fetal death in one twin do not appear to be at increased risk of infection due to a retained twin. Dystocia secondary to the demised fetus has been reported infrequently. Cesarean delivery rates seem to be increased in patients with single intrauterine fetal death because of nonreassuring fetal status.

PROBLEMS SPECIFIC TO MONOCHORIONIC TWINS

The general obstetrician–gynecologist rarely encounters monochorionic twins complicated by the twin–twin transfusion syndrome, monoamnionicity, conjoined twins, and acardia. Consultation with an obstetrician–gynecologist with expertise in the management of high-risk pregnancies, such as a maternal–fetal medicine specialist, is advised (9).

Twin–Twin Transfusion Syndrome

Twin–twin transfusion syndrome is a complication of monochorionic pregnancies characterized by an imbalance in the blood flow across the shared placenta of 2 fetuses. Although all monochorionic twins share a por-

tion of their vasculature, approximately 15% will develop twin–twin transfusion syndrome. The syndrome can become manifest at any gestational age. Earlier onset often is associated with poor prognosis.

Twin–twin transfusion syndrome can be chronic or acute. In chronic cases, the transfer of blood occurs little by little throughout the entire pregnancy. The net effect of this blood flow imbalance is a large, hyperperfused, recipient twin and a small, hypoperfused, anemic donor twin. (See also "Fetal Therapy.")

Monoamnionicity

Monoamniotic twins are a rare form of monozygous twins where both fetuses occupy the same amniotic sac. Less than 1% of monozygotic twins are monoamniotic (3). The diagnosis is made using ultrasonography. An amniotic membrane is not visualized in a same-sex pregnancy with 1 placental mass. The diagnosis of mono-amniotic twins can be confirmed by cord entanglement.

Monoamniotic twins have been associated with a high rate of perinatal mortality. Past studies have indicated a fetal mortality rate greater than 50%. More recent studies indicate a perinatal mortality rate ranging from 10% to 21% (15, 16). Preterm delivery, growth restriction, congenital anomalies, cord entanglement, and cord accidents are common in monochorionic pregnancies.

The management of these pregnancies is controversial, particularly regarding the optimal protocol for antenatal surveillance and the optimal timing for delivery. Intrauterine fetal demise can occur at any gestational age. With this in mind, some experts suggest early delivery (17). Other investigators have suggested that early delivery is not prudent secondary to the risks of prematurity (18).

Because of the unpredictability of acute cord compression, the optimal frequency of antenatal testing is controversial. The nonstress test has the ability to show cord compression.

Twin Reversed Arterial Perfusion Syndrome

Twin reversed arterial perfusion syndrome (TRAP), also known as acardia, is defined by the absence of a normally functioning heart in 1 fetus of a multiple pregnancy. The incidence is estimated to be 1% among monozygotic twins. The true incidence is unknown because many cases of TRAP may result in early pregnancy loss. The normal fetus perfuses the acardiac twin by an umbilical artery to umbilical artery anatomosis at the placental surface. Blood flow in the umbilical artery of the recipient twin is reversed, and deoxygenated blood is brought from the pump twin to the acardiac twin. As a result, there is a normal twin and an amorphous twin. A range of anomalies can be seen in the acardiac twin, including anencephaly, absent limbs, intestinal atresia, abdominal wall defects, and absent organs. Because of the increased cardiac workload, the normal twin can develop heart failure.

The diagnosis is made by ultrasonography, and the differential diagnosis of acardia includes intrauterine fetal death or anencephaly in one twin. The etiology is thought to be the development of arterial-to-arterial vascular anastomoses between the umbilical arteries of twins in early embryogenesis. Approximately 75% of cases are monochorionic diamniotic gestations, and 25% of cases are monochorionic monoamniotic. The pump twin generally is morphologically normal, but approximately 9% have trisomy. Of acardiac twins, 33% have an abnormal karyotype, including monosomy, trisomy, deletions, mosaicism, and polyploidy.

The goal of management is to maximize the outcome of the normal twin. Poor prognosis has been associated with polyhydramnios and congestive heart failure in the pump twin. Prognosis for the pump twin depends on the ratio of the weight of the perfused twin to the weight of the pump twin. The normal biometric measurements cannot be used to measure the acardiac twin. As a result, a second-order regression equation has been devised: weight in grams = $[-1.66 \times \text{length}] + [1.21 \times \text{length}^2]$. When the twin weight ratio is greater than 0.70, there is a 30% risk of congestive heart failure for the pump twin.

In the absence of poor prognostic indicators (congestive heart failure, polyhydramnios, and a twin weight ratio of less than 0.70), expectant management with serial ultrasonography is suggested. Administration of steroids is advised if delivery is anticipated between 24 and 34 weeks, and tocolysis is suggested to stop preterm labor to optimize the outcome of the pump twin.

Medical management with indomethacin and digoxin have been reported (14). More invasive management has included hysterotomy of the acardiac twin followed by interval delivery of the pump twin. Percutaneous interruption of the circulation in the acardiac twin also has been described. Procedures have included insertion of a thrombogenic coil into the recipient twin's umbilical cord, endoscopic ligation of the cord, injection of silk soaked in alcohol into the cord, injection of absolute alcohol into the cord, and radioablation (14, 19). These methods usually are reserved for cases where the pump twin has already developed cardiac failure at a previable age.

Management

The management of multiple pregnancy includes adequate nutrition, avoidance of strenuous physical activity, and frequent prenatal visits. Patients should be counseled regarding the increased risk of complications associated with multiple pregnancy. It currently is recommended that women with multifetal pregnancies increase their daily caloric intake to approximately 300 kcal more than women with singleton pregnancies. Iron and folic acid supplements also are recommended. Women with normal BMI who are pregnant with twins should gain between 35 and 45 pounds.

Genetic screening in multiple gestations is different from that used in singleton gestations because multiple gestations have higher levels of serum analytes. Maternal serum alpha-fetoprotein levels can be corrected and used for NTD screening in twins. Alpha-fetoprotein screening for high-order multiple gestations and serum screening for Down syndrome in high-order multiple gestations has not been validated. At this point, nuchal translucency screening for Down syndrome remains investigational, although preliminary reports are encouraging.

Because of the greater number of fetuses, multiple gestations have a higher risk for aneuploidy than singleton gestations. As a result, invasive genetic testing should be considered at earlier maternal ages. A 35-year-old woman with a singleton gestation has the same risk for aneuploidy as a 33-year-old woman with twins and a 31-year-old woman with triplets (20). Amniocentesis is an appropriate option for women carrying multiple gestations. Chorionic villus sampling of 2 or more fetuses also is suitable in experienced hands, and there is low risk for cross-contamination. Monozygotic fetuses can be discordant for both genetic and anatomic abnormalities.

Routine antepartum surveillance of uncomplicated multifetal pregnancies has not been shown to be of benefit. Fetal testing is suggested in complicated twin pregnancies, such as those with growth abnormalities, abnormal fluid volumes, fetal anomalies, monoamnionicity, and other pregnancy complications. Antenatal surveillance includes the nonstress test or the standard or modified biophysical profile. Doppler studies may be indicated for growth restriction or for the twin–twin transfusion syndrome (9).

Route of delivery in multiple gestations depends on fetal presentation in labor and provider experience. Time interval between deliveries of the twins is not important, provided that reassuring fetal status is evident by continuous fetal heart rate monitoring or by ultrasonography. If the presenting twin is nonvertex, cesarean delivery is suggested. If the first twin is vertex, vaginal delivery can be anticipated. Cesarean delivery may be the preferred route of delivery if there is significant growth discordance between the twins or if the provider does not have adequate experience with such deliveries. Some obstetricians have had favorable experiences delivering triplets vaginally. Nonetheless, most providers deliver triplets and high-order multiple gestations by cesarean birth because continuous fetal heart rate monitoring of triplets and high-order multiple gestations in labor is challenging (9, 10).

Neurologic Outcome

An association between multiple pregnancy and cerebral palsy has been established for more than a century. In 1897, Sigmund Freud suggested that multiple birth was a greater cause of spastic diplegia than asphyxia. Studies on the etiology of cerebral palsy have substantiated Freud's report and have demonstrated that the prevalence of cerebral palsy in multiple gestations ranges from 5.4% to 10.8%. Although many of these studies were not of the highest scientific quality, the fact that they all came to the same conclusion supports the association between multiple birth and cerebral palsy (9, 21).

Epidemiologic studies on the prevalence of cerebral palsy in multiple gestations and studies on multiple pregnancies complicated by cerebral palsy have been conducted. In these reports, the prevalence of cerebral palsy ranges from 6.7 to 12.6 per 1,000 surviving infants. The variation in reports is derived from the population studied and methods of identification, in addition to potential regional differences, medical care variations, and population ascertainment bias. Only 1 study included a control group of twins. Low birth weight, first-born birth order, and monochorionicity were more common in twins with cerebral palsy than in twins without the condition. Another group of investigators reported that the risk of producing 1 child with cerebral palsy in twin, triplet, and quadruplet gestations was 15 per 1,000 twins, 80 per 1,000 triplets, and 429 per 1,000 quadruplets (22).

Multifetal Pregnancy Reduction

Ovulation induction and assisted reproductive technology have been associated with increasing numbers of high-order multiple gestations. The purpose of first-trimester multifetal pregnancy reduction is to improve perinatal outcomes by decreasing maternal complications secondary to multiple gestations and by decreasing adverse fetal outcomes associated with preterm delivery. Reducing high-order multiple gestations to twins reduces the risk of preterm labor and delivery and increases birth weight and gestational age at delivery (10). In some cases, such as a history of a previous second-trimester loss, reduction from a twin gestation to a singleton gestation may be indicated.

Nonetheless, multifetal reduction is an ethical dilemma (23, 24). The starting number of fetuses needed to justify the procedure is controversial. Studies have been conflicting regarding whether or not multifetal reduction from triplets to twins results in better perinatal outcomes than expectant management (25–27). In addition, although most women do not regret their decision, women undergoing multifetal pregnancy reduction may have feelings of loss, guilt, and sadness.

The procedure most commonly is performed transabdominally under ultrasound guidance between 10 and 13 weeks of gestation. A dizygotic gestation is confirmed by ultrasonography. Potassium chloride is injected into the fetal heart until asystole is achieved. If chorionic villus sampling is performed before the procedure and one fetus is found to have a genetic anomaly, that fetus is targeted for selective termination. Otherwise, the fetus with a smaller crown–rump length than expected for gestational age or the easiest-to-reduce fetus is chosen. The fetus over the cervix usually is avoided.

This procedure is reserved for dichorionic pregnancies. The acute death of one twin in a monozygotic gestation can produce acute hemodynamic changes in the surviving fetus with devastating neurologic sequelae. In monochorionic pregnancies, selectively reducing 1 fetus using intracardiac potassium chloride is contraindicated because of the presence of communicating placental anastomoses.

Several studies document pregnancy loss rates associated with multifetal pregnancy reduction. With extensive experience, the current loss rate is approximately 6% (28). There is little maternal risk associated with the procedure. The terminated fetus usually is resorbed or becomes a small papyraceous fetus. There have been no reports of coagulation disorders following this procedure. Maternal serum alpha-fetoprotein is always elevated following this procedure and cannot be used as a screening tool in these pregnancies.

Selective Reduction

Patients with diagnosed discordant anomalies may choose selective reduction. Most selective reductions have been performed in twins, but they also have been undertaken in high-order multiple gestations. In dichorionic pregnancies, ultrasound-guided intracardiac injection of potassium chloride is used.

A recent study reported favorable outcomes on selective reduction in 200 cases, including 164 cases of twins, 32 cases of triplets, and 4 cases of quadruplets. The average gestational age at the time of the procedure was 19 2/7 weeks with a range of 12 0/7 to 23 6/7 weeks. Selective reduction procedures generally are performed later in gestation than multifetal reduction because the anomaly often is undetected until the second trimester. Indications for selective reduction included genetic abnormalities, structural abnormalities, placental insufficiency, and cervical incompetence. The unintended pregnancy loss rate was 4%. The average gestational age at delivery was 36 1/7 weeks of gestation. Approximately 84% of these women gave birth after 32 weeks of gestation. The investigators concluded that selective fetal reduction for an abnormal pregnancy is safe when performed by experienced practitioners (29).

If selective fetal reduction is desired in a monochorionic pregnancy, complete ablation of the umbilical cord of the anomalous fetus is recommended to avoid multiorgan morbidity in the remaining normal fetus. Techniques used have included ultrasound-guided coagulation of the umbilical cord using bipolar cautery, fetoscopic cord ligation, fetoscopic laser ablation of umbilical vessels, percutaneous injection of alcohol or occlusive materials into the umbilical cord or into the umbilical vein, and radioablation (30–32). Preterm rupture of membranes complicates approximately 20% of these cases. Maternal coagulopathy secondary to fetal demise with either technique has not been reported.

Multiple Pregnancy and Postterm Pregnancy

Current ACOG recommendations suggest that uncomplicated twins be delivered by 40 weeks of gestation (9). When managing patients with multiple gestations, there is a temptation to be reassured by increasing gestational age in the third trimester as the potential complications of prematurity recede. Recent studies, however, suggest that multiple pregnancies may benefit from delivery before 40 weeks of gestation (33, 34). The underlying theory is that uteroplacental insufficiency in multiple pregnancies at advanced gestational ages may place the fetuses at risk for intrauterine fetal death (34). Several studies have focused on "the prospective risk of fetal death" to help determine by which gestational age a multiple pregnancy should be delivered (33, 34). With this statistic, the fetal death rate is calculated from the number of fetal deaths occurring at a particular gestational age divided by the number of fetuses at risk (all fetuses in all ongoing pregnancies). A more accurate impression for risk of intrauterine fetal death can be obtained with this statistic than the classic definition of fetal death rate (number of fetal deaths at a particular gestational age divided by the number of live births and fetal deaths during the same period).

For twins, the prospective risk of fetal death appears to be equivalent to that of postterm singletons at approximately 36–37 weeks of gestation. Delivering these pregnancies at such a gestational age could lead to complications secondary to prematurity. As a result, gestational-age-specific prospective risk of fetal death must be taken into context with gestational-specific neonatal death rates. If the rate of neonatal death at a given gestational age is less than that of prospective risk of fetal death if the pregnancy continues, then delivery should be considered. The prospective risk of fetal death for twins intersects with the neonatal death rate at approximately 39 weeks of gestation, indicating that it may be reasonable to consider delivery of uncomplicated twins at 39 weeks of gestation rather than at 40 weeks of gestation.

References

1. Martin JA, Hamilton BE, Ventura SJ, Menacker F, Park MM, Sutton PD. Births: final data for 2001. Natl Vital Stat Rep 2002;51:1–102.

2. Devine PC, Malone FD, Athanassiou A, Harvey-Wilkes K, D'Alton ME. Maternal and neonatal outcome of 100 consecutive triplet pregnancies. Am J Perinatol 2001;18: 225–35.

3. D'Alton ME, Simpson LL. Syndromes in twins. Semin Perinatol 1995;19:375–86.

4. Dube J, Dodds L, Armson BA. Does chorionicity or zygosity predict adverse perinatal outcomes in twins? Am J Obstet Gynecol 2002;186: 579–83.

5. Benirschke K. The biology of the twinning process: how placentation influences outcome. Semin Perinatol 1995;19: 342–50.

6. Chow JS, Benson CB, Racowsky C, Doubilet PM, Ginsburg E. Frequency of a monochorionic pair in multiple gestations: relationship to mode of conception. J Ultrasound Med 2001;20:757–60; quiz 761.

7. Schachter M, Raziel A, Friedler S, Strassburger D, Bern O, Ron-El R. Monozygotic twinning after assisted reproductive techniques: a phenomenon independent of micromanipulation. Hum Reprod 2001;16:1264–9.

8. Norton ME, D'Alton ME, Bianchi DW. Molecular zygosity studies aid in the management of discordant multiple gestations. J Perinatol 1997;17:202–7.

9. Multiple gestation: complicated twin, triplet, and higher-order multifetal pregnancy. ACOG Practice Bulletin No. 56. American College of Obstetricians and Gynecologists. Obstet Gynecol 2004;104:869–83.

10. American Academy of Pediatrics, American College of Obstetricians and Gynecologists. Guidelines for perinatal care. 5th ed. Elk Grove Village (IL): AAP; Washington, DC: ACOG; 2002.

11. Goldenberg RL, Iams JD, Miodovnik M, vanDorsten JP, Thurnau G, Bottoms S, et al. The preterm prediction study: risk factors in twin gestations. National Institute of Child Health and Human Development Maternal-Fetal Medicine Units Network: Am J Obstet Gynecol 1996;175: 1047–53.

12. Malone FD, Craigo SD, Chelmow D, D'Alton ME. Outcome of twin gestations complicated by a single anomalous fetus. Obstet Gynecol 1996;88:1–5.

13. Weiss JL, Cleary-Goldman J, Tanji K, Budorick N, D'Alton ME. Multicystic encephalomalacia after first-trimester intrauterine fetal death in monochorionic twins. Am J Obstet Gynecol 2004;190:563–5.

14. Malone FD, D'Alton ME. Anomalies peculiar to multiple gestations. Clin Perinatol 2000;27:1033–46, x.

15. Rodis JF, McIlveen PF, Egan JF, Borgida AF, Turner JW, Campbell WA. Monoamniotic twins: improved perinatal survival with accurate prenatal diagnosis and antenatal fetal surveillance. Am J Obstet Gynecol 1997;177: 1046–9.

16. Allen VM, Windrim R, Barrett J, Ohlsson A. Management of monoamniotic twin pregnancies: a case series and systematic review of the literature. BJOG 2001;108:931–6.

17. House M, Harney K, D'Alton ME, Chelmow D, Craigo S. Intensive management of monoamniotic twin pregnancies improves perinatal outcome [abstract]. Am J Obstet Gynecol 2001;185:S113.

18. Tessen JA, Zlatnik FJ. Monoamniotic twins: a retrospective controlled study. Obstet Gynecol 1991;77:832–4.

19. Tsao K, Feldstein VA, Albanese CT, Sandberg PL, Lee H, Harrison MR, et al. Selective reduction of acardiac twin by radiofrequency ablation. Am J Obstet Gynecol 2002;187: 635–40.

20. American College of Obstetricians and Gynecologists. Prenatal diagnosis of fetal chromosomal abnormalities. ACOG Practice Bulletin No. 27. Washington, DC: ACOG; 2001.

21. American College of Obstetricians and Gynecologists, American Academy of Pediatrics. Neonatal encephalopathy and cerebral palsy: defining the pathogenesis and pathophysiology. Washington, DC: ACOG; 2003.

22. Yokoyama Y, Shimizu T, Hayakawa K. Prevalence of cerebral palsy in twins, triplets and quadruplets. Int J Epidemiol 1995;24:943–8.

23. Berkowitz RL, Lynch L, Stone J, Alvarez M. The current status of multifetal pregnancy reduction. Am J Obstet Gynecol 1996;174:1265–72.

24. Berkowitz RL. Ethical issues involving multifetal pregnancies. Mt Sinai J Med 1998;65:185–90; discussion, 215–23.

25. Boulot P, Vignal J, Vergnes C, Dechaud H, Faure JM, Hedon B. Multifetal reduction of triplets to twins: a prospective comparison of pregnancy outcome. Hum Reprod 2000;15:1619–23.

26. Leondires MP, Ernst SD, Miller BT, Scott RT Jr. Triplets: outcomes of expectant management versus multifetal reduction for 127 pregnancies. Am J Obstet Gynecol 2000; 183:454–9.

27. Yaron Y, Bryant-Greenwood PK, Dave N, Moldenhauer JS, Kramer RL, Johnson MP, et al. Multifetal pregnancy reductions of triplets to twins: comparison with nonreduced triplets and twins. Am J Obstet Gynecol 1999;180:1268–71.

28. Stone J, Eddleman K, Lynch L, Berkowitz RL. A single center experience with 1000 consecutive cases of multifetal pregnancy reduction. Am J Obstet Gynecol 2002;187: 1163–7.

29. Eddleman K, Stone JL, Lynch L, Berkowitz RL. Selective termination of anomalous fetuses in multifetal pregnancies: two hundred cases at a single center. Am J Obstet Gynecol 2002;187:1168–72.

30. Nicolini U, Poblete A, Boschetto C, Bonati F, Roberts A. Complicated monochorionic twin pregnancies: experience with bipolar cord coagulation. Am J Obstet Gynecol 2001;185:703–7.

31. Challis D, Gratacos E, Deprest JA. Cord occlusion techniques for selective termination in monochorionic twins. J Perinat Med 1999;27:327–38.

32. Sydorak RM, Feldstein V, Machin G, Tsao K, Hirose S, Lee H, et al. Fetoscopic treatment for discordant twins. J Pediatr Surg 2002;37:1736–9.

33. Sairam S, Costeloe K, Thilaganathan B. Prospective risk of stillbirth in multiple-gestation pregnancies: a population-based analysis. Obstet Gynecol 2002;100:638–41.

34. Kahn B, Lumey LH, Zybert PA, Lorenz JM, Cleary-Goldman J, D'Alton ME, et al. Prospective risk of fetal death in singleton, twin, and triplet gestations: implications for practice. Obstet Gynecol 2003;102:685–92.

INTRAUTERINE GROWTH RESTRICTION

A small-for-gestational-age (SGA) fetus is one whose biometric measurements or estimated weight is below a chosen threshold at a given gestational age. The threshold usually is arbitrarily chosen as 10th percentile, 5th percentile –2 SD, and the like, but its actual value also will depend on the population from which it was derived. Although such norms are easy to obtain and apply clinically, many such defined SGA fetuses will be constitutionally small and otherwise normal. Growth will be restricted in only a small proportion (approximately 20%). Intrauterine growth restriction refers, therefore, to those fetuses whose growth is truly impaired, preventing them from achieving their individual growth potential. This group of fetuses is significantly more difficult to identify, but it is also the group whose pathologic processes underlying growth impairment contribute to adverse outcomes of pregnancy.

There is an overlap between SGA and IUGR fetuses (Fig. 14). Of SGA fetuses defined as birth weight below the 10th percentile, 30–70% are thought to have IUGR (1). This proportion is estimated to increase with lower cutoffs for SGA. This seems to be further supported by increasing perinatal mortality with declining percentile of birth weight. However, a fetus with IUGR may not be SGA; its growth might be severely impaired but still above a chosen cutoff.

The accurate identification of IUGR is critical because the condition poses significant risk to the fetus, not only in utero but also after delivery, and the consequences seem to imprint themselves on the life span of the individual. Fetuses that are small for gestational age and specifically, those with IUGR are at increased risk of stillbirth (odds ratio [OR], 6.1, 95% confidence interval [CI], 5.0–7.5), neonatal death (OR, 4.1, 95% CI, 2.4–4.8) (1), and neonatal encephalopathy (OR, 4.37, 95% CI, 1.4–13.4) (2), as well as birth hypoxia, neonatal morbidity (3), cerebral palsy, impaired neurodevelopment (4), cognitive function (IQ) (5), and possibly type 2 (nonin-

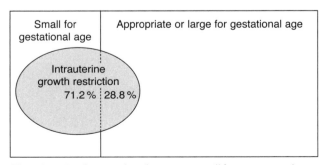

■ **FIG. 14.** The overlap between small-for-gestational-age (SGA) fetuses and fetuses with intrauterine growth restriction (IUGR).

sulin dependent) diabetes, hypertension, and coronary artery disease in adult life (6).

Accumulating evidence strongly indicates that at least a portion of IUGR originates in the first months of preg-

---

BOX 6

Factors Associated With Intrauterine Growth Restriction

Maternal

Smoking

Low prepregnancy weight

Poor weight gain

Malnutrition (<1,500 kcal/d)

Age <16 or >35 years

Diabetes

Chronic renal disease

Systemic lupus erythematosus

Cyanotic heart disease

Sickle cell anemia

Antiphospholipid syndrome

Chronic hypertension

Preeclampsia

Hypercoagulable states (controversial)

Medications

Antiseizure

Corticosteroids

Folic acid antagonists (methotrexate)

Warfarin

Low maternal socioeconomic status

Fetal

Multiple gestation

Anomalies

Chromosomal

Structural

Infections

Viral—cytomegalovirus

Protozoal—toxoplasmosis

Spirochetal—syphilis

Previous intrauterine growth restriction

Placental

Abruption

Previa

Confined placental mosaicism

---

nancy. This has been well recognized for a subset of fetuses with IUGR that have chromosomal abnormalities and some congenital malformations. However, recent studies demonstrate that even normally formed fetuses with IUGR are already smaller than their normally growing counterparts during the first trimester (7). In the first trimester, these IUGR pregnancies produce decreased amounts of placental proteins implicated in fetal growth (8). The multiple risk factors for IUGR (Box 6), together with the early onset of growth impairment in pregnancy, make IUGR a clinical problem that is difficult both to diagnose and to manage.

Diagnosis

The diagnosis of SGA and IUGR, as with other disorders, relies on the principles of Bayes' theorem. The chance of the disease increases with positive results of tests performed. The size of this increase in probability depends on how good the test is in detecting the disease. Physicians are intuitively proficient in combining these probabilities. It is not necessary for clinical purposes to conduct calculations of the probabilities before making a diagnosis and a clinical decision. However, it is useful to appreciate the magnitude to which the test we apply increases the probability of the disease. The Bayesian approach uses for this purpose the likelihood ratio (LR): the sensitivity of the test divided by its reciprocal of specificity or a false-positive rate. It is a useful value because a single number expresses the validity of the test represented by its sensitivity and specificity. It also helps to estimate the posttest odds of the disease by simply multiplying the pretest odds, derived from the prevalence of the disease in the population, by the likelihood ratio of a given test.

As a result, multiple tests employed to detect SGA or IUGR will diagnose it with higher probability than each of the tests applied alone. The size of this increase in the probability of the disease theoretically could be a result of multiplication of all LRs of tests performed. Practically, however, the tests are frequently correlated and not independent, thereby decreasing the final accuracy of detecting this disease.

Also, repeating the same test over time (to demonstrate a trend in growth) will provide additional information that translates into separate LRs, which will further refine (increase or decrease) the probability of a disease. As a result, a trend has more predictive value than a single measurement.

Methods employed to diagnose SGA and IUGR evaluate either biometric measurements of the fetus or biophysical parameters of fetal well-being. The first include abdominal palpation, fundal height measurement, and ultrasound biometry. Biophysical parameters include amniotic fluid volume estimates and uterine artery Doppler impedance.

Both types of tests crucially depend on an accurate estimate of gestational age. This dependence always has to be considered in interpreting the results of these tests and, consequently, in clinical decision making.

ABDOMINAL PALPATION

Abdominal palpation is of limited value in detecting a fetus that is SGA or has IUGR. Sensitivity to detect an SGA fetus is only 44–50%. Palpation is, however, a part of the routine examination, and the cost and effort required are minimal. When a small fetus is suspected during abdominal palpation, further evaluation is indicated.

FUNDAL HEIGHT

Similarly, fundal height measurement is a part of a routine prenatal examination requiring only minimal effort and costs. The diagnostic accuracy of fundal height measurement also is limited, translating to an LR of approximately 2.3. Serial fundal height measurements perform better (LR = 3.6). The value of fundal height measurement in improving perinatal mortality is unclear. A single study to investigate this relationship demonstrated no significant improvement (9). The limited accuracy of fundal height measurement should be kept in mind when interpreting its results.

However, the accuracy of fundal height measurement can be improved by appropriate measuring technique, demonstration of a trend in serial measurements, and use of customized norms. Correct measuring technique relies on measurement from the fundus to the symphysis pubis (from a changing to a fixed point) with the distance marks hidden from the examiner.

Customized fundal height norms define an individual growth trajectory for each fetus based on physiologic variables that are known to determine fetal birth weight. These variables include maternal weight, height, parity, ethnicity, fetal sex, and gestational age. Because they are different for each fetus, they determine an individual optimal growth curve for each fetus.

In one study, the use of customized charts improved sensitivity in detecting SGA at birth from 29% to 48% (10, 11). Although specificities were not calculated in this study due to its design, they were likely similar or better when customized norms were used. This assumption is based on a reduction in hospital admissions and ultrasound examinations (corresponding to a false-positive rate) with the use of a customized fundal height norm.

ULTRASOUND BIOMETRY

Abdominal circumference and estimated fetal weight are the 2 most accurate ultrasound biometrical parameters for prediction of SGA fetuses at birth. The 10th percentile appears to be the best cutoff for both parameters in this respect. Published LRs for abdominal circumfer-

ences less than the 10th percentile range from 1.9 to 4.5; estimated fetal weight less than the 10th percentile has a median LR of 2.8. Various formulae to calculate estimated fetal weight are used. Most demonstrate high validity and the tendency to underestimate the actual birth weight (12). Among the formulae, the equation by Hadlock was reported to perform especially well in small fetuses (12, 13). It appears that similar to fundal height measurements, the performance of ultrasound biometry can be improved by serial examinations to demonstrate growth velocity and by individualization of the norms.

Serial measurements of abdominal circumference and estimated fetal weight better predict impairment of fetal growth than a single measurement. They are more accurate in prediction of IUGR identified postnatally as an abnormal: ponderal index, subscapular skinfold thickness, or mid-arm circumference. Decreased estimated fetal weight growth rate additionally correlates with adverse pregnancy outcomes, including perinatal mortality (14). A decline in abdominal circumference and estimated fetal weight predict IUGR (abnormal ponderal index) with an LR of 2.1 and 3.9, respectively. Conversely, head circumference to abdominal circumference ratios (HC/AC), frequently found in standard ultrasound examination reports, perform worse than abdominal circumference or estimated fetal weight alone in predicting an SGA fetus or IUGR.

The use of individualized birth weight norms, based on physiologic determinants, results in better prediction of adverse pregnancy outcomes than traditional population norms. This also appears to be true for antenatal ultrasound assessment of fetal growth. Such norms used prenatally result in better identification of SGA fetuses (LR = 4.0–6.2). This is a result of both better sensitivity and a lower false-positive rate (15, 16). The optimal cutoff for individualized norms appears to be the 8th percentile for identification of SGA fetuses and adverse outcomes of pregnancy (15). These norms, although not available yet for the U.S. population, have been reported to be superior to national population birth weight norms in prediction of adverse pregnancy outcomes.

A systematic review and meta-analysis published by the Cochrane Database of Systematic Reviews demonstrated that the use of routine ultrasound examinations after 24 weeks of gestation in a low-risk population is not associated with improvement of perinatal mortality. This might reflect a true lack of benefit, as well as a high false-positive rate of the population norms used in those studies, especially in low-risk pregnancies (17).

Biophysical tests do not appear to be good predictors of SGA fetuses or even growth restriction. This is most likely a consequence of their reflection of fetal well-being independent of fetal growth. The 2 parameters most likely to be associated with impaired fetal growth are low amniotic fluid index and Doppler impedance in umbilical and uterine arteries; they demonstrate moderately predictive accuracy. Low amniotic fluid index has an LR of 1.2 in predicting an abnormal ponderal index at birth (18). A meta-analysis of uterine artery Doppler studies has shown its modest predictive accuracy of SGA fetuses at birth, with an LR of 3.6 in the low-risk population and 2.7 in the high-risk population (19).

Management

A significant proportion, up to 19%, of SGA fetuses have chromosomal abnormalities. These pregnancies frequently are associated with structural malformations, normal or increased amount of amniotic fluid, and normal umbilical artery Doppler impedance. In a large study of pregnancies with SGA fetuses, ultrasound examination demonstrated structural malformations in 96% of the chromosomally abnormal SGA fetuses (20). The LR of a chromosomally abnormal fetus in the presence of structural malformation on ultrasound examination is approximately 9.1. Likelihood ratios for structural anomalies and markers of chromosomal abnormalities in the general population also have been published (20). The finding of normal or an increased amount of amniotic fluid in an SGA fetus increases the likelihood of chromosomal abnormalities almost 3 times (LR = 2.7), whereas the presence of end diastolic flow in the umbilical artery increases the likelihood by 60% (LR = 1.6). Therefore, targeted ultrasound examination with evaluation of amniotic fluid volume and umbilical artery Doppler impedance should constitute the initial step in evaluating a fetus that is small for gestational age.

Umbilical artery Doppler impedance is well suited to be a pivotal test in the management of the SGA fetus. It is the only fetal surveillance method that, when used in a high-risk population, is associated with a trend toward improvement of perinatal mortality. Umbilical artery Doppler is the only test that can predict neonatal morbidity in SGA fetuses. It is superior in this respect to fetal heart rate variability and biophysical profile (21).

Because intervention in fetuses with positive test results will lead to further testing and, frequently, preterm delivery, it is important that abnormal umbilical artery impedance have a low false-positive rate. Therefore, it is reassuring that absent end-diastolic flow is rare (only 2.7%) in SGA fetuses. Additionally, the use of umbilical artery Doppler in SGA pregnancies reduces false-positive results, which decreases the rate of hospital admissions, labor inductions, and cesarean delivery for fetal distress (22). It also has few false-negative results. A persistently abnormal biophysical profile is reported to always be associated with the absence of diastolic flow. Although absent and reversed end-diastolic flow are associated with significant risk of stillbirth (14% and 24%, respectively) and neonatal death (27% and 51%, respectively), the time interval from identification of abnormal umbili-

cal artery impedance to onset of abnormalities of fetal heart rate or biophysical profile varies from 2 to 25 days (23). Therefore, after identification of the absent end-diastolic flow, the decision to deliver must be based on other modes of fetal surveillance.

Fetal heart rate monitoring and biophysical profile are the 2 methods most commonly applied in this capacity, although fetal venous Doppler examination shows promise in this respect. The benefit of umbilical artery impedance testing lies mainly in identification of a high-risk group of SGA fetuses that will require intensive surveillance. Women with fetuses with normal end-diastolic flow can be managed safely on an outpatient basis (24). These patients also can be monitored adequately with testing performed less frequently (25). Abnormal umbilical artery Doppler studies reflect earlier onset and more severe growth restriction (26).

Although there are very limited data on the management of these pregnancies, it appears that these women can be managed as outpatients with frequent fetal surveillance. Conversely, patients with absent or reversed end-diastolic flow of the umbilical artery (Fig. 15) require hospitalization and daily fetal monitoring. The recommendation for daily fetal surveillance is based on the reported short period within which fetal heart rate and biophysical profile become abnormal in those patients (27).

The effects of both nonstress tests and biophysical profiles on reduction of perinatal mortality in a high-risk population have been evaluated by meta-analyses of interventional trials. Neither test procedure demonstrated a significant improvement of this outcome. There was actually a trend toward increased perinatal mortality in pregnancies monitored with nonstress testing (28). However, it is important to keep in mind that these analyses included far too few patients to determine if a clinically significant improvement in perinatal mortality exists. For example, because of the very low incidence of

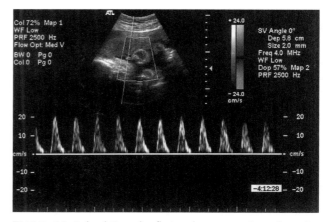

■ FIG. 15. Pulsed Doppler flow velocity waveform from the umbilical artery of a growth-restricted fetus. There is absence of end diastolic flow. (Courtesy of Joshua A. Copel, MD)

perinatal mortality, the meta-analysis of biophysical profile surveillance trials was powered sufficiently to detect only a reduction in perinatal mortality in excess of 4-fold (29), whereas the meta-analysis of nonstress testing was powered to detect only an even greater effect. What transpires, however, from these studies is a very low false-positive rate, a rarity of perinatal death among monitored pregnancies. The high false-positive rate of these tests is likely to be ameliorated by using them in conjunction with umbilical artery impedance, which has a lower false-positive rate.

Interventions aimed to treat IUGR do not demonstrate a significant effect on perinatal outcome. Ultimately, delivery is the single intervention currently available. The question of timing of delivery, however, remains unresolved. If we knew at what gestational age the incidence of stillbirth exceeds the incidence of neonatal death for fetuses with and without abnormal umbilical artery impedance, we could determine appropriate recommendations for timing of delivery. Unfortunately, such data can be obtained only by very large studies. Meanwhile, a recent study of stillbirths demonstrates that most unexplained SGA stillbirths occur after 33 weeks of gestation. Many clinicians, therefore, deliver SGA pregnancies with absent or reversed end-diastolic flow in the umbilical artery at 34 weeks of gestation despite otherwise normal fetal surveillance. Fetuses small for gestational age with increased umbilical artery impedance frequently are delivered at 37 weeks of gestation (30).

References

1. Clausson B, Gardosi J, Francis A, Cnattingius S. Perinatal outcome in SGA births defined by customised versus population-based birthweight standards. BJOG 2001;108:830–4.

2. Badawi N, Kurinczuk JJ, Keogh JM, Alessandri LM, O'Sullivan F, Burton PR, et al. Antepartum risk factors for newborn encephalopathy: the Western Australian case-control study. BMJ 1998;317(7172):1549–53.

3. McIntire DD, Bloom SL, Casey BM, Leveno KJ. Birth weight in relation to morbidity and mortality among newborn infants. N Engl J Med 1999;340:1234-8.

4. Taylor DJ, Howie PW. Fetal growth achievement and neurodevelopmental disability. Br J Obstet Gynaecol 1989;96:789–94.

5. Goldenberg RL, DuBard MB, Cliver SP, Nelson KG, Blankson K, Ramey SL, et al. Pregnancy outcome and intelligence at age five years. Am J Obstet Gynecol 1996;175:1511–5.

6. Barker DJ, Eriksson JG, Forsen T, Osmond C. Fetal origins of adult disease: strength of effects and biological basis. Int J Epidemiol 2002;31:1235–9.

7. Smith GC, Smith MF, McNay MB, Fleming JE. First-trimester growth and the risk of low birth weight. N Engl J Med 1998;339:1817–22.

8. Smith GC, Stenhouse EJ, Crossley JA, Aitken DA, Cameron AD, Connor JM. Early-pregnancy origins of low birth weight. Nature 2002;417:916.

9. Neilson JP. Symphysis-fundal height measurement in pregnancy. The Cochrane Database of Systematic Reviews 1998, Issue 2. Art. No.: CD000944. DOI: 10.1002/14651858.CD000944.

10. Mongelli M, Gardosi J. Symphysis-fundus height and pregnancy characteristics in ultrasound-dated pregnancies. Obstet Gynecol 1999;94:591–4.

11. Gardosi J, Francis A. Controlled trial of fundal height measurement plotted on customised antenatal growth charts. Br J Obstet Gynaecol 1999;106:309–17.

12. Chien PF, Owen P, Khan KS. Validity of ultrasound estimation of fetal weight. Obstet Gynecol 2000;95:856–60.

13. Kaaij MW, Struijk PC, Lotgering FK. Accuracy of sonographic estimates of fetal weight in very small infants. Ultrasound Obstet Gynecol 1999;13:99–102.

14. de Jong CL, Francis A, van Geijn HP, Gardosi J. Fetal growth rate and adverse perinatal events. Ultrasound Obstet Gynecol 1999;13:86–9.

15. de Jong CL, Francis A, van Geijn HP, Gardosi J. Customized fetal weight limits for antenatal detection of fetal growth restriction. Ultrasound Obstet Gynecol 2000;15:36–40.

16. Mongelli M, Gardosi J. Reduction of false-positive diagnosis of fetal growth restriction by application of customized fetal growth standards. Obstet Gynecol 1996;88:844–8.

17. Bricker L, Neilson JP. Routine ultrasound in late pregnancy (after 24 weeks gestation). The Cochrane Database of Systematic Reviews 2000, Issue 1. Art. No.: CD001451. DOI: 10.1002/14651858.CD001451.

18. Owen P, Khan KS, Howie P. Single and serial estimates of amniotic fluid volume and umbilical artery resistance in the prediction of intrauterine growth restriction. Ultrasound Obstet Gynecol 1999;13:415–9.

19. Chien PF, Arnott N, Gordon A, Owen P, Khan KS. How useful is uterine artery Doppler flow velocimetry in the prediction of pre-eclampsia, intrauterine growth retardation and perinatal death? An overview. BJOG 2000;107:196–208.

20. Soothill PW, Ajayi RA, Campbell S, Nicolaides KH. Prediction of morbidity in small and normally grown fetuses by fetal heart rate variability, biophysical profile score and umbilical artery Doppler studies. Br J Obstet Gynaecol 1993;100:742–5.

21. Nicolaides KH. Screening for chromosomal defects. Ultrasound Obstet Gynecol 2003;21:313–21.

22. Neilson JP, Alfirevic Z. Doppler ultrasound for fetal assessment in high risk pregnancies. The Cochrane Database of Systematic Reviews 1996, Issue 2. Art. No.: CD000073. DOI: 10.1002/14651858.CD000073.

23. Forouzan I. Absence of end-diastolic flow velocity in the umbilical artery: a review. Obstet Gynecol Surv 1995;50:219–27.

24. Nienhuis SJ, Vles JS, Gerver WJ, Hoogland HJ. Doppler ultrasonography in suspected intrauterine growth retarda-

tion: a randomized clinical trial. Ultrasound Obstet Gynecol 1997;9:6–13.

25. McCowan LM, Harding JE, Roberts AB, Barker SE, Ford C, Stewart AW. A pilot randomized controlled trial of two regimens of fetal surveillance for small-for-gestational-age fetuses with normal results of umbilical artery doppler velocimetry. Am J Obstet Gynecol 2000;182:81–6.

26. McCowan LM, Harding JE, Stewart AW. Umbilical artery Doppler studies in small for gestational age babies reflect disease severity. BJOG 2000;107:916–25.

27. Baschat AA, Gembruch U, Harman CR. The sequence of changes in Doppler and biophysical parameters as severe fetal growth restriction worsens. Ultrasound Obstet Gynecol 2001;18:571–7.

28. Pattison N, McCowan L. Cardiotocography for antepartum fetal assessment. The Cochrane Database of Systematic Reviews 1999, Issue 1. Art. No.: CD001068. DOI: 10.1002/14651858.CD001068.

29. Alfirevic Z, Neilson JP. Biophysical profile for fetal assessment in high risk pregnancies. The Cochrane Database of Systematic Reviews 1996, Issue 1. Art. No.: CD000038. DOI: 10.1002/14651858.CD000038.

30. Royal College of Obstetricians and Gynaecologists. The investigation and management of the small-for-gestational-age fetus. RCOG Guideline No. 31. London, UK: RCOG; 2002.

PRETERM LABOR AND DELIVERY

Preterm birth, which occurs before the end of 37 weeks of gestation, has increased in the past few years to approximately 12% of all births (1, 2). Much of the increase is a result of an increase in the number of multiple gestations as a consequence of fertility treatment. One study found that among high-order births (triplets or more), 43% resulted from assisted reproductive technology, 38% were the result of ovulation-inducing drugs, and only 20% were conceived spontaneously (3).

Preterm births account for more than 60% of non-anomaly-related neonatal mortality and morbidity. Most neonatal deaths occur in infants born between 20 and 32 weeks of gestation and whose birth weight is below 1,500 g. Prematurity-related conditions were the second most common cause of infant mortality (deaths from birth to 1 year old) with a rate of 130.5 per 100,000 live births among all races in 2000 (4). For black infants, prematurity-related diagnoses were the leading causes of infant mortality (340.5 per 100,000 live births) from 1989 to 1997 (5).

Significant increases in survival rates occur at 25–26 weeks of gestation (from 20% at 24 weeks to more than 60% at 26 weeks of gestation). Most of the survivors born at 26 weeks of gestation or more will survive without major disability (6), but long-term impairment remains high for surviving infants delivered at 25 weeks of gestation and earlier. Infants born at 30 weeks of gestation have survival rates that approach 97% in most perinatal centers and display short- and long-term outcomes that are better than is generally appreciated (7).

Pathophysiology

Most preterm deliveries occur as a result of 1 or more of 4 primary pathogenic processes. Each has unique biochemical mediators, but all 4 share a common final biologic pathway that leads to cervical changes and uterine contractions with or without membrane rupture:

1. *Activation of maternal–fetal hypothalamic–pituitary–adrenal axis due to fetal or maternal stress:* There is increasing epidemiologic, clinical, and experimental evidence that uteroplacental vascular abnormalities accompanied by IUGR are present in up to one third of preterm deliveries. Similarly, maternal psychosocial and physiologic indicators of stress have been increasingly linked to preterm delivery (8). The pathway promoting stress-associated preterm delivery is likely to be similar to that for physiologic parturition.

2. *Decidual–chorioamniotic or systemic inflammation caused by genitourinary tract or systemic infection:* There are abundant epidemiologic, clinical, histologic, cell culture, and microbiologic data linking genital tract infections with preterm delivery via the activation of cervical, decidual, and fetal membrane cytokine networks.

3. *Decidual hemorrhage:* Decidual hemorrhage (abruptio placentae), regardless of whether it results in recurrent vaginal bleeding, has been strongly associated with a 3-fold to 7-fold increased risk of prematurity, particularly preceded by preterm rupture of membranes. The biochemical pathway by which such hemorrhage leads to preterm delivery appears to be mediated by thrombin generation. Thrombin binds to cellular receptors in the decidua to stimulate the production of various proteases (eg, plasminogen activators, matrix metalloproteases–collagenases) that ripen the cervix. Thrombin also may exert direct effects on the myometrium to stimulate contractions.

4. *Pathologic uterine distention:* Distention of the uterus activates the myometrium and increases the expression of fetal membrane cytokines.

Each of these 4 pathogenic mechanisms converges on a common pathway involving increased uterotonin and protease expression. More than one cascade may operate to produce preterm delivery in a given patient. The role of individual, genetically determined variations in inflammatory response is an active area of research that may explain the occurrence of preterm birth in some but not all women with common risk factors.

Risk Factors

It is difficult to identify women who are destined to give birth preterm (see Box 7). Vaginal infections, such as bacterial vaginosis, have been linked to a greater risk of preterm birth, but it is not clear whether screening and treatment are effective in preventing preterm birth (9, 10). Sociodemographic risk factors linked to preterm birth include low socioeconomic status and African-American race.

Scoring systems based on historical risk factors have low sensitivities in identifying women who give birth preterm. Clinical symptoms and signs such as uterine contractions, measured by self-perception or tocodynamometry, have low sensitivity and positive predictive value, even in women with historical risk factors for preterm delivery (11).

Markers for the risk of preterm birth are present as early as 18–24 weeks of gestation. These markers include cervicovaginal fetal fibronectin, cervical length of less than 25 mm by transvaginal ultrasonography, a Bishop score of 4 or more, and maternal bacterial vaginosis. All of these tests have low sensitivities to predict preterm delivery (Table 9).

Screening and Prevention

No efficient strategy exists to identify risk of preterm birth in the absence of clinical risk factors. A history of preterm birth and multifetal gestation are the strongest clinical predictors of preterm delivery. Tests to predict preterm birth, such as bacterial vaginosis screening, endovaginal ultrasonography, and fetal fibronectin testing, are not sufficiently sensitive to apply to routine prenatal care. Cervical ultrasonography and fetal fibronectin assessment may be useful to evaluate women with clinical risk factors who, if test results are negative, may not benefit from traditional interventions such as reduced physical or sexual activity.

Screening and treatment for bacterial vaginosis may be considered for women at high risk for preterm labor. The use of cervical cerclage for women with incompetent cervix is warranted, but cerclage for women with a prior preterm birth is controversial. An NIH study is evaluating this procedure in women who have had a previous preterm birth. Randomized trials have reached opposite conclusions about the role of cerclage in this group of women (12, 13).

Women with a history of preterm birth treated with supplemental progesterone had a reduced risk of recurrent preterm delivery in 2 randomized trials (14, 15). Weekly intramuscular injections of 250 mg of 17 α-hydroxy-progesterone caproate (14) and nightly administration of a 100-mg progesterone vaginal suppository (15) both reduced the rate of preterm birth by approximately 35–40% compared with placebo-treated controls. Currently, no evidence exists to support recommending supplemental progesterone in other at-risk women, such as those with multiple gestation, cervical cerclage, a positive fibronectin, or a short cervix determined by ultrasonography.

Diagnosis

The symptoms and signs of early preterm labor may include mild, menstruallike cramps; constant low backache; uterine contractions, which are often painless; and a recent increase in vaginal discharge or presence of a pink-stained discharge. Because these symptoms are subtle, they may not be recognized until the labor process and cervical dilation is in an advanced stage (>4 cm). The diagnosis of preterm labor early in its course is difficult. Women who are treated after a diagnosis of preterm labor based on persistent contractions accompanied by cervical change are often (up to 40%) not actually in labor. Persistent contractions without additional evidence of labor are not sufficient to begin treatment. Ruptured membranes, bleeding, and clear evidence of cervical effacement (80% or more) or dilation (more than 2 cm) are the most reliable clinical signs (16, 17). When measured in women with contractions whose cervical dilation is less than 3 cm, a negative fetal fibronectin test or a transvaginal ultrasonographic cervical length of 30 mm or more identify women who are not in labor, thus reducing the chance of false-positive diagnosis and overtreatment.

Treatment

The initial evaluation of patients with suspected preterm labor should include determination of the presence and frequency of uterine contractions, the cervical status, a sterile speculum examination to exclude ruptured membranes, and an assessment of gestational age. Before tocolysis is considered, a search should be made for treat-

---

> ### BOX 7
>
> ### Risk Factors for Preterm Birth
>
> - Multiple gestation (40–50%)
> - Previous preterm birth (15–40% recurrence)
> - Second-trimester bleeding
> - Hydramnios
> - Uterine anomalies
> - Previous cone biopsy
> - Previous second-trimester losses
> - Cervical dilation and effacement before 32 weeks of gestation
> - Excessive preterm uterine activity
> - Placenta previa

TABLE 9. Value of Tests in Predicting Spontaneous Delivery at Less Than 35 Weeks of Gestation

Test	Weeks of Gestation at Time of Testing		
	22–24	27–28	31–32
	Percentage		
Maximal Nighttime Contraction Frequency ≥4/h			
Sensitivity	8.6	28.1	27.3
Specificity	96.4	88.7	82.0
Positive predictive value	25.0	23.1	11.3
Negative predictive value	88.3	91.1	93.0
Maximal Daytime Contraction Frequency ≥4/h			
Sensitivity	0	12.9	13.6
Specificity	98.4	93.9	84.9
Positive predictive value	0	20.0	7.1
Negative predictive value	87.0	90.2	92.1
Cervicovaginal Fibronectin ≥50 ng/mL			
Sensitivity	18.9	21.4	41.2
Specificity	95.1	94.5	92.5
Positive predictive value	35.0	30.0	30.4
Negative predictive value	92.6	94.1	98.1
Cervical Length ≤25 mm			
Sensitivity	47.2	53.6	82.4
Specificity	89.2	82.2	74.9
Positive predictive value	37.0	25.0	20.9
Negative predictive value	92.6	94.1	98.1
Bishop Score ≥4*			
Sensitivity	35.1	46.4	82.4
Specificity	91.0	77.9	61.8
Positive predictive value	35.1	18.8	14.7
Negative predictive value	91.0	92.9	97.8

*The Bishop score is a composite measure of cervical length, dilatation, position, consistency, and the degree of descent (station) of the presenting part of the fetus. The results indicate the degree of readiness for labor; values from 0 to 4 indicate not ready for labor, and values from 9 to 13 indicate ready for labor.

Iams JD, Newman RB, Thom EA, Goldenberg RL, Mueller-Heubach E, Moawad A, et al. Frequency of uterine contractions and the risk of spontaneous preterm delivery. N Engl J Med 2002;346:250–5. Copyright © 2002 Massachusetts Medical Society. All rights reserved.

able factors of preterm labor, such as pyelonephritis, and an evaluation made to determine whether there are maternal or fetal contraindications to a specific tocolytic treatment. Relative contraindications include mild hypertension, IUGR, and cervical dilation greater than 4 cm. A urine culture often is obtained, and cultures for group B hemolytic streptococcus, *Chlamydia trachomatis*, and *Neisseria gonorrhoeae* are recommended by some. Amniocentesis for fetal lung maturity and a Gram stain as well as culture may be appropriate, depending on gestational age and the presenting clinical situation. Some of these factors may be contraindications for one drug but not for another. The risk–benefit ratio of tocolysis must be considered for each patient. Although many clinicians feel that tocolytic drugs should be used when possible,

considerable debate remains as to their efficacy and safety. The principal value of arresting labor is to gain sufficient time before delivery to achieve 3 goals:

1. Transfer the mother to a facility that can care for her preterm infant.

2. Administer prophylactic antibiotics to reduce the chance of neonatal group B streptococcus (GBS) infection in the infant.

3. Administer antenatal corticosteroids to improve neonatal survival and reduce neonatal morbidity.

The benefits of the use of tocolytics to prolong pregnancy when premature labor occurs is not clearly proved beyond the initial 24–48 hours. The benefits of tocolytic therapy apparently are derived more from ancillary treatments such as corticosteroids, antibiotic prophylaxis against GBS, and maternal transportation to a facility with more advanced high-risk nursery care. It also promotes a regionalized approach to maternal care based on risk factors. Several drugs are currently in use as follows.

Magnesium sulfate often is chosen as the initial drug regardless of gestational age because of its safety, particularly in the presence of diabetes. A loading dose of 4–6 g is given intravenously over 30 minutes followed by a continuous maintenance dose of 2–4 g/h, usually resulting in a maternal serum concentration of 6–8 mg/dL. The infusion rate is titrated to the uterine response, with careful maternal monitoring for toxicity. If contractions persist after 1–2 hours at the 4-g/h rate, alternate management should be considered. Before 32 weeks of gestation, many centers use indomethacin as an alternative (18). After 32 weeks of gestation, terbutaline (one subcutaneous dose of 0.25 mg) may be added to magnesium sulfate as a supplement. Terbutaline, as a supplement, should not be continued more than 4 hours (ie, one additional dose after 4 hours) because of the side effects of the combined therapy (19, 20).

Prostaglandin synthetase inhibitors (eg, indomethacin) have been reported to be the most effective tocolytic agents. These agents may produce oligohydramnios and narrowing of the ductus arteriosus, but research has shown that these effects are both rare and reversible if the drug is given before 32 weeks of gestation and the duration of therapy is limited to 48–72 hours. Amniotic fluid volume and ductal flow assessment are not needed when these guidelines are followed. The advantages of indomethacin are its efficacy and relative safety. Unlike other agents, it rarely causes cardiovascular side effects. Asthma may occur in aspirin-sensitive women, and platelet function may be affected. Indomethacin should be avoided when either the mother or the fetus has a renal disorder. The initial dose is 50–100 mg orally, followed by 25–50 mg every 6 hours.

Calcium channel-blocking drugs cause a decrease in intracellular free calcium and, hence, inhibition of myometrial contractility. Nifedipine is as effective as β-mimetics in stopping contractions. The drug is given orally, not parenterally, and has an onset of action of 20–30 minutes. Sublingual use is not appropriate because it may cause profound hypotension. Side effects, including hypotension and headache, are common and may be reduced with adequate pretreatment hydration. However, because pulmonary edema may occur with any tocolytic, including nifedipine, fluid balance should be carefully monitored. Calcium channel blockers should not be combined with magnesium sulfate because of the risk of respiratory depression due to muscle blockade (21).

Beta-adrenergic drugs are less commonly used today because of side effects. Furthermore, randomized trials have not demonstrated effectiveness in prolonging pregnancy when compared with controls. When using these drugs (ritodrine and terbutaline) the following concerns must be considered:

- Hypotension
- Excessive tachycardia
- Myocardial ischemia
- Pulmonary edema
- Restriction of fluid administration to less than 2,500 mL/d
- Careful monitoring of urinary output
- Evaluation by electrocardiogram of any occurrence of chest pain
- Occurrence of hypokalemia
- Occurrence of hypoglycemia

Using therapeutic tocolysis only after the onset of contractions has not been shown to prolong latency. No studies have demonstrated that the use of tocolytic agents improves neonatal outcome, but none has evaluated tocolysis when corticosteroids and antibiotics are given concurrently. It could be that short-term pregnancy prolongation with tocolysis would enhance the potential for corticosteroid effect. Given evidence of short-term pregnancy prolongation without evident risk in some studies, it is not unreasonable to initiate tocolysis in women at high risk for infant morbidity should there be concurrent attempts to prevent infection, prolong pregnancy, and induce fetal pulmonary maturity. However, in the absence of data demonstrating neonatal benefit of such intervention, this approach should not be considered an expected practice.

Corticosteroid Therapy

Maternal administration of betamethasone or dexamethasone has been shown in many controlled trials to decrease both neonatal mortality and neonatal morbidity, including respiratory distress syndrome and intraventricular hemorrhage. The 2000 NIH Consensus Conference reaffirmed the clinical recommendations of the 1994 NIH Consensus Conference on the use of antenatal corticosteroids and addressed the issue of repeat courses of antenatal steroids (22). Specifically, the panel concluded that any women who are at risk of preterm delivery within 7 days between 24 and 34 weeks of gestation should receive a single course of either betamethasone or dexamethasone for fetal maturation. They concluded that there were no data to support the use of any other steroid regimen.

The panel further concluded that there was insufficient evidence of either the safety or the efficacy of repeated courses of corticosteroids. The American College of Obstetricians and Gynecologists endorsed these recommendations (22) and recommended that antenatal corticosteroids not be used after 34 weeks of gestation unless there was laboratory evidence of fetal lung immaturity.

Controversy has emerged as to whether neonatal mortality is increased with betamethasone versus dexamethasone. Specifically, a meta-analysis indicated that neonatal mortality was decreased with betamethasone but not with dexamethasone (23). It has been reported that betamethasone was more efficacious than dexamethasone in preventing periventricular leukomalacia (24).

It is appropriate to conclude that a single course of antenatal corticosteroids should be given at 24–34 weeks of gestation in the presence of threatened preterm delivery. Moreover, such therapy appears to be of benefit in women with preterm premature rupture of membranes. Current data would suggest there are no apparent benefits of repeat courses of antenatal steroids, and such therapy may prove to be harmful. Treatment with corticosteroids for less than 24 hours is associated with a significant reduction in neonatal mortality, respiratory distress syndrome, and intraventricular hemorrhage.

References

1. Martin JA, Hamilton BE, Ventura SJ, Menacker F, Park MM, Sutton PD. Births: final data for 2001. Natl Vital Stat Rep 2002;51:1–102.

2. Martin JA, Hamilton BE, Ventura SJ, Menacker F, Park MM. Births: final data for 2000. Natl Vital Stat Rep 2002; 50:1–101.

3. Contribution of assisted reproductive technology and ovulation-inducing drugs to triplet and higher-order multiple births—United States, 1980–1997. MMWR Morb Mortal Wkly Rep 2000;49:535–8.

4. Minino AM, Smith BL. Deaths: preliminary data for 2000. Natl Vital Stat Rep 2001;49:1–40.

5. Demissie K, Rhoads GG, Ananth CV, Alexander GR, Kramer MS, Kogan MD, et al. Trends in preterm birth and neonatal mortality among blacks and whites in the United States from 1989 to 1997. Am J Epidemiol 2001;154: 307–15.

6. MacDonald H. Perinatal care at the threshold of viability. American Academy of Pediatrics. Committee on Fetus and Newborn. Pediatrics 2002;110:1024–7.

7. Lemons JA, Bauer CR, Oh W, Korones SB, Papile LA, Stoll BJ, et al. Very low birth weight outcomes of the National Institute of Child Health and Human Development Neonatal Research Network, January 1995 through December 1996. NICHD Neonatal Research Network. Pediatrics 2001; 107:E1.

8. Challis JR, Smith SK. Fetal endocrine signals and preterm labor. Biol Neonate 2001;79:163–7.

9. Carey JC, Klebanoff MA, Hauth JC, Hillier SL, Thom EA, Ernest JM, et al. Metronidazole to prevent preterm delivery in pregnant women with asymptomatic bacterial vaginosis. National Institute of Child Health and Human Development Network of Maternal-Fetal Medicine Units. N Engl J Med 2000;342:534–40.

10. Klebanoff MA, Carey JC, Hauth JC, Hillier SL, Nugent RP, Thom EA, et al. Failure of metronidazole to prevent preterm delivery among pregnant women with asymptomat-ic Trichomonas vaginalis infection. N Engl J Med 2001;345:487–93.

11. Iams JD, Newman RB, Thom EA, Goldenberg RL, Mueller–Heubach E, Moawad A, et al. Frequency of uterine contractions and the risk of spontaneous preterm delivery [published erratum appears in N Engl J Med 2003;349: 513]. N Engl J Med 2002;346:250–5.

12. Rust OA, Atlas RO, Reed J, van Gaalen J, Balducci J. Revisiting the short cervix detected by transvaginal ultrasound in the second trimester: why cerclage therapy may not help. Am J Obstet Gynecol 2001;185:1098–105.

13. Althuisius SM, Dekker GA, van Geijn HP, Bekedam DJ, Hummel P. Cervical incompetence prevention randomized cerclage trial (CIPRACT): study design and preliminary results. Am J Obstet Gynecol 2000;183:823–9.

14. Meis PJ, Klebanoff M, Thom E, Dombrowski MP, Sibai B, Moawad AH, et al. Prevention of recurrent preterm delivery by 17 alpha-hydroxyprogesterone caproate [published erratum appears in N Engl J Med 2003;349:1299]. N Engl J Med 2003;348:2379–85.

15. da Fonseca EB, Bittar RE, Carvalho MH, Zugaib M. Prophylactic administration of progesterone by vaginal suppository to reduce the incidence of spontaneous preterm birth in women at increased risk: a randomized placebo-controlled double-blind study. Am J Obstet Gynecol 2003; 188:419–24.

16. Macones GA, Segel SY, Stamilo DM, Morgan MA. Predicting delivery within 48 hours in women treated with parenteral tocolysis. Obstet Gynecol 1999;93:432–6.

17. Macones GA, Segel SY, Stamilo DM, Morgan MA. Prediction of delivery among women with early preterm labor by means of clinical characteristics alone. Am J Obstet Gynecol 1999;181:1414–8.

18. Macones GA, Marder SJ, Clothier B, Stamilio DM. The controversy surrounding indomethacin for tocolysis. Am J Obstet Gynecol 2001;184:264–72.

19. Hatjis CG, Swain M, Nelson LH, Meis PJ, Ernest JM. Efficacy of combined administration of magnesium sulfate and ritodrine in the treatment of premature labor. Obstet Gynecol 1987;69:317–22.

20. Management of preterm labor. ACOG Practice Bulletin No. 43. American College of Obstetricians and Gynecologists. Obstet Gynecol 2003;101:1039–47.

21. Ben-Ami M, Giladi Y, Shalev E. The combination of magnesium sulfate and nifedipine: a cause of neuromuscular blockade. Br J Obstet Gynaecol 1994;101:262–3.

22. Antenatal corticosteroids revisited: repeat courses. NIH Consens Statement 2000;17(2):1–18.

23. Antenatal corticosteroid therapy for fetal maturation. ACOG Committee Opinion No. 273. American College of Obstetrics and gynecology. Obstet Gynecol 2002;99:871–3.

24. Ballard PL, Ballard RA. Scientific basis and therapeutic regimens for use of antenatal glucocorticoids. Am J Obstet Gynecol 1995;173:254–62.

25. Baud O, Foix-L'Helias L, Kaminski M, Audibert F, Jarreau PH, Papiernik E, et al. Antenatal glucocorticoid treatment and cystic periventricular leukomalacia in very premature infants. N Engl J Med 1999;341:1190–6.

PREMATURE RUPTURE OF MEMBRANES

Rupture of membranes that occurs before the onset of labor is described as premature rupture of membranes (PROM). At term, PROM complicates approximately 8% of pregnancies. Membrane rupture occurring before 37 weeks of gestation, referred to as preterm PROM, occurs in 3% of pregnancies and is responsible for approximately one third of all preterm births (1). Midtrimester PROM that occurs at or before 26 weeks of gestation complicates 0.6–0.7% of pregnancies. Although this delineation was clinically relevant in the 1970s and 80s, the limit of potential neonatal survival ("viability") continues to decrease. Currently, it is more clinically relevant to differentiate preterm PROM into "previable PROM," which occurs before the limit of viability, "preterm PROM remote from term" (from viability to approximately 32 weeks of gestation), and "preterm PROM near term" (approximately 32–36 weeks of gestation).

Because PROM is associated with delivery, perinatal infection, and umbilical cord compression due to oligohydramnios, term and preterm PROM are important causes of perinatal morbidity and mortality. Near term, delivery of a noninfected and nonasphyxiated infant is associated with a high likelihood of survival and a low risk of severe morbidity. As such, management should be directed toward delivery with attention to risk factors for perinatal infection. Alternatively, when preterm PROM occurs remote from term, immediate delivery will be associated with a significant risk of significant perinatal morbidity and mortality that decreases with advancing gestational age at delivery. In the absence of contraindications, management should be directed toward conserving the pregnancy and reducing perinatal morbidity. When "previable PROM" occurs, immediate delivery will lead to neonatal death. Conservative management may lead to previable or periviable birth, but also may lead to extended latency and delivery of a potentially viable infant. Regardless of the gestational age, the patient should be well informed regarding the potential maternal, fetal, and neonatal complications of PROM.

Etiology

Early membrane rupture may occur for a variety of reasons, including the following:

- Physiologic weakening, occurring at or near term, associated with apoptosis (programmed cell death), increased collagenase activity, and dissolution of the amniochorionic extracellular matrix exacerbated by contraction-induced shearing forces
- Ascending genital tract infection, a leading cause of preterm PROM, which initiates a cytokine cascade that enhances amniochorionic apoptosis, protease production, and dissolution of the extracellular matrix

- Placental abruption, which enhances decidual thrombin expression and triggers thrombin–thrombin receptor interactions to increase decidual–chorionic protease production and dissolution of the extracellular matrix C
- Mechanical stretch, which appears to enhance expression of amniochorionic cytokines to increase protease production

Other risk factors associated with PROM include low socioeconomic status, low BMI, prior preterm birth, cigarette smoking, urinary tract and sexually transmitted infections, cervical conization or cerclage, preterm labor or symptomatic contractions in the current gestation, uterine overdistention (eg, twins, polyhydramnios), amniocentesis, and vaginal bleeding in pregnancy. Each of these risk factors likely is associated with PROM through membrane degradation or loss of elastic tensile strength, chorio–decidual inflammation, or decreased maternal resistance to ascending bacterial colonization. The ultimate cause of PROM often is not evident.

Clinical Course

A hallmark of PROM is early delivery; latency is inversely proportional to gestational age at membrane rupture. At term, one half of expectantly managed pregnant women give birth within 5 hours and 95% give birth within 28 hours of membrane rupture (2). Of all patients with membranes ruptured before 34 weeks of gestation, 93% will give birth in less than 1 week (3). Even with conservative management, 50–60% of women with preterm PROM remote from term will give birth within 1 week of membrane rupture. When PROM occurs near or before the limit of viability, up to 1 in 4 women will not give birth for at least 1 month. With conservative management, a small proportion of women with membrane rupture can anticipate cessation of fluid leakage (2.6–13%), except patients experiencing membrane rupture subsequent to amniocentesis, who commonly heal.

Risks

MATERNAL RISKS

Amnionitis is the most common maternal complication after PROM. The risk of infection decreases with increasing gestational age at membrane rupture and increases with increasing "latency" from membrane rupture to delivery. With PROM at term, 9% of pregnant women will develop intrauterine infection. The risk increases to 24% with membrane rupture longer than 24 hours. Intraamniotic infection complicates 13–60% of pregnancies, and endometritis occurs in approximately 2–13% of pregnancies after PROM remote from term. Abruptio placentae may lead to preterm PROM or may result secondarily, affecting 4–12% of these pregnancies. Retained placenta and postpartum hemorrhage necessitating dilation and curettage, maternal sepsis, and death are uncommon but serious complications of expectantly managed PROM near or before the limit of viability.

FETAL AND NEONATAL RISKS

The frequency and severity of neonatal complications after PROM vary with the gestational age at which rupture and delivery occur and are increased with perinatal infection, placental abruption, and umbilical cord compression. At term, the fetus is at risk for umbilical cord compression from oligohydramnios and is susceptible to ascending infection.

Complications of preterm birth are the most significant risks to the infant born after preterm PROM. Respiratory distress syndrome (RDS) is the most common serious complication after preterm PROM at any gestational age. Other serious acute morbidities, including necrotizing enterocolitis, intraventricular hemorrhage (IVH), and sepsis, are common with early preterm birth but relatively uncommon near term. Remote from term, serious perinatal morbidity that may lead to long-term sequelae or death is common. Current community-based survival and morbidity curves based on gestational age at delivery have been published (4). However, data specific to infants delivered after preterm PROM are not available. It has been found that perinatal sepsis is 2-fold more common in the setting of preterm PROM than preterm birth after preterm labor with intact membranes. In some circumstances, the risk of these complications may outweigh the 1–2% risk of stillbirth due to umbilical cord compression after preterm PROM (3).

Lethal pulmonary hypoplasia occurs when alveolar development is arrested when PROM occurs at the critical phase of development, generally before 20 weeks of gestation (5, 6). Although lethal pulmonary hypoplasia rarely occurs with PROM after 24–26 weeks of gestation, presumably because alveolar development growth is adequate to support postnatal life, there remains the potential for nonlethal pulmonary hypoplasia, predisposing the infant to pulmonary complications such as pneumothorax and pneumomediastinum related to poor pulmonary compliance and the need for high ventilatory pressures. Restriction deformities can occur after oligohydramnios subsequent to PROM, and are similar to those seen with Potter's syndrome.

Prediction of Preterm PROM

Prior preterm birth and preterm birth resulting from preterm PROM are associated with subsequent preterm PROM. This risk increases with decreasing gestational age of prior delivery. Those with a prior preterm birth at 23–27 weeks have a 27.1% risk of subsequent preterm birth ($P < .001$), and those with a prior history of preterm PROM have a 3.3-fold higher risk of preterm birth after PROM (13.5% versus 4.1%, $P < .01$) and a 13.5-fold higher risk of preterm PROM before 28 weeks of gestation (1.8 versus 0.13%, $P < .01$) in a subsequent gestation.

One study has suggested ancillary testing with transvaginal cervical ultrasonography or cervicovaginal onco-fetal fibronectin screening, or both, to be useful in differentiating women at high or low risk for subsequent preterm birth (7). The presence of a short cervix (<25 mm) and a positive fetal fibronectin test result at 23–24 weeks of gestation have been associated with preterm birth due to PROM. Nulliparous women with a positive cervicovaginal fetal fibronectin test result and a short cervix had a 16.7% risk of preterm birth due to preterm PROM, whereas multiparous women with a history of preterm PROM, a short cervix, and a positive fetal fibronectin test result had a 25% risk of preterm PROM, a 31-fold increased risk of PROM with delivery before 35 weeks of gestation over those without risk factors (25 versus 0.8%, $P = .001$). Although the ability to identify women at increased risk for preterm PROM through ancillary testing is increasing, such testing is expensive and inconvenient, will identify only a fraction of those destined to give birth preterm, and has not yet led to an effective preventive intervention. As such, routine screening cannot be recommended for this indication.

Diagnosis

The textbook description of use of sterile techniques for examination, testing for pH of vaginal fluid, microscopic evaluation for ferning, obtaining of cervical cultures, and avoidance of cervical digital examination all remain current. When a diagnostic dilemma occurs, injection of dilute sterile indigo carmine into a pocket of amniotic fluid with ultrasonographic assistance is an acceptable technique.

Management

Preterm PROM has been classified as previable, remote from term, and near term. The purpose of the classification system presented is to better target management options.

PREVIABLE (<23 WEEKS OF GESTATION)

Immediate delivery almost always will result in death of the fetus. Even conservative therapy most likely will result in the delivery of a previable or extremely premature infant. Based on the estimated gestational age and fetal weight, factual information should be given to the parents as to the probability of delaying delivery for a significant interval of time. They also should be given the most current information at that facility as to the possibility for survival and the associated morbidity, both short term and long term, for a fetus delivered within that time frame. If expectant management is chosen, a detailed ultrasound study of the fetus is indicated to look for anomalies. Hospitalization for a period of maternal observation and fetal monitoring is recommended initially, but there is no consensus as to the advantages of continued inpatient versus outpatient management. The risks of infection, abruption, and cord complications need to be addressed in the monitoring plan. The risk of pulmonary hypoplasia as a complication, especially when amniotic fluid index remains low, can be followed by serial ultrasonogram studies. Measurement of lung length, chest circumference, chest–abdominal circumference ratio, and chest–circumference–femur length ratio, with ultrasonography or with Doppler studies, have a high predictive value for lethal pulmonary hypoplasia (5). Experimental measures to reseal the membranes and to perform cerclage have been explored but cannot be recommended (8–10). When the parents elect not to pursue expectant management, the pregnancy can be terminated by dilation and evacuation, or induction of labor with oxytocin or with prostaglandins.

PRETERM PROM REMOTE FROM TERM (23–32 WEEKS OF GESTATION)

Advances in neonatal care have made possible the survival of very premature infants. However, the immediate and long-term morbidity of such early birth makes prolongation of pregnancy an important goal of conservative therapy after PROM. Initial therapy is bed rest and continuous maternal and fetal monitoring. The risks of premature labor, abruption, amnionitis, and umbilical cord complications are the targets of monitoring. Prolonged bed rest adds additional maternal risk for thrombophlebitis (see "Deep Vein Thrombosis"). Prevention of DVT should be considered when bed rest is ordered (11). Following the initial evaluation, daily evaluation of the fetal heart rate (FHR) pattern is advised because abnormalities are common (32–76%) as a result of cord compression. When this has been demonstrated, continuous FHR monitoring is advised. Evaluation of fetal well-being can be assessed by nonstress and biophysical profile tests. However, FHR monitoring offers the opportunity to concurrently evaluate for the presence of and fetal response to uterine contractions.

The value of antibiotic therapy following diagnosis of PROM at these gestational ages has been the subject of many prospective studies and was explored by a prospective NIH-sponsored study that showed a positive effect in prolonging pregnancy and reducing fetal morbidity. Details of the study indicate that short-term (7-day), aggressive therapy with ampicillin, erythromycin, and amoxicillin showed statistically positive effects. Ampicillin-clavulanic acid was not beneficial and could be harmful because of an increase in necrotizing enterocolitis in the neonate (12).

Recognizing the current concept of the value of antibiotic use resulting in greater prolongation of pregnancy, the administration of corticosteroids concurrently has been studied, with promising results. Although perinatal and maternal infection was not increased, a meta-analysis showed reduction in RDS, IVH, and necrotizing enterocolitis (13).

PRETERM PROM NEAR TERM (32–36 WEEKS OF GESTATION)

The interval between PROM and the onset of labor becomes gradually shorter as term is approached. Management should be based on individual assessment of the estimated risk for maternal, fetal, and neonatal complications associated with conservative therapy versus expeditious delivery. Intrapartum prophylaxis against GBS is recommended for women giving birth preterm and for those with PROM at term when the interval until delivery is expected to be 18 hours or more, unless recent anovaginal GBS cultures were negative (14). A test for fetal lung maturity can be done. If the test result is positive, there is no apparent neonatal benefit for further conservative management; delivery is indicated.

The presence of evidence for advanced labor, intrauterine infection, significant uterine bleeding, or nonreassuring fetal testing are indications for delivery regardless of the gestational age. When prolongation of pregnancy permits it, maternal transfer to a facility with the resources to provide the care necessary for both the mother and a premature neonate should be arranged. The facility should be capable of providing 24-hour neonatal resuscitation and intensive care because generally, conservative management should be pursued for only those pregnancies in which there is a significant risk of neonatal morbidity and mortality should delivery occur immediately. If adequate facilities for maternal and neonatal care do not exist, patient transfer should be undertaken early in the course of management to avoid emergent transfer once complications arise.

The use of tocolysis in the face of PROM has not been demonstrated to provide independent fetal benefit. However, in the absence of factors requiring prompt delivery, tocolysis may be useful in providing the opportunity to use antibiotic and corticosteroid therapy but is as yet unproved. The question remains whether or not the complication of PROM can be safely managed in an outpatient setting to reduce the cost of prolonged hospitalization. The information currently available is insufficient to assess the effects of outpatient versus inpatient management and cannot be recommended.

Special Considerations

ANTIBIOTIC ADMINISTRATION

There may be a role for adjunctive antibiotic therapy with erythromycin and amoxicillin or ampicillin during conservative management of preterm PROM remote from term. Antibiotics prolong the latency period and improve perinatal outcomes in patients with preterm PROM and should be administered according to one of several published protocols if expectant management is to be pursued before 35 weeks of gestation. The combination of oral erythromycin and extended broad-spectrum ampicillin–clavulanic acid in a lower risk population near term does not appear to be beneficial and may be harmful. This latter regimen is not recommended. Several recent studies have attempted to determine whether antibiotic therapy for a brief duration is adequate after preterm PROM (15, 16). These studies are of inadequate size and power to demonstrate equivalent effectiveness against infant morbidity. As such, a National Institute of Child Health and Human Development Maternal–Fetal Medicine Units (NICHD MFMU) protocol of 7 days of therapy is recommended.

CORTICOSTEROID ADMINISTRATION

During conservative management of preterm PROM before 30–32 weeks of gestation, a single course of betamethasone (12 mg intramuscularly every 24 hours for 2 doses) or dexamethasone (6 mg intramuscularly every 12 hours for 4 doses) should be given because of the potential for reduction of IVH. It has been suggested that the use of antenatal corticosteroids may not be appropriate after preterm PROM because women with this condition would give birth too quickly to accrue the potential benefits, because preterm PROM might induce fetal pulmonary maturation, and because antenatal corticosteroid treatment might delay the diagnosis or increase the risk of perinatal infection. However, with antibiotic treatment, most women with conservatively managed preterm PROM will remain pregnant for at least 24–48 hours and the risk of infection is decreased. Furthermore, despite any potential maturational effect of PROM, RDS remains the most common acute morbidity in this setting (41% in the NICHD MFMU trial) (17).

Two recent randomized clinical trials have evaluated antenatal corticosteroid administration concurrent with antibiotic administration. One study found less RDS (18.4% versus 43.6%, P = .03) with no obvious increase in perinatal infection (3% versus 5%, P = NS) with antenatal corticosteroids after preterm PROM at 24–34 weeks of gestation (18). In the second trial, although there was no significant reduction in RDS with antenatal corticosteroids, there was no increase in maternal or neonatal infectious morbidity with treatment. Those women remaining pregnant after at least 24 hours of treatment had fewer perinatal deaths (1.3% versus 8.3%, P = .05) (19). In the most recent meta-analysis, antenatal corticosteroid administration after preterm PROM substantially reduced the risks of RDS (20% versus 35.4%), IVH (7.5% versus 15.9%), and necrotizing enterocolitis (0.8% versus 4.6%) without significantly increasing the risks of maternal infection (9.2% versus 5.1%) or neonatal infection (7.0% versus 6.6%) (13).

ANTEPARTUM PATIENT DISCHARGE

Generally, hospitalization for bed rest and pelvic rest is indicated after preterm PROM. Because latency frequently is brief, intrauterine and fetal infection may occur, and the fetus is at risk for umbilical cord compression, ongoing surveillance of both mother and fetus is necessary.

One clinical trial of patient discharge after preterm PROM has suggested that pregnant women who are stable can be discharged before delivery to reduce health care costs. However, this trial lacked the necessary power for adequately evaluating the effect of discharge on these outcomes. Although the potential for a reduction in health care costs with antepartum patient discharge is enticing, it is important to establish that such management will not be associated with increased risks and costs related to perinatal morbidity. Any cost savings from antenatal discharge will be rapidly lost with a small increase in stays in the neonatal intensive care unit as a result of infectious or gestational age-dependent morbidity.

CERCLAGE REMOVAL

Cervical cerclage is a known risk factor for PROM, which complicates about 1 in 4 pregnancies with a cerclage and about half of pregnancies having emergent cerclage placement. No prospective studies exist on the management of women with preterm PROM and a cervical cerclage in situ. Retrospective studies have suggested that when cerclage is removed on admission, the risk of adverse perinatal outcomes is not higher than after preterm PROM without a cerclage. Studies comparing pregnancies with cerclage retained or removed after preterm PROM have been small and have yielded conflicting results (20–22). Each has found insignificant trends toward increased maternal infection with retained cerclage, and 1 study found increased infant mortality and death from sepsis with retained cerclage, despite brief pregnancy prolongation. One study, comparing different practices at 2 institutions, found significant pregnancy prolongation with cerclage retention. However, it is possible that this finding reflects population or practice differences rather than those related solely to cerclage retention. No controlled study has found a significant reduction in infant morbidity with cerclage retention after preterm PROM. Given the potential risk without evident neonatal benefit, the general approach to management should include early cerclage removal after preterm PROM. The role for short-term cerclage retention while attempting to enhance fetal maturation with antenatal corticosteroids in the periviable gestation has not been determined.

CEREBRAL PALSY AND ADVERSE NEUROLOGIC OUTCOME

Data are accumulating linking perinatal infection to neurologic complications. Because preterm PROM is associated with early delivery and with perinatal infection, it is a potential risk factor for long-term neurologic morbidity. Cerebral palsy and cystic periventricular leukomalacia have been linked to amnionitis, which is commonly seen after preterm PROM (23). Similarly, elevated amniotic fluid cytokines and fetal systemic inflammation, which may accompany or reflect maternal or fetal infection, have been associated with preterm PROM, as well as brain lesions, such as periventricular leukomalacia and the subsequent development of cerebral palsy (24–26). However, no data suggest that immediate delivery of the candidate for conservative management after preterm PROM remote from term will prevent these sequelae.

References

1. Ventura SJ, Martin JA, Taffel SM, Mathews TJ, Clarke SC. Advance report of final natality statistics, 1993. Monthly vital statistics report from the Centers for Disease Control and Prevention. 1995;44(3S)1–88.

2. Hannah ME, Ohlsson A, Farine D, Hawson SA, Hodnett ED, Myhr TL, et al. Induction of labor compared with expectant management for prelabor rupture of the membranes at term. TERMPROM Study Group. N Engl J Med 1996;334:1005–10.

3. Mercer BM, Arheart KL. Antimicrobial therapy in expectant management of preterm premature rupture of the membranes [published erratum appears in Lancet 1996;347:410]. Lancet 1995;346:1271–9.

4. Mercer BM. Preterm premature rupture of the membranes. Obstet Gynecol 2003;101:178–93.

5. Laudy JA, Tibboel D, Robben SG, de Krijger RR, de Ridder MA, Wladimiroff JW. Prenatal prediction of pulmonary hypoplasia: clinical, biometric, and Doppler velocity correlates. Pediatrics 2002;109:250–8.

6. Rizzo G, Capponi A, Angelini E, Mazzoleni A, Romanini C. Blood flow velocity waveforms from fetal peripheral pulmonary arteries in pregnancies with preterm premature rupture of the membranes: relationship with pulmonary hypoplasia. Ultrasound Obstet Gynecol 2000;15:98–103.

7. Mercer BM, Goldenberg RL, Meis PJ, Moawad AH, Shellhaas C, Das A, et al. The Preterm Prediction Study: prediction of preterm premature rupture of the membranes through clinical findings and ancillary testing. The National Institute of Child Health and Human Development Maternal–Fetal Medicine Units Network. Am J Obstet Gynecol 2000;183:738–45.

8. Sciscione AC, Manley JS, Pollock M, Maas B, Shlossman PA, Mulla W, et al. Intracervical fibrin sealants: a potential treatment for early preterm premature rupture of the membranes. Am J Obstet Gynecol 2001;184:368–73.

9. Quintero RA, Morales WJ, Bornick PW, Allen M, Garabelis N. Surgical treatment of spontaneous rupture of membranes: the amniograft—first experience. Am J Obstet Gynecol 2002;186:155–7.

10. O'Brien JM, Barton JR, Milligan DA. An aggressive interventional protocol for early midtrimester premature rupture of the membranes using gelatin sponge for cervical plugging. Am J Obstet Gynecol 2002;187:1143–6.

11. Kovacevich GJ, Gaich SA, Lavin JP, Hopkins MP, Crane SS, Stewart J, et al. The prevalence of thromboembolic events among women with extended bed rest prescribed as part of the treatment for premature labor or preterm premature rupture of membranes. Am J Obstet Gynecol 2000;182:1089–92.

12. Kenyon SL, Taylor DJ, Tarnow-Mordi W; Oracle Collaborative Group. Broad spectrum antibiotics for preterm, prelabor rupture of fetal membranes: the ORACLE I Randomized trial. Lancet 2001;357:979–88.

13. Harding JE, Pang J, Knight DB, Liggins GC. Do antenatal corticosteroids help in the setting of preterm rupture of membranes? Am J Obstet Gynecol 2001;184:131–9.

14. Prevention of early-onset group B streptococcal disease in newborns. ACOG Committee Opinion No. 279. American College of Obstetricians and Gynecologists. Obstet Gynecol 2002;100:1405–12.

15. Lewis DF, Adair CD, Robichaux AG, Jaekle RK, Moore JA, Evans AT, et al. Antibiotic therapy in preterm premature rupture of membranes: are seven days necessary? A preliminary, randomized clinical trial. Am J Obstet Gynecol 2003;188:1413–6; discussion 1416–7.

16. Segel SY, Miles AM, Clothier B, Parry S, Macones GA. Duration of antibiotic therapy after preterm premature rupture of fetal membranes. Am J Obstet Gynecol 2003;189:799–802.

17. Mercer BM, Miodovnik M, Thurnau G, Goldenberg RL, Das AF, Ramsey RD, et al. Antibiotic therapy for reduction of infant morbidity after preterm premature rupture of the membranes. A randomized controlled trial. National Institute of Child Health and Human Development Maternal-Fetal Medicine Units Network. JAMA 1997;278:989–95.

18. Lewis DF, Brody K, Edwards MS, Brouillette RM, Burlison S, London SN. Preterm premature ruptured membranes: a randomized trial of steroids after treatment with antibiotics. Obstet Gynecol 1996;88:801–5.

19. Pattinson RC, Makin JD, Funk M, Delport SD, Macdonald AP, Norman K, et al. The use of dexamethasone in women with preterm premature rupture of membranes—a multicentre, double-blind, placebo-controlled, randomised trial. Dexiprom Study Group. S Afr Med J 1999;89:865–70.

20. Ludmir J, Bader T, Chen L, Lindenbaum C, Wong G. Poor perinatal outcome associated with retained cerclage in patients with premature rupture of membranes. Obstet Gynecol 1994;84:823–6.

21. Jenkins TM, Berghella V, Shlossman PA, McIntyre CJ, Maas BD, Pollock MA, Wapner RJ. Timing of cerclage removal after preterm premature rupture of membranes: maternal and neonatal outcomes. Am J Obstet Gynecol 2000;183:847–52.

22. McElrath TF, Norwitz ER, Lieberman ES, Heffner LJ. Perinatal outcome after preterm premature rupture of membranes with in situ cervical cerclage. Am J Obstet Gynecol 2002;187:1147–52.

23. Wu YW, Colford JM Jr. Chorioamnionitis as a risk factor for cerebral palsy: a meta-analysis. JAMA 2000;284:1417–24.

24. Yoon BH, Jun JK, Romero R, Park KH, Gomez R, Choi JH, et al. Amniotic fluid inflammatory cytokines (interleukin-6, interleukin-1beta, and tumor necrosis factor-alpha), neonatal brain white matter lesions, and cerebral palsy. Am J Obstet Gynecol 1997;177:19–26.

25. Yoon BH, Romero R, Kim CJ, Koo JN, Choe G, Syn HC, et al. High expression of tumor necrosis factor-alpha and

interleukin-6 in periventricular leukomalacia. Am J Obstet Gynecol 1997;177:406–11.

26. Yoon BH, Romero R, Yang SH, Jun JK, Kim IO, Choi JH, et al. Interleukin-6 concentrations in umbilical cord plasma are elevated in neonates with white matter lesions associated with periventricular leukomalacia. Am J Obstet Gynecol 1996;174:1433–40.

POSTTERM GESTATION

By definition, postterm pregnancy refers to a gestation that has extended to or beyond 42 weeks (ie, 294 days or estimated date of delivery plus 14 days). The incidence of postterm pregnancy is approximately 7% (1), and postterm pregnancy is associated with increased perinatal morbidity and mortality. Significant morbidity is related to oligohydramnios, meconium aspiration, macrosomia, and dysmaturity. Maternal complications include labor dystocia, cesarean delivery, perineal trauma, and postpartum hemorrhage.

Antepartum, intrapartum, and neonatal deaths are increased at 42 weeks of gestation. At 43 weeks of gestation, perinatal mortality is doubled; by 44 weeks of gestation, it is increased 4-fold to 6-fold. In a review of 181,524 births in Sweden occurring at 40 weeks of gestation or beyond, there were 251 intrauterine deaths (2). The odds ratio for fetal death increased with increasing gestational age (1.5, 1.8, and 2.9 at 41, 42, and 43 weeks of gestation, respectively). Postterm pregnancy may be secondary to inaccurate pregnancy dating; however, many cases are a true prolongation of gestation. Accurate pregnancy dating is critical to the diagnosis.

Several risk factors are linked to postterm pregnancy. The most common are nulliparity and prior postterm pregnancy, male sex, and genetic predisposition.

If the cervix is considered favorable for induction at 41–42 weeks of gestation, it seems reasonable to induce labor. Considerable controversy exists as to the most judicious mode of management in the presence of an unfavorable cervix. It is recommended that some form of antenatal testing be initiated by 42 weeks of gestation to assess fetal well-being (3). No data from randomized trials demonstrate the superiority of biophysical profile to weekly or twice-weekly fetal heart rate monitoring and ultrasound estimates of amniotic fluid volume. Amniotic fluid volume should be considered decreased if the 4-quadrant amniotic fluid index is less than 5 cm. Regardless of the assessment modality, delivery should be effected in the presence of fetal compromise, oligohydramnios, or both.

Induction of labor is considered when the benefits of delivery outweigh the risks of continuing the pregnancy. In high-risk pregnancies, this generally is thought to be near 38 weeks of gestation. In uncomplicated singleton pregnancies, it is unclear and controversial where this threshold lies (4). In recent years, the risk of stillbirth late in gestation has been refined (5, 6). Initially, the risk of stillbirth at each gestational age was estimated using all deliveries as the denominator. Actually, only all ongoing pregnancies are at risk. Consequently, the initial estimation of risk for stillbirth late in gestation was an underestimation because most pregnancies end before 42 weeks of gestation. Three recent epidemiologic studies have evaluated the risk of stillbirth in pregnancies near term and have demonstrated that the risk of stillbirth beyond 41 weeks of gestation was greater than previously reported. Furthermore, cervical ripening methods have improved, and current data suggest that the risk of cesarean delivery associated with induction at term may be lower than previously reported (7).

Results from the Canadian Multicentre Postterm Pregnancy Trial group would suggest that induction of labor compared with serial antenatal monitoring results not only in better outcomes but also in less cost (8). How this might apply to the U.S. population is unclear at this time. In a recent meta-analysis of 16 randomized clinical trials of induction of labor versus expectant management in pregnancies at 41 or more weeks of gestation, labor induction was associated with a lower cesarean delivery rate without an increase in adverse outcomes (9).

References

1. Martin JA, Hamilton BE, Sutton PD, Ventura SJ, Menacker F, Munson ML. Births: final data for 2002. Natl Vital Stat Rep 2003;52(10):1–113.

2. Divon MY, Haglund B, Nisell H, Otterblad PO, Westgren M. Fetal and neonatal mortality in the postterm pregnancy: the impact of gestational age and fetal growth restriction. Am J Obstet Gynecol 1998;178:726–31.

3. Management of postterm pregnancy. ACOG Practice Bulletin No. 55. American College of Obstetricians and Gynecologists. Obstet Gynecol 2004;104:639–46.

4. Rand L, Robinson JN, Economy KE, Norwitz ER. Post-term induction of labor revisited. Obstet Gynecol 2000;96:779–83.

5. Hilder L, Costeloe K, Thilaganathan B. Prolonged pregnancy: evaluating gestation, specific risks of fetal and infant mortality. Br J Obstet Gynaecol 1998;105:169–73.

6. Cotzias CS, Paterson-Brown S, Fisk NM. Prospective risk of unexplained stillbirth in singleton pregnancies at term: population based analysis. BMJ 1999;319:287–8.

7. Yeast JD, Jones A, Poskin M. Induction of labor and the relationship to cesarean delivery: a review of 7001 consecutive inductions. Am J Obstet Gynecol 1999;180:628–33.

8. Goeree R, Hannah M, Hewson S. Cost-effectiveness of induction of labour versus serial antenatal monitoring in the Canadian Multicentre Postterm Pregnancy Trial. CMAJ 1995;152:1445–50.

9. Sanchez-Ramos L, Olivier F, Delke I, Kaunitz AM. Labor induction versus expectant management for postterm pregnancies: a systematic review with meta-analysis. Obstet Gynecol 2003;101:1312–8.

Medical Complications of Pregnancy

CARDIAC DISEASE

Optimal care of a patient with cardiac disease in pregnancy is predicated on the obstetrician's understanding of the pathophysiologic changes of pregnancy, coupled with knowledge of the effects of pregnancy on the specific cardiac lesion. Care of patients with significant cardiac disease often is best accomplished by a team approach, in consultation with a cardiologist and anesthesiologist.

The general categorization of cardiac disease presented in Box 8 may be useful in counseling patients who are contemplating initiating or continuing a pregnancy (1). Patients in Group I should, with appropriate care, have minimal risk to maternal life. In patients in Group II, the risk of adverse pregnancy outcome or significant illness is increased significantly despite optimal management. For most patients in Group III, there is an unacceptable risk of death, even with optimal management. For such patients, averting or terminating pregnancy is the treatment of choice. Maternal outcome correlates with the functional classification of the patient's condition based on the criteria of the New York Heart Association (Box 9).

Recent statistics and maternal mortality estimates suggest that with appropriate care in developed countries, maternal death generally is confined to patients with pulmonary hypertension, endocarditis, ischemic cardiac disease, cardiomyopathy, and cardiac dysrhythmia (2). Women with cardiac disease face 4 hemodynamic challenges during pregnancy, the first of which is the increased intravascular volume associated with pregnancy. This increase begins early and approaches 50% by the early third trimester. Thereafter, intravascular volume reaches a plateau. Patients with fixed cardiac output may be unable to tolerate such increases in intravascular volume, and pulmonary edema may result.

Second, patients experience a decline in systemic vascular resistance as pregnancy progresses. For some lesions, such as aortic stenosis, this decrease in cardiac afterload has the potential to improve cardiac function. However, the condition of patients with right-to-left shunts (such as ventriculoseptal defect with Eisenmenger's syndrome) may deteriorate as systemic vascular resistance decreases in the face of fixed and elevated pulmonary vascular resistance. This results in shunting of blood away from the lungs, desaturation, and clinical decompensation.

Third, the estrogen-induced hypercoagulability that is associated with pregnancy poses specific hazards for some patients with atrial fibrillation or mechanical cardiac valves. Such patients are prone to systemic thromboembolism, and this risk is increased during pregnancy. Both of these conditions may require full anticoagulation

therapy. Women with mechanical cardiac devices retain a risk of embolism even with heparin therapy. For such patients, coumarin derivatives may be superior in preventing thromboembolism. Given the gravity of systemic thromboembolism in pregnancy, therapy with warfarin may be considered. With appropriate informed

---

BOX 8

Maternal Risk of Cardiac Disease Complications Associated with Pregnancy

Group I: Minimal Risk of Complications (Mortality <1%)

  Atrial septal defect*

  Ventricular septal defect*

  Patent ductus arteriosus*

  Pulmonic/tricuspid disease

  Corrected tetralogy of Fallot

  Bioprosthetic valve

  Mitral stenosis, New York Heart Association classes I and II

  Marfan's syndrome with normal aorta

Group II: Moderate Risk of Complications (Mortality 5–15%)

  Mitral stenosis with atrial fibrillation[†]

  Artificial valve[†]

  Mitral stenosis, New York Heart Association classes III and IV

  Aortic stenosis

  Coarctation of aorta, uncomplicated

  Uncorrected tetralogy of Fallot

  Previous myocardial infarction

Group III: Major Risk of Complications or Death (Mortality >25%)

  Pulmonary hypertension

  Coarctation of aorta, complicated

  Marfan's syndrome with aortic involvement

*If unassociated with pulmonary hypertension

[†]If anticoagulation with heparin, rather than warfarin, is elected

Reprinted from Foley MR. Cardiac disease. Dildy GA 3d, Belfort MA, Svade GR, Phelan JP, Hankins GD, Clark SL, editors. Critical care obstetrics. 4th ed. Malden (MA): Blackwell Science; 2004.

consent, an option is the use of full anticoagulation therapy with low-molecular-weight heparin for the duration of pregnancy or the substitution of warfarin during the middle trimester. The former approach eliminates any significant fetal risk but may incur an increased risk of maternal systemic thromboembolism; the latter will reduce but may not eliminate fetal risk while minimizing maternal risk, at least during the middle trimester.

Finally, normal pregnancy is associated with marked fluctuations in cardiac output during labor, delivery, and the postpartum period. Patients with fixed cardiac output may be unable to tolerate such sudden shifts, and pulmonary edema may result.

With an appropriate understanding of these clinical issues, the obstetrician can be prepared, in consultation with a cardiologist and anesthesiologist, to develop a management scheme that minimizes the risk of complications. For example, with patients in whom increased preload may not be well tolerated, diuresis and heart rate control (in cases of mitral stenosis) may improve the chances for a successful pregnancy outcome. In a similar fashion, appropriate conduction anesthesia during labor and delivery may minimize cardiac output fluctuations for patients whose cardiac lesions otherwise may not allow them to tolerate the delivery process.

BOX 9

New York Heart Association Classification of Cardiovascular Disease

Class I: Patients who are not limited by cardiac disease in their physical activity. Ordinary physical activity does not precipitate the occurrence of symptoms such as fatigue, palpitations, dyspnea, and angina.

Class II: Patients in whom the cardiac disease causes a slight limitation in physical activity. These patients are comfortable at rest, but ordinary physical activity will precipitate symptoms.

Class III: Patients in whom the cardiac disease results in a marked limitation of physical activity. They are comfortable at rest, but less than ordinary physical activity will precipitate symptoms.

Class IV: Patients in whom the cardiac disease results in the inability to carry on physical activity without discomfort. Symptoms may be present even at rest, and discomfort is increased by any physical activity.

Reprinted from Obstetric anesthesia, 2nd ed. Camann WR, Thornhill ML. Cardiovascular disease. Chestnut DH, editor. p. 776–808. Copyright 1999, with permission from Elsevier.

Prophylaxis Against Subacute Bacterial Endocarditis

It remains controversial whether patients with valvular cardiac disease who undergo uncomplicated vaginal delivery benefit from prophylaxis against subacute bacterial endocarditis (SBE). The American Heart Association (AHA) does not recommend prophylaxis for delivery of low-risk patients (Box 10). However, because predicting the absence of complications is almost impossible and because for optimal effectiveness the antibiotics should be administered 30 minutes before the anticipated bacteremia, many authorities administer SBE prophylaxis during labor and delivery for patients who would otherwise be candidates for such therapy. This would include most patients with structural cardiac abnormalities or valvular disease. The recommended treatment is ampicillin, 2 g intravenously, and gentamicin, 1 mg/kg intravenously, administered 30–60 minutes before delivery. Vancomycin is an alternative for patients who are allergic to penicillin. The value of 1 or 2 repeat doses of antibiotics at 8-hour intervals after delivery is uncertain.

Maternal Conditions

RIGHT-SIDED LESIONS

Right-sided structural cardiac lesions, when not associated with pulmonary hypertension, generally are tolerated well during pregnancy, labor, and delivery. Attention to appropriate fluid balance and prophylaxis against SBE are important management principles.

LEFT-SIDED LESIONS

Left-sided lesions are more complex than right-sided ones. In patients with mitral stenosis, control of heart rate with β-blockers and, at times, judicious diuresis to avoid pulmonary edema are essential (3). Both of these treatments generally can be carried out without fear of adverse fetal effects. During labor and delivery in patients with severe mitral stenosis, pulmonary artery catheterization may sometimes be helpful in allowing the clinician to reduce preload through cautious diuresis while maintaining cardiac output. Patients who deliver with pulmonary capillary wedge pressure levels exceeding 14–16 mm Hg appear to have an increased likelihood of postpartum pulmonary edema.

In patients with aortic stenosis, the problem is somewhat different. In the presence of an intact mitral valve, pulmonary edema is uncommon. Rather, these patients are at risk of sudden hypotension, arrhythmia, and death should preload fall. Thus, avoidance of hypovolemia or hypotension is essential. In addition, for patients with significant aortic stenosis, activity restriction during pregnancy is essential. Intrapartum fluid and blood component replacement should be geared to avoiding

Medical Complications

American Academy of Dermatology
www.aad.org

American Autoimmune Related Diseases Association
www.aarda.org

American Cancer Society
www.cancer.org

American College of Obstetricians and Gynecologists
www.acog.org

American College of Rheumatology
www.rheumatology.org

American Diabetes Association
www.diabetes.org

American Heart Association
www.americanheart.org

American Lung Association
www.lungusa.org

American Society for Dermatologic Surgery
www.asds-net.org

American Thyroid Association
www.thyroid.org

ClinicalTrials.gov
clinicaltrials.gov

MEDLINEplus
medlineplus.gov

National Cancer Institute
www.nci.nih.gov

National Center for Infectious Diseases
www.cdc.gov/ncidod

National Heart, Lung, and Blood Institute
www.nhlbi.nih.gov

National Institute of Allergy and Infectious Diseases
www.niaid.nih.gov

National Institute of Arthritis and Musculoskeletal
and Skin Diseases
www.niams.nih.gov

National Institute of Diabetes and Digestive and
Kidney Diseases
www.niddk.nih.gov

National Institute of Neurological Disorders and Stroke
www.ninds.nih.gov

Society of Gynecologic Oncologists
www.sgo.org

hypotension. As in patients with mitral stenosis, SBE prophylaxis is essential.

Patients with isolated mitral or aortic insufficiency generally tolerate labor and delivery without significant complication; again, careful attention to intake and output as well as SBE prophylaxis is essential. Most patients with significant cardiac disease will benefit from the intrapartum administration of oxygen and epidural anesthesia during labor.

Pulmonary Hypertension

Pulmonary hypertension, which remains one of the most dangerous complications of pregnancy, may be either primary or secondary to long-standing valvular lesions, such as mitral stenosis. Although patients with pulmonary hypertension may develop shortness of breath and cardiovascular decompensation during the antepartum period, the most critical time for these women is the peripartum period. During this time, any event that decreases cardiac preload, such as blood loss or, at times, conduction anesthesia, may dramatically and abruptly reduce pulmonary perfusion, resulting in desaturation and cardiovascular collapse. Thus, during labor in these patients, any fall in cardiac preload must be scrupulously avoided and blood volume maintained, even at the cost of pulmonary edema. In severe cases, pulmonary artery catheterization may be

BOX 10

American Heart Association Recommendations on Prophylaxis of Bacterial Endocarditis

The American Heart Association does not recommend prophylactic treatment for the following genitourinary tract procedures:

- Vaginal hysterectomy*
- Vaginal delivery*
- Cesarean delivery*
- In uninfected tissue:
  — Urethral catheterization
  — Uterine dilation and curettage
  — Therapeutic abortion
  — Sterilization procedure
  — Insertion or removal of intrauterine device

*Prophylaxis is optional for high-risk patients.

Dajani AS, Taubert KA, Wilson W, Bolger AF, Bayer A, Ferrieri P, et al. Prevention of bacterial endocarditis. Recommendations by the American Heart Association. JAMA 1997;277:1794–801. Copyrighted 1997, American Medical Association.

of assistance in ensuring adequate cardiac output and intravascular volume. Such patients also may decompensate and develop intractable and ultimately fatal right heart failure in the postpartum period. Although the exact cause of this event is unknown, a rebound worsening of pulmonary hypertension associated with the loss of placental hormones is suspected.

Ischemic Cardiac Disease

Ischemic cardiac disease carries a significant risk during pregnancy because of the increased oxygen demand on the heart (4). Thus, patients with a history of coronary artery cardiac disease should be counseled against pregnancy. If pregnancy is to be undertaken, bed rest often is essential to minimize myocardial oxygen demands as the fetus grows. The use of nitrates for angina is acceptable during pregnancy, as is the use of β-blocking agents and clopidogrel. The prevalence of ischemic heart disease seems to be increasing possibly because more women are becoming pregnant at an older age.

Mitral Valve Prolapse

Mitral valve prolapse, a relatively common and generally benign syndrome, affects up to 17% of women of childbearing age. The diagnosis is suspected by auscultation of a systolic murmur and click and can be confirmed by echocardiography. Patients may develop troublesome palpitations, which are amenable to treatment with β-blocking agents. Patients with evidence of mitral valve regurgitation should receive SBE prophylaxis during pregnancy.

Fetal Considerations

Patients with cyanotic heart disease or those with reduced cardiac output are at risk for IUGR and stillbirth. In such patients, delivery for fetal rather than maternal deterioration is relatively common. Thus, serial ultrasonography to assess fetal growth and antepartum fetal heart rate assessment in the third trimester are important in any woman with cardiac disease complicated by maternal hypoxia or reduced cardiac output.

The risk of fetal cardiac defects is increased in women with congenital cardiac anomalies. This risk is on the order of 5% but may approach 10% or higher in women with congenital outflow tract obstruction. Thus, in any woman with congenital cardiac disease, fetal echocardiography is essential.

Peripartum Cardiomyopathy

Cardiomyopathy is a relatively common cause of death during pregnancy. Peripartum cardiomyopathy is defined as the development of cardiac failure with echocardiographic evidence of left ventricular dysfunction in the last month of pregnancy or within 5 months of delivery in the absence of both an identifiable cause of cardiac failure and recognizable cardiac disease prior to the last month of pregnancy (5). In practice, deviation from this definition often leads to overdiagnosis. Maternal mortality from peripartum cardiomyopathy approaches 20% (6). Treatment is nonspecific and may include inotropic support, diuresis, and afterload reduction in addition to delivery. In survivors, subclinical reductions in contractile reserve generally persist, increasing the maternal risk during future pregnancies (7).

References

1. Cardiac disease. In: Clark SL, Cotton DB, Hankins GD, Phelan JP, editors. Critical care obstetrics. 3rd ed. Malden (MA): Blackwell Science; 1997.

2. Berg CJ, Atrash HK, Koonin LM, Tucker M. Pregnancy-related mortality in the United States, 1987–1990. Obstet Gynecol 1996;88:161–7.

3. Desai DK, Adanlawo M, Naidoo DP, Moodley J, Kleinschmidt I. Mitral stenosis in pregnancy: a four-year experience at King Edward VIII Hospital, Durban, South Africa. BJOG 2000;107:953–8.

4. Roth A, Elkayam U. Acute myocardial infarction associated with pregnancy. Ann Intern Med 1996;125:751–62.

5. Pearson GD, Veille JC, Rahimtoola S, Hsia J, Oakley CM, Hosenpud JD, et al. Peripartum cardiomyopathy: National Heart, Lung, and Blood Institute and Office of Rare Diseases (National Institutes of Health) workshop recommendations and review. JAMA 2000;283:1183–8.

6. Witlin AG, Mabie WC, Sibai BM. Peripartum cardiomyopathy: an ominous diagnosis. Am J Obstet Gynecol 1997; 176:182–8.

7. Lampert MB, Weinert L, Hibbard J, Korcarz C, Lindheimer M, Lang RM. Contractile reserve in patients with peripartum cardiomyopathy and recovered left ventricular function. Am J Obstet Gynecol 1997;176:189–95.

CHRONIC HYPERTENSION

Chronic hypertension is preexisting hypertension or hypertension present before the 20th week of pregnancy. Hypertension is defined as a systolic blood pressure of 140 mm Hg or more or a diastolic blood pressure of 90 mm Hg or more or both. Chronic hypertension is classified as mild (≥140/90 mm Hg) or severe (≥180/110 mm Hg) (1). Preeclampsia superimposed on chronic hypertension is discussed in the section on preeclampsia.

Chronic hypertension appearing for the first time during pregnancy, especially after 20 weeks of gestation, can be difficult (if not impossible) to distinguish from preeclampsia or gestational hypertension. In some cases, the diagnosis cannot be confirmed until after 12 weeks postpartum when there is persistent hypertension (1, 2).

Effects in Pregnancy

Pregnant women with chronic hypertension have increased complications, the most common of which is the development of superimposed preeclampsia. This complication occurs in approximately 25% or more of women with preexisting hypertension (3). Other potential complications include intrauterine growth restriction, placental abruption, and fetal demise. These risks are far higher in the presence of superimposed preeclampsia. The cesarean delivery rate also is increased. Maternal complications such as stroke, dilated cardiomyopathy and heart failure, and myocardial infarction are uncommon in pregnancy unless the patient has severe, uncontrolled hypertension. The development of superimposed preeclampsia in these women is associated with an increased risk of both perinatal death and placental abruption (3).

Treatment

The only compelling reason to treat women with chronic hypertension is to prevent maternal catastrophic cardiovascular complications. Thus there appears to be little, if any, benefit to treat pregnant women with mild hypertension unless the patient has other complications such as preexisting renal or cardiovascular disease (1). In 2 meta-analyses of antihypertensive therapy versus no therapy, not only was there no fetal benefit of therapy, but the incidence of growth restriction was increased (4, 5). It is recommended, however, that women with severe chronic hypertension (1, 6) be treated, although the benefit to the fetus of such therapy is less than clear (7).

Probably the two most commonly used antihypertensive agents to treat pregnant women are methyldopa and labetalol. Various antihypertensives for the treatment of chronic hypertension during pregnancy are summarized in Table 10 (1–3). The angiotensin-converting enzyme (ACE) inhibitors should be avoided during pregnancy because of the potential for both teratogenic effects and subsequent fetal and neonatal effects from their use (1, 2). Atenolol use in the first trimester is associated with low birth weight (8).

The treatment of superimposed preeclampsia in women with chronic hypertension is the same as that for preeclampsia (see "Preeclampsia").

References

1. Chronic hypertension in pregnancy. ACOG Practice Bulletin No. 29. American College of Obstetricians and Gynecologists. Obstet Gynecol 2001;98:177–85.

2. Report of the National High Blood Pressure Education Program Working Group on High Blood Pressure in Pregnancy. Am J Obstet Gynecol 2000;183:S1–S22.

3. Sibai BM, Lindheimer M, Hauth J, Caritis S, vanDorsten P, Klebanoff M, et al. Risk factors for preeclampsia, abruptio placentae, and adverse neonatal outcomes among women with chronic hypertension. National Institute of Child Health and Human Development Network of Maternal-Fetal Medicine Units. N Engl J Med 1998;339:667–71.

4. von Dadelszen P, Ornstein MP, Bull SB, Logan AG, Koren G, Magee LA. Fall in mean arterial pressure and fetal growth restriction in pregnancy hypertension: a meta-analysis. Lancet 2000;355:87–92.

5. Magee LA, Ornstein MP, von Dadelszen P. Fortnightly review: management of hypertension in pregnancy. BMJ 1999;318:1332–6.

6. Sibai BM. Chronic hypertension in pregnancy. Obstet Gynecol 2002;100:369–77.

7. Roberts JM, Pearson GD, Cutler JA, Lindheimer MD; National Heart, Lung and Blood Institute. Summary of the NHLBI Working Group on Research on Hypertension During Pregnancy. Hypertens Pregnancy 2003;22:109–27.

8. Bayliss H, Churchill D, Beevers M, Beevers DG. Antihypertensive drugs in pregnancy and fetal growth: evidence for "pharmacological programming" in the first trimester? Hypertens Pregnancy 2002;21:161–74.

DEEP VEIN THROMBOSIS AND PULMONARY EMBOLISM

Thromboembolism is a leading cause of maternal mortality. The prevalence of DVT has been reported to be 0.13 per 1,000 in the antepartum period and 0.61 per 1,000 in the postpartum period (within 4 weeks of delivery). The occurrence of coexistent pulmonary embolism depends on whether treatment for DVT has been initiated expeditiously. If patients with DVT remain untreated, up to 25% will develop pulmonary embolism, with 15% dying of their illness. In contrast, fewer than 5% of patients receiving anticoagulant treatment for DVT will develop pulmonary embolism and less than 1% will die.

All elements of Virchow's triad (stasis, hypercoagulability, vascular derangements) are present in pregnancy, contributing to the enhanced risk of venous thrombosis seen in pregnant women. Stasis of blood in the lower extremities results from estrogen-mediated stimulation of nitric oxide production, which induces increased deep venous capacitance. In addition, position-related uterine compression can lead to varying degrees of progressive deep venous stasis (1). Delivery, especially operative vaginal delivery and cesarean delivery, and puerperal infections are associated with vascular damage and induction of endothelial tissue factor expression and thus increased risk for DVT (2).

Other pregnancy-related clinical risk factors for DVT include varicosities with venous vascular insufficiency and increased parity. Finally, many clinical risk factors for DVT observed in nonpregnant individuals also may be present. These include trauma, orthopedic injury, nephrotic syndrome, obesity, increased bed rest, age older than 35 years, and previous thromboembolic event.

In addition to clinical risk factors, pregnancy-associated changes in hemostatic and fibrinolytic proteins pro-

TABLE 10. Antihypertensive Therapy for Pregnant Women With Chronic Hypertension

Agent*	Dosage	Comments
Central sympatholytic agents: methyldopa	Oral: 250 mg at bedtime increasing to twice daily, or every 6 h (max = 500 mg every 6 h) IV: 250–500 mg every 6 h	Drowsiness, dry mouth, nasal congestion, rebound hypertension, sedation, lethargy, dizziness, nausea, diarrhea, depression, sodium and water retention, drug-induced hepatitis; excreted by kidneys, half-life = 1.8 h.
Diuretic (thiazide): hydrochlorothiazide	Oral: 12.5 mg daily increasing to 25 mg daily	Decreased potassium sodium, magnesium, zinc; increased uric acid, glucose, BUN/Cr, Ca+, cholesterol.
Diuretic (loop): furosemide	Oral: 20–40 mg daily increasing to 160 mg twice daily IV: 40–80 mg (4 mg/min)	Monitor for fluid and increasing electrolyte imbalances. Increased glucose, uric acid; decreased potassium, magnesium. Patients allergic to sulfonamides may be allergic to furosemide. Dizziness, headache, gastrointestinal irritation, hypotension.
β-Adrenergic blocker: atenolol	Oral: 25 mg increasing to 100 mg daily	Bradycardia, fatigue, nausea and vomiting, dizziness, depression. May increase cholesterol, rebound hypertension. Not for use in patients with diabetes, hyperthyroidism, or intermittent claudication. Intrauterine growth restriction.
α/β-Adrenergic blocker: labetalol	Oral: 100 mg twice daily increasing to 400 mg twice daily IV: 20 mg over 10 min (max = 2 mg/min infusion)	Gastrointestinal distress, fluid retention, dry mouth, orthostatic hypotension; half-life = 5.8 h, excreted by kidneys (55–60%), 30% in feces.
Calcium antagonist: felodipine	Oral: 5–10 mg daily increasing to 10 mg twice daily	99% bound to plasma proteins. Hepatic metabolism; reflex increase in heart rate; selective effects on vascular smooth muscle much greater than those on cardiac muscle. Peripheral edema, headache.

IV indicates intravenous(ly); BUN, blood urea nitrogen; Cr, creatinine.

*All medications are pregnancy category C, except hydrochlorothiazide (category D). Angiotensin-converting enzyme inhibitors are contraindicated in pregnancy because of the risk of fetal effects starting in the second trimester. Pregnancy interruption is not advised when exposure has occurred in the early first trimester.

mote thromboembolism. Pregnancy is associated with a 20–200% increase in levels of fibrinogen, prothrombin (factor II), and clotting factors VII, VIII, X, and XII. In contrast, levels of the endogenous anticoagulant protein S decrease significantly during pregnancy, while concentrations of the antifibrinolytic type 1 plasminogen activator inhibitor increase by up to 3-fold. These hemostatic alterations likely reduce the risk of antepartum, intrapartum, and postpartum hemorrhage, but their net effect is to promote clot formation, extension, and stability, thus contributing significantly to the 10-fold increase in pregnancy-associated venous thrombosis. The risk of venous thrombosis is increased further in pregnant women with antiphospholipid syndrome or inherited thrombophilias (3, 4).

Antiphospholipid Syndrome

Antiphospholipid syndrome is the most common acquired thrombophilia and accounts for 14% (2–20%) of venous thrombosis in pregnancy (3, 4). Additionally, antiphospholipid syndrome is associated with thrombocytopenia and recurrent fetal loss. In antiphospholipid syndrome, antiphospholipid antibodies are directed against proteins bound to negatively charged (anionic) phospholipids. The most commonly encountered forms of the syndrome are isolated lupus anticoagulant antibodies, anticardiolipin antibodies, and anti-β_2-glycoprotein-I antibodies.

For a diagnosis of antiphospholipid syndrome, the patient must meet 1 of 2 clinical criteria and at least 1 of 2 laboratory criteria (Box 11). None of the many other

BOX 11

International Consensus Statement on Preliminary Criteria for the Classification of the Antiphospholipid Syndrome*

Clinical Criteria

Vascular thrombosis

One or more clinical episodes of arterial, venous, or small-vessel thrombosis, occurring within any tissue or organ

Complications of pregnancy

One or more unexplained deaths of morphologically normal fetuses at or after the 10th week of gestation; or

One or more premature births of morphologically normal neonates at or before the 34th week of gestation; or

Three or more unexplained consecutive spontaneous abortions before the 10th week of gestation

Laboratory Criteria[†]

Anticardiolipin antibodies

Anticardiolipin IgG or IgM antibodies present at moderate or high levels in the blood on 2 or more occasions at least 6 weeks apart[‡]

Lupus anticoagulant antibodies

Lupus anticoagulant antibodies detected in the blood on 2 or more occasions at least 6 weeks apart, according to the guidelines of the International Society on Thrombosis and Hemostasis[§]

*A diagnosis of definite antiphospholipid syndrome requires the presence of at least 1 of the clinical criteria and at least one of the laboratory criteria. No limits are placed on the interval between the clinical event and the positive laboratory findings.

[†]The following antiphospholipid antibodies are currently not included in the laboratory criteria: anticardiolipin IgA antibodies, anti-β_2-glycoprotein I antibodies, and antiphospholipid antibodies directed against phospholipids other than cardiolipin (eg, phosphatidylserine and phosphatidylethanolamine) or against phospholipid-binding proteins other than cardiolipin-bound β_2-glycoprotein I (eg, prothrombin, annexin V, protein C, or protein S).

[‡]The threshold used to distinguish moderate or high levels of anticardiolipin antibodies from low levels has not been standardized and may depend on the population under study. Many laboratories use 15 or 20 international "phospholipid" units as the threshold separating low from moderate levels of anticardiolipin antibodies. Others define the threshold as 20 or 2.5 times the median level of anticardiolipin antibodies or as the 99th percentile of anticardiolipin levels within a normal population. Until an international consensus is reached, any of these 3 definitions seems reasonable.

[§]Guidelines are from Brandt JT, Triplett DA, Alving B, Scharrer I. Criteria for the diagnosis of lupus anticoagulants: an update. Thromb Haemost 1995;74:1185–90.

Levine JS, Branch DW, Rauch J. The antiphospholipid syndrome. N Engl J Med 2002;346:752–63. Copyright © 2002 Massachusetts Medical Society. All rights reserved.

clinical manifestations of the disorder need be present. Although other antiphospholipid antibodies may be present, their clinical significance (other than those directed against anticardiolipin IgG and IgM) remains unclear.

Inherited Thrombophilias

The inherited forms of thrombophilia include a wide variety of relatively common genetic conditions that predispose women to DVT (Table 11). They also have been clearly implicated in fetal loss (spontaneous abortion and stillbirth). The role of DVT in IUGR is unclear.

Inherited thrombophilias increase the risk of thromboembolism in pregnancy 8-fold. These episodes include not only typical lower-extremity DVT and pulmonary embolism, but also unusual thrombotic manifestations such as sagittal, mesenteric, and portal vein thromboses.

Excluding hyperhomocysteinemia, only 8–14% of the Caucasian population meets laboratory criteria for a thrombophilic disorder; however, they account for 70% of venous thromboses diagnosed in pregnancy (5, 6). A pregnant patient with an inherited thrombophilia of low thrombogenic potential (ie, heterozygotes or compound heterozygotes for the Factor V Leiden and prothrombin G20210A mutations, as well as protein C or protein S deficiencies, or the rare patient with hyperhomocysteinemia unresponsive to folate and vitamin B_{12} therapy) and a history of thromboembolism should be treated with prophylactic unfractionated or low-molecular-weight heparin during pregnancy. However, patients with highly thrombogenic thrombophilias (ie, antithrombin deficiency or homozygotes for the Factor V Leiden or prothrombin G20210A mutations) appear to require therapeutic heparin (see "Prevention" for details).

TABLE 11. Inheritance, Diagnosis, Prevalence, and Relative Pathogenicity of the Inherited Thrombophilias

Disorder	Genetics	Assays	Prevalence	Risk of VTE
Factor V Leiden	AD	DNA	3–15%	3–8-fold (0.2%)
Prothrombin G20210A	AD	DNA	2–3%	3-fold (0.5%)
Antithrombin	AD	Activity assay	0.02%	25–50-fold (50%)
Protein C	AD	Activity assay	0.2–0.3%	10–15-fold (4%)
Protein S	AD	Activity assay If low, assess total & free antigen	0.1–2.1%	2-fold (4%)
Hyperhomocysteinemia	AR	Fasting homocysteine level ± MTHFR mutation screen	11%	2.5-fold (levels >18.5 µmol/L) and 3–4-fold (>200 µmol/L) (0.25–0.35%)

AD indicates autosomal dominant; AR, autosomal recessive; MTHFT, methylene tetrahydrofolate reductase.

Data from Haemostasis and Thrombosis Task Force, British Committee for Standards in Haematology. Investigation and management of heritable thrombophilia. Brit J Haematol 2001;114:512–28.

Diagnosis

DEEP VEIN THROMBOSIS

The clinical diagnosis of DVT in pregnancy is often inaccurate and unreliable. Of patients exhibiting the classic features of DVT (ie, calf or thigh tenderness, pain, erythema, and edema), more than one half do not have the condition. Thus, compression color Doppler ultrasonography of the femoral and popliteal veins and calf trifurcation should be performed to confirm the diagnosis. This approach has been found to be highly sensitive (>98%) and specific (>96%) in detecting thromboses of the deep femoral and popliteal veins (7). If ultrasound findings are abnormal, venous thrombosis is diagnosed and treatment initiated. A follow-up scan is required within 3 days to confirm the results. If ultrasound findings are normal but there is a high index of suspicion (positive history, clinical progression), contrast venography is indicated. Venography with an abdominal lead shield exposes the fetus to low levels of radiation (<0.0005 Gy [0.05 rad])— far lower than the dose associated with childhood cancers (> 0.04 Gy [4 rads]) and teratogenicity (>1.6 Gy [160 rads]). Contrast venography is the most accurate method of diagnosing DVT in pregnancy. Alternatively, magnetic resonance imaging (MRI) or computed tomography (CT) can be used to secure a diagnosis, although experience with these modalities is limited.

PULMONARY EMBOLISM

The classic clinical triad of dyspnea, pleuritic chest pain, and hemoptysis occurs in only one quarter of patients with documented pulmonary embolism. Although patients may display hypoxia, 17% of patients will have normal PaO_2 laboratory values. Echocardiographic findings in severe cases may include right ventricular dilation and hypokinesis, tricuspid regurgitation, and pulmonary artery dilation. An electrocardiogram may reveal right bundle branch block, right axis shift, Q wave in leads III and aVF, S wave in leads I and aVL greater than 1.5 mm, T wave inversions in leads III and aVF, or new onset atrial fibrillation.

A ventilation and perfusion scan (V/Q scan) should be the initial evaluation if available, but results must be interpreted based on a high degree of suspicion. The amount of radiation exposure from a V/Q scan is less than 0.005 Gy (0.5 rad) of radiation, whereas spiral CT scans and pulmonary angiography, with appropriate abdominal shielding, expose the fetus to less than 0.0005 Gy (0.05 rad) for the entire examination. Magnetic resonance imaging or spiral volumetric computed tomography (SVCT) pulmonary angiography can be employed as noninvasive substitutes. Thus, a pulmonary angiogram should be obtained in a high-risk patient with a negative compression ultrasound result. However, the reported sensitivities of these techniques vary between 60% and 90%. Although SVCT is relatively sensitive and specific for diagnosing central pulmonary artery thrombi, it is insensitive for diagnosing subsegmental clots. Thus, SVCT appears to have a role as a "rule-in" test for large central emboli but cannot exclude smaller peripheral lesions. A high-risk patient with a positive spiral CT requires therapy, but a negative spiral CT should prompt pulmonary angiography.

Prevention

If there is a high degree of suspicion of DVT, treatment with heparin should be considered pending availability of results (Box 12).

As noted previously, women with high-risk thrombophilias (ie, antithrombin deficiency and homozygosity for the Factor V Leiden and prothrombin G20210A mutations), regardless of personal history of venous thrombosis, should be treated with full therapeutic anticoagulation

---

BOX 12

Prophylactic Heparin Regimens in Pregnancy

Unfractionated Heparin

Low-dose prophylaxis:

1. 5,000–7,500 U every 12 hours during the first trimester

   7,500–10,000 U every 12 hours during the second trimester

   10,000 U every 12 hours during the third trimester unless the APTT is elevated. The APTT may be checked near term and the heparin dose reduced if prolonged

OR

2. 5,000–10,000 U every 12 hours throughout pregnancy, adjusting dose to ≥10,000 U twice to three times a day to achieve APTT of 1.5–2.5 × control, 6 hours after treatment

Low-Molecular-Weight Heparin

Low-dose prophylaxis:

Dalteparin, 5,000 U once or twice daily, or enoxaparin, 40 mg once daily or 30 mg twice daily

Adjusted-dose prophylaxis:

Dalteparin, 5,000–10,000 U every 12 hours, or enoxaparin, 30–80 mg every 12 hours, adjusting the dose to achieve an anti-factor Xa level of 0.1–0.2 U/mL 4 hours after treatment

APTT indicates activated partial thromboplastin time.

Data from Colvin BT, Barrowcliffe TW. The British Society for Haematology guidelines on the use and monitoring of heparin 1992: second revision. J Clin Pathol 1993;46:97–103. Ginsberg JS, Hirsh J. Use of antithrombotic agents during pregnancy. Chest 1998;114:524S-530S. Guidelines on the presentation, investigation and management of thrombosis associated with pregnancy. Maternal and Neonatal Haemostasis Working Party of the Haemostasis and Thrombosis Task. J Clin Pathol 1993;46: 489–96.

Modified from American College of Obstetricians and Gynecologists. Thromboembolism in pregnancy. ACOG Practice Bulletin 19. Washington, DC: ACOG; 2000.

---

during pregnancy and maintained on anticoagulation for at least 6 weeks postpartum and up to 3 months if they have a history of prior venous thromboembolism. In contrast, pregnant women with low-risk thrombophilias (ie, heterozygotes for the Factor V Leiden and prothrombin G20210A mutations, as well as protein C or protein S deficiencies, or hyperhomocysteinemia unresponsive to folate and vitamin B_{12} therapy) and no personal history of DVT have a low incidence of DVT in pregnancy (0.2–4%) and do not appear to require antepartum antico-

agulation therapy (8). However, they should receive anticoagulation therapy postpartum if they require a cesarean delivery, because the vast majority of fatal pulmonary emboli occur during this period, or if they have other major risk factors for thrombosis (eg, obesity, prior prolonged bed rest, strong family history) (9, 10). Although controversial, patients without an identifiable thrombophilia whose prior thrombosis occurred during pregnancy should probably be given low-dose heparin as antenatal prophylaxis.

Treatment

The mainstays of therapy for DVT are anticoagulation, elevation of the extremity, and analgesia. For pulmonary embolism, therapy includes initiation of anticoagulation therapy and maintenance of adequate cardiac output and oxygenation. When DVT occurs during pregnancy or the puerperium or when a pregnant woman requires anticoagulation based on risk factors (eg, orthopedic surgery, immobilization, mechanical heart valve) or history (prior DVT), heparin is the anticoagulant of choice. It does not cross the placenta, appears to be safe for the fetus, and does not enter breast milk.

The maternal side effects of heparin therapy include hemorrhage, thrombocytopenia, and osteoporosis. Hemorrhage is more common with concomitant aspirin use or in the face of thrombocytopenia or liver disease and occurs less frequently when low-molecular-weight heparin preparations are employed. Heparin-induced thrombocytopenia occurs in 3% of patients and has 2 forms: 1) early-onset, transient, heparin-induced platelet aggregation, for which therapy need not be interrupted; and 2) immunoglobulin G (IgG)–mediated, heparin-induced, potentially severe, thrombotic thrombocytopenia occurring within 2 weeks of initiating therapy, which mandates cessation of therapy. Heparin-induced osteoporosis is far more common when doses of more than 15,000 units per day are given for more than 6 months. These patients might benefit from dietary supplementation with 1,500 mg of calcium per day. Low-molecular-weight preparations are associated with lower risks of heparin-induced thrombocytopenia and osteoporosis.

The dose of unfractionated heparin required may vary secondarily to differences in heparin-binding proteins in pregnancy. The aPTT, heparin, or anti-factor Xa level should be evaluated every 4 hours during the initial phase of therapy and dosages adjusted as needed to maintain an activated partial thromboplastin time (aPTT) between 1.5 and 2.5 times control. Intravenous therapeutic unfractionated heparin should be continued for at least 5 days or until clinical improvement is noted. Unfractionated heparin may then be administered subcutaneously every 8–12 hours to maintain the aPTT at 1.5–2 times control, 6 hours after the injection.

Women with DVT diagnosed during a pregnancy should receive therapeutic anticoagulation for at least

3 months during the pregnancy followed by prophylactic therapy (11). However, one study found that 6 months of anticoagulation treatment after a first episode of idiopathic DVT substantially reduced the recurrence rate (1.3% per patient year compared with 23% for patients on a 3-month regimen) (12). Women with a history of DVT remote from pregnancy and the puerperium that was associated with a nonrecurrent risk factor (eg, surgery, orthopedic immobilization) but without acquired or inherited thrombophilias appear to be at very low risk for recurrence. Although anticoagulation during the antepartum period appears unnecessary in such patients, DVT prophylaxis should be employed during the postpartum period.

Postpartum anticoagulation therapy should be continued for 6–12 weeks after DVT and for 4–6 months after pulmonary embolism or complex iliofemoral DVT. Oral anticoagulant therapy can be initiated postpartum by titrating the warfarin dose to maintain the patient's international normalized ratio (INR) at approximately 2. Because warfarin exerts a more rapid inhibitory effect on levels of protein C than on the procoagulant factors and given that protein S levels are suppressed during pregnancy, heparin should be maintained during the initial 4 days of warfarin therapy or until a therapeutic INR is reached to avoid warfarin-induced skin necrosis and paradoxical thromboembolism.

LOW-MOLECULAR-WEIGHT HEPARIN

Low-molecular-weight heparin has been shown to be a safe and effective alternative to traditional unfractionated heparin for both acute treatment and thromboprophylaxis of venous thromboembolism in pregnant patients (13). Like unfractionated heparin, low-molecular-weight heparin does not cross the placenta and has no teratogenic effects. However, compared with unfractionated heparin, low-molecular-weight heparin has a longer half-life and bioavailability, a more predictable dose–response relationship, and decreased risk of thrombocytopenia and hemorrhagic complications. Growing experience with the use of low-molecular-weight heparin during pregnancy suggests that it also can be used in pregnancy to treat patients with venous thrombosis, pulmonary embolism, or thrombophilic disorders. The goal of therapy is to maintain the anti-factor Xa activity between 0.5 and 1.2 units/mL and the heparin level between 0.2 and 0.4 units/mL (11).

WARFARIN

The anticoagulant activity of warfarin is a result of its inhibition of vitamin K, which is a cofactor in the synthesis of factors VII, IX, X, and prothrombin (factor II). Carrying a 33% risk of embryopathy (ie, nasal hypoplasia, stippled epiphysis, and central nervous system abnormalities) when exposure is between gestational weeks 7 and 12, it is loosely bound to albumin and crosses the placenta. Fetal and placental bleeding is also a serious complication with warfarin use throughout pregnancy. Vitamin K or fresh frozen plasma can be used to reverse the effect of warfarin. Warfarin use during pregnancy is normally contraindicated. However, pregnant women with mechanical heart valves may constitute a group that warrant warfarin use during the second trimester of pregnancy because current studies suggest an increase in thrombogenic complications using unfractionated heparin (14). Warfarin does not accumulate in breast milk or have an anticoagulant effect on the infant and is not contraindicated in breastfeeding mothers.

Special Considerations

GREENFIELD FILTER PLACEMENT

Placement of a Greenfield filter in the inferior vena cava may be mandated by the following events:

- Recurrent pulmonary embolism despite adequate anticoagulant therapy
- Pulmonary embolism or iliofemoral DVT in a patient with a contraindication to anticoagulation therapy
- Development of serious hemorrhagic sequelae with anticoagulant therapy

EPIDURAL ANESTHESIA IN PATIENTS RECEIVING LOW-MOLECULAR-WEIGHT HEPARIN

Epidural hematoma formation has been reported in patients receiving regional anesthesia while receiving low-molecular-weight heparin. To avoid this untoward event, patients may be switched from low-molecular-weight heparin to unfractionated heparin at or near term. Alternatively, if the last dose of low-molecular-weight heparin was more than 24 hours before the administration of regional anesthesia, the risk of hematoma formation should be low. Consultation with an experienced anesthesiologist is indicated (15).

MECHANICAL HEART VALVES

Long-term anticoagulant therapy is indicated in most patients with mechanical heart valve prostheses. Compared to unfractionated heparin use throughout pregnancy, the use of warfarin in these women was associated with the "greatest maternal protection" (14). The risk of thrombosis in the heparin group and the warfarin group was 25% and 3.9%, respectively, while the risks of maternal mortality were 7% and 1.8%, respectively (16). Among the women in this study, the use of warfarin between gestational weeks 6 and 12 was associated with a doubling of the fetal loss rate to 30% and observation of stigmata of the fetal warfarin syndrome in 6% of cases. Thus, with appropriate informed consent, it may be an appropriate option to use full anticoagulation with unfractionated heparin in the first and third trimesters and to substitute warfarin during the middle trimester. However, although this approach may reduce fetal risk, this risk is not eliminated. Thus, therapeutic doses of heparin should be used in these patients seeking to maintain therapeutic anticoagulation during trough times. Because platelet aggregation on the mechanical valve may contribute to valve thrombosis, low-dose aspirin also should be employed in these patients.

References

1. Macklon NS, Greer IA, Bowman AW. An ultrasound study of gestational and postural changes in the deep venous system of the leg in pregnancy. Br J Obstet Gynaecol 1997; 104:191–7.

2. McColl MD, Ramsay JE, Tait RC, Walker ID, McCall F, Conkie JA, et al. Risk factors for pregnancy associated venous thromboembolism. Thromb Haemost 1997;78: 1183–8.

3. Girling JC, de Swiet M. Thromboembolism in pregnancy: an overview. Curr Opin Obstet Gynecol 1996;8:458–63.

4. Levine JS, Branch DW, Rauch J. The antiphospholipid syndrome. N Engl J Med 2002;346:752–63.

5. Investigation and management of heritable thrombophilia. Haemostasis and Thrombosis Task Force, British Committee for Standards in Haematology. Br J Haematol 2001;114:512–28.

6. Greer IA. The challenge of thrombophilia in maternal-fetal-medicine. N Engl J Med 2000;342:424–5.

7. Douketis JD, Ginsberg JS. Diagnostic problems with venous thromboembolic disease in pregnancy. Haemostasis 1995;25:58–71.

8. Lockwood CJ. Inherited thrombophilias in pregnant patients: detection and treatment paradigm. Obstet Gynecol 2002;99:333–41.

9. Ginsberg JS, Hirsh J. Use of antithrombotic agents during pregnancy. Chest 1998;114(Suppl):524S–30S.

10. Barbour LA, Pickard J. Controversies in thromboembolic disease during pregnancy: a critical review. Obstet Gynecol 1995;86:621–33.

11. American College of Obstetricians & Gynecologists. Thromboembolism in pregnancy. ACOG Practice Bulletin 19. Washington, DC: ACOG; 2000.

12. Kearon C, Gent M, Hirsh J, Weitz J, Kovacs MJ, Anderson DR, et al. A comparison of three months of anticoagulation with extended anticoagulation for a first episode of idiopathic venous thromboembolism [published erratum appears in N Engl J Med 1999;341:298]. N Engl J Med 1999;340:901–7.

13. Chan WS, Ray JG. Low molecular weight heparin use during pregnancy: issues of safety and practicality. Obstet Gynecol Surv 1999;54:649–54.

14. Reimold SC, Rutherford JD. Clinical practice. Valvular heart disease in pregnancy. N Engl J Med 2003;349:52–9.

15. Horlocker TT, Wedel DJ, Benzon H, Brown DL, Enneking KF, Heit JA, et al. Regional anesthesia in the anticoagulated patient: defining the risks. American Society of Regional Anesthesia and Pain Medicine. Reg Anesth Pain Med 2004; 29(suppl):1–12.

16. Chan WS, Anand S, Ginsberg JS. Anticoagulation of pregnant women with mechanical heart valves: a systematic review of the literature. Arch Intern Med 2000;160:191–6.

PULMONARY DISORDERS

The pregnant woman undergoes unique physiologic changes that may predispose her to more severe sequelae from any given insult when compared with the same result when not pregnant. Included are reductions in total lung volume that, by the third trimester, result in her tidal volume virtually overlapping her critical closing volume and a tendency to develop atelectasis even at base line, further exacerbated by disease states. This should translate into a need for closer observation of the pregnant woman as well as her fetus than is necessary when she is not pregnant.

Asthma

Asthma may complicate up to 4% of pregnancies, and its prevalence appears to be increasing. Pregnancies affected by asthma are also at increased risk for preterm birth, preeclampsia, low birth weight, and perinatal mortality. Severe disease is more likely to become worse during pregnancy. The course of asthma in an earlier pregnancy often predicts the course of asthma in a subsequent pregnancy.

Controlling asthma during pregnancy is important for the health and well-being of the mother and fetus. The Working Group on Asthma During Pregnancy of the NIH has concluded that asthma should be treated as aggressively in pregnancy as in the nonpregnant adult. That group identified four components of a management program for pregnant women with asthma:

1. Assessing and monitoring asthma monthly, with objective measures of lung function

2. Avoidance or control of asthma triggers

3. Patient education

4. Stepwise approach to pharmacologic therapy

Known environmental irritants, of which cigarette smoke may be the most common, may trigger asthma attacks. Other common irritants include dust mites, indoor mold, pollen, cockroaches, and animal dander. Patients with asthma should try to limit their exposure to these triggers, especially during exacerbations. Measures such as changing filters in the home heating and cooling systems, avoiding smokers, moving pets outside, staying indoors to prevent exposure to outdoor allergens, encasing mattresses and pillows in impermeable covers, and avoiding the home for 1 hour after vacuuming or dusting may help prevent exacerbations.

Management of an asthma exacerbation requires assessment of its severity (Fig. 16). Subjective assessments are notoriously inaccurate. Objective measures of lung function are necessary to assess the severity of disease and to tailor appropriate therapy for ongoing symptoms. The best measure is forced expiratory volume in 1 second (FEV_1); however, the peak expiratory flow rate correlates with FEV_1 and can be measured with an inexpensive, hand-held flow meter. Home monitoring of the peak expiratory flow rate provides a daily assessment of lung function and response to ongoing therapy. Peak expiratory flow rate and FEV_1 do not change during a normal pregnancy. The patient with asthma should establish a "personal best" during an asymptomatic period.

Adjustments of therapy and interventions are based on reductions from the patient's personal best benchmark.

First-trimester ultrasound confirmation of gestational age allows comparison for eventual fetal growth. Additional ultrasound examinations may be warranted if IUGR is suspected. In the third trimester, the need for fetal surveillance should be based on the severity of asthma.

Pharmacologic therapy for asthma should be individualized based on severity of disease. The patient should not be undertreated because of pregnancy. Inhaled medications are preferred because they deliver the agent directly to the bronchial tree, thus decreasing the potential for systemic side effects (Table 12). Inhaled bronchodilators (β_2-agonists) are the generally accepted first-line therapy for patients with mild asthma (ie, those with an FEV_1 of $\geq 80\%$; mild persistent, $FEV_1 > 70\%$).

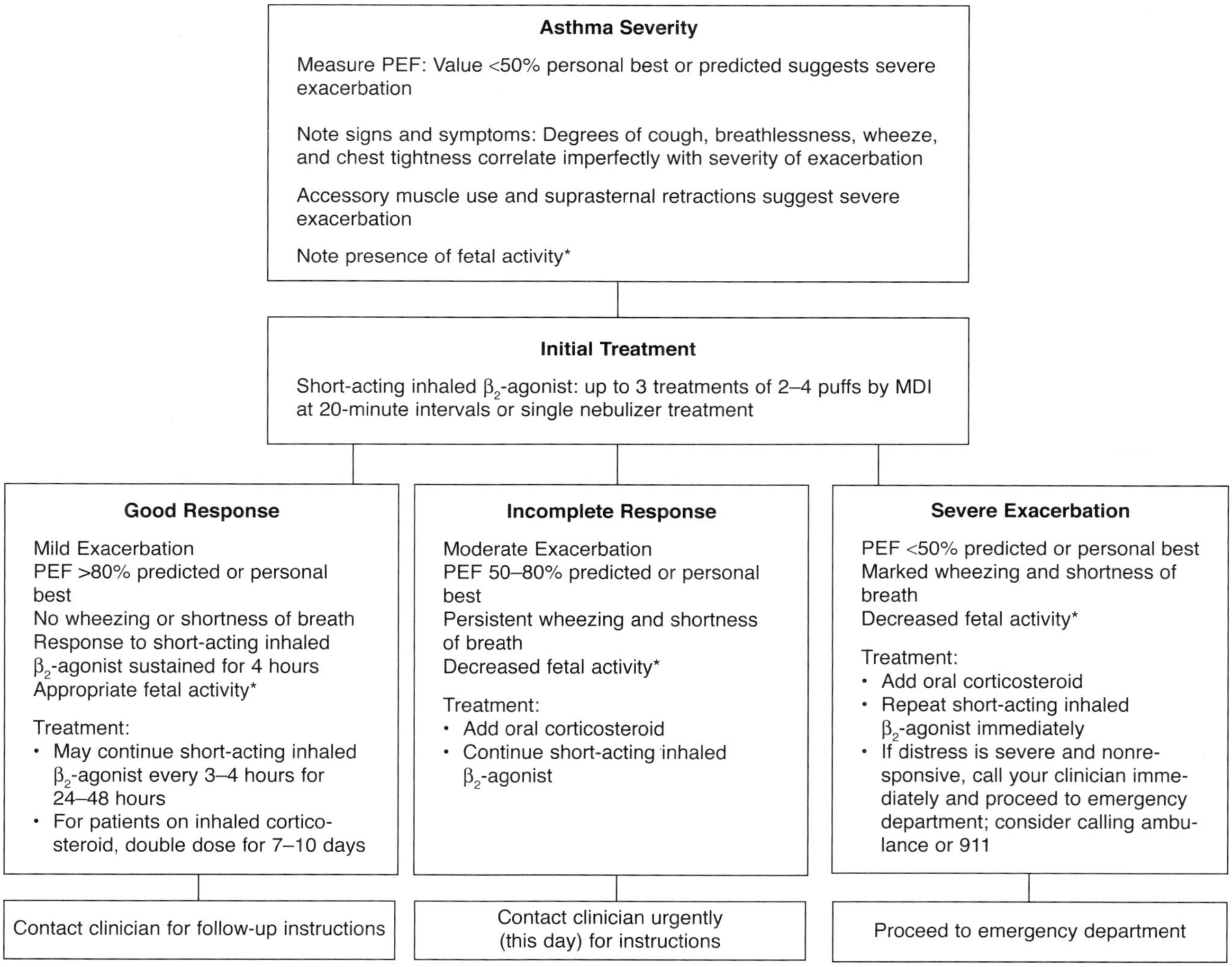

Asthma Severity

Measure PEF: Value <50% personal best or predicted suggests severe exacerbation

Note signs and symptoms: Degrees of cough, breathlessness, wheeze, and chest tightness correlate imperfectly with severity of exacerbation

Accessory muscle use and suprasternal retractions suggest severe exacerbation

Note presence of fetal activity*

Initial Treatment

Short-acting inhaled β_2-agonist: up to 3 treatments of 2–4 puffs by MDI at 20-minute intervals or single nebulizer treatment

Good Response

Mild Exacerbation
PEF >80% predicted or personal best
No wheezing or shortness of breath
Response to short-acting inhaled β_2-agonist sustained for 4 hours
Appropriate fetal activity*

Treatment:
• May continue short-acting inhaled β_2-agonist every 3–4 hours for 24–48 hours
• For patients on inhaled corticosteroid, double dose for 7–10 days

Contact clinician for follow-up instructions

Incomplete Response

Moderate Exacerbation
PEF 50–80% predicted or personal best
Persistent wheezing and shortness of breath
Decreased fetal activity*

Treatment:
• Add oral corticosteroid
• Continue short-acting inhaled β_2-agonist

Contact clinician urgently (this day) for instructions

Severe Exacerbation

PEF <50% predicted or personal best
Marked wheezing and shortness of breath
Decreased fetal activity*

Treatment:
• Add oral corticosteroid
• Repeat short-acting inhaled β_2-agonist immediately
• If distress is severe and nonresponsive, call your clinician immediately and proceed to emergency department; consider calling ambulance or 911

Proceed to emergency department

■ **FIG. 16.** Algorithm for management of acute asthma exacerbation. FEV_1 indicates forced expiratory volume in 1 second; MDI, metered-dose inhaler; PEF, peak expiratory flow. *Fetal activity is monitored by observing whether fetal kick counts decrease over time. (National Institutes of Health. Working Group report on managing asthma during pregnancy: recommendations for pharmacologic treatment: update 2004. National Asthma Education Program Working Group on Asthma During Pregnancy. National Heart, Lung, and Blood Institute. Bethesda (MD): NIH; 2005. NIH Publication No. 05-3279. Available at: http://www.nhlbi.nih.gov/health/prof/lung/asthma/astpreg/astpreg_full.pdf. Retrieved February 8, 2005.

Inhaled antiinflammatory agents (corticosteroids) should be added to the daily regimen of patients with persistent asthma (symptoms at least 2 days/wk or 2 nights/month) or who do not respond to bronchodilators. If low doses of inhaled corticosteroid do not control persistent asthma, the dose should be increased or a long-acting β_2-agonist added. Pregnant women who do not respond to maximal doses of both inhaled corticosteroids and bronchodilators are considered to have severe asthma ($FEV_1 \leq 60\%$) and usually require systemic corticosteroids. Although these medications may produce troublesome side effects, their use is warranted because uncontrolled asthma poses a greater threat to the pregnancy and fetus than do the medications necessary to control it.

TABLE 12. Selected Medications for the Treatment of Asthma

Generic Name	Available Strengths	Usual Dosage	Side Effects
Short-acting Inhaled β_2-Agonists			
Albuterol	MDI: 90 µg per puff	2 puffs every 4–6 hours as needed	Tachycardia, nervousness, tremor, headache, insomnia, nausea
Pirbuterol	Autohaler: 200 µg per puff	2 puffs every 4–6 hours as needed	
Long-acting Inhaled β_2-Agonists			
Formoterol	Aerolizer: 12 µg per inhalation	1 capsule twice daily	Headache, tremor, restlessness, dizziness
Salmeterol	Diskus: 50 µg per inhalation	1 inhalation twice daily	
Inhaled Corticosteroids			
Beclomethasone	MDI: 40 or 80 µg per puff	40–240 µg twice daily or higher	Sore throat, dry mouth, hoarseness, oral candidiasis
Budesonide	Turbuhaler: 200 µg per inhalation	200 µg daily–600 µg twice daily or higher	
Flunisolide	MDI: 250 µg per puff	250–1,000 µg twice daily or higher	
Fluticasone	MDI: 44, 110, or 220 µg per puff	MDI: 44–330 µg twice daily or higher	
	Rotadisk: 50, 100, or 250 µg per inhalation	Rotadisk: 50–500 µg twice daily or higher	
Triamcinolone	MDI: 100 µg per puff	400–2,000 µg per day or higher divided into 2–4 doses	
Mast Cell Stabilizer			
Cromolyn	MDI: 1 mg per puff	2–4 puffs 3–4 times daily	Cough, sore throat, hoarseness, bad taste, nausea
Leukotriene Modifiers			
Montelukast	10-mg tablet	10 mg nightly	Nausea, headache, diarrhea
Zafirlukast	10- or 20-mg tablets	20 mg twice daily	
Methylxanthine			
Theophylline	Various regular and extended release tablets, capsules, and liquids	300–800 mg daily	Headache, tachycardia, insomnia, tremor, restlessness
Combination Product			
Fluticasone/Salmeterol	100/50, 250/50 or 500 µg/50 µg per inhalation	1 inhalation twice daily	Pharyngitis, oral candidiasis, tremor

*Inhaled medications are available in the following devices: Autohaler is breath-activated; Aerolizer is used to inhale contents of a capsule, patients must load device before each use; Diskus is used to inhale contents of a capsule, doses are preloaded; MDI is a metered dose inhaler, the traditional type of inhaler; Turbuhaler is used to inhale a dry powder, doses are preloaded. Albuterol, budesonide, and cromolyn are also available in nebulizer formulations.

Pneumonia

Pulmonary disorders in pregnancy often require management of acute symptoms. Patients may require stabilization in a hospital setting to ensure adequate oxygenation. The safety and efficacy of antileukotrienes have not been evaluated in pregnancy, although they have an emerging role in management.

Influenza A and B viruses, respiratory syncytial virus, and parainfluenza virus can cause viral pneumonia. Influenza outbreaks occur yearly on a seasonal basis. These viruses usually are spread by aerosolized droplets produced from talking, sneezing, or coughing, which then quickly infect the epithelium of the respiratory tract. The incubation period is typically 1–3 days, and symptoms usually resolve spontaneously within 7–10 days. Roughly 1% of cases of influenza develop into pneumonia; mortality is reported to be as high as 25–30%. Treatment generally is symptomatic, but the antiviral drug amantadine (pregnancy class C) may reduce the severity and duration of symptoms (typical dosage, 200 mg/d). The best prevention for influenza is vaccination with the trivalent vaccine. Vaccination is recommended for women who will be in the second or third trimester of pregnancy during the flu season and women who have problems during pregnancy regardless of the stage. It is an inactive virus vaccine approved for any person (pregnant or nonpregnant) requesting it.

The most common of the bacterial pneumonias is that caused by *Streptococcus pneumoniae* (pneumococcal pneumonia), followed in frequency by *Haemophilus influenzae, Klebsiella pneumoniae,* and a host of other gram-negative and anaerobic bacteria. Etiologic agents of atypical pneumonia include *Mycoplasma pneumonias,* viruses, *Legionella* pneumonia, and *Chlamydia pneumoniae*. Treatment should be based on the organism.

Management of typical bacterial pneumonia should include both supportive measures for symptoms and pharmacologic agents directed at the responsible pathogen, if possible. Sputum Gram stain and culture may prove beneficial. An adequate specimen should contain more than 25 neutrophils and fewer than 10 epithelial cells. Because identifying the exact pathogen is the exception rather than the rule, initial antibiotic treatment is usually empirical. Most pneumonias in adults are caused by pneumococci or mycoplasma, making erythromycin an ideal first choice, especially in pregnancy. The usual dosage of erythromycin is 500 mg orally or intravenously every 6 hours. The long-acting, better-tolerated macrolide antibiotics clarithromycin and azithromycin are appropriate, although more expensive, alternatives. In women who appear very ill or are suspected to be infected with more unusual bacterial agents, a second- or third-generation cephalosporin or β-lactam antibiotic with a β-lactamase inhibitor may be necessary.

Sarcoidosis

Sarcoidosis occurs in only 40 people per 100,000 and affects men and women equally, but there is a 10–20-fold increase in the attack rate for African Americans. Most women will experience symptoms for the first time between ages 20 and 40 years. Sarcoidosis is a chronic condition of unknown etiology characterized by accumulation of noncaseating granulomas. More than 90% of the patients afflicted with this condition will have an abnormal chest X-ray in which interstitial pneumonitis is the classic finding. Mediastinal lymphadenopathy, which can be seen on a chest X-ray, is present in up to 90% of cases.

Generally, the prognosis for patients with sarcoidosis is good. In almost 50% of patients, the condition resolves spontaneously; in the remaining 40–50% of patients some permanent organ dysfunction persists. Corticosteroids are the hallmark of therapy. Their use generally is based on patient symptoms, chest X-ray findings, and pulmonary function testing. Unless there is severe pre-existing disease, sarcoidosis seldom affects pregnancy adversely. In the largest series reported to date in Finland, there was no evidence of disease progression in those pregnancies where sarcoid was active (1). Additionally, in women with inactive sarcoid, pregnancy outcome was good, and there was no evidence of increased disease activation. Severe sarcoidosis in pregnancy warrants careful assessment and serial determinations of pulmonary function. Deterioration of lung function should prompt the use of prednisone 1 mg/kg/d for 4–6 weeks.

Cystic Fibrosis

Cystic fibrosis is a chronic progressive disorder due to a genetic mutation on the long arm of chromosome 7. This disorder results in exocrine gland dysfunction and the overproduction of thick viscid secretions. As a rule, all affected patients will demonstrate some form of pulmonary involvement, which will ultimately lead to their death in most cases. Hypertrophy of the bronchial glands, along with thick mucus plugging, results in small airway obstruction. *Pseudomonas aeruginosa* typically colonizes the respiratory tract and leads to chronic bronchitis and bronchiectasis. Acute and chronic inflammation results in extensive pulmonary fibrosis and finally pulmonary insufficiency.

In pregnancy, the maternal and perinatal mortality is increased. Outcomes for both the fetus and the mother are directly related to the degree of pulmonary disease at the time of conception. When the FEV_1 is less than 60% predicted in the prepregnant state, there is a substantially increased risk of preterm delivery, maternal pulmonary complications, and early death of the mother (2, 3). In contrast, successful pregnancy outcomes can be expected when the prepregnancy FEV_1 is more than 80% predicted and prepregnancy treatments, including pancreatic enzyme replacements, oral antibiotics, aerosolized bronchodilators, chest physiotherapy, and nutritional support, are continued.

All cystic fibrosis patients considering pregnancy should be encouraged to have preconceptional and genetic counseling. Once pregnancy is confirmed, serial pulmonary function testing should be performed on a regular basis. Frequent surveillance and early intervention is recommended for superimposed pulmonary infection, development of diabetes, and heart failure as a consequence of cor pulmonale. Meticulous attention should be paid to postural drainage and bronchodilator therapy to help maintain pulmonary function and prevent infection. Inhaled recombinant human deoxyribonuclease improves lung function by decreasing sputum viscosity (4). In labor, epidural anesthesia is recommended, especially in the event that operative delivery is indicated. Intubation should be avoided in patients with asthma.

Tuberculosis

The number of cases of tuberculosis in women of childbearing age in the United States increased 40% between 1985 and 1992 (5). Tuberculosis in foreign-born persons has increased 50% and in 1998 represented 40% of the 18,000 cases in the United States (6). Tuberculosis is increasing in frequency because of: 1) immigration from areas where tuberculosis is endemic, such as Mexico and Southeast Asia; 2) the emergence of multidrug-resistant organisms; and 3) increased numbers of adults who are HIV seropositive (7). In the United States, most cases of active tuberculosis during pregnancy occur as reactivation of old disease or in women with chronic diseases leading to immunosuppression, such as AIDS. See Box 13 for a list of high-risk groups recommended for tuberculosis screening.

The infection is spread by inhalation of *Mycobacterium tuberculosis*, which produces a granulomatous pulmonary reaction. In roughly 90% of patients, the infection is confined to the lungs and becomes contained and remains dormant for long periods. In a small percentage, especially in patients who are immunocompromised, tuberculosis can become reactivated to produce clinical disease. Active clinical infection usually causes cough with minimal sputum production, fever, hemoptysis, and weight loss. On chest X-ray, an infiltrate is typical, which also may be associated with cavitation and mediastinal lymphadenopathy. Acid-fast bacilli are seen in roughly two thirds of infected patients.

Tuberculosis infection in pregnancy is associated with increased incidences of growth restriction, low birth weight, preterm delivery, and a 6-fold increase in the perinatal mortality rate. Adverse outcomes are correlated with late diagnosis, incomplete treatment, and advanced pulmonary lesions.

If the intracutaneous skin test is negative, no further testing is warranted. However, a positive test should be interpreted according to a patient's risk factors for infec-

tion or immunocompromise. In women who are from the low-risk groups, a 15-mm zone of induration is considered positive. In these women, treatment is often withheld until after delivery if their chest X-ray is normal. A chest X-ray should be performed in patients with a tuberculin reaction and an indeterminate history of prior reactivity, as well as in those with history or physical findings consistent with active disease. A definite diagnosis depends on demonstration of *M tuberculosis* by culture of sputum, tissue, or other body fluids. Because culture techniques take several weeks, therapy may be started if specimen test results are positive for acid-fast bacilli. Treatment regimens for tuberculosis are based on the presence or absence of active disease. In the presence of active disease, determinations are based primarily on chest X-ray and, in the absence of active disease, on the duration of purified protein derivative (PDD), or tuberculin, positivity (Fig. 17).

BOX 13

High-Risk Groups Recommended for Tuberculosis Screening

- Close contacts of persons known or suspected to have tuberculosis, sharing the same household or other enclosed environment

- Persons infected with the human immunodeficiency virus

- Persons who inject illicit drugs or other locally identified high-risk substance users, such as crack cocaine users and users of alcohol

- Persons with medical risk factors (eg, diabetes, chronic renal failure, hematologic disorders) known to increase the risk of disease if infection has occurred

- Residents of long-term-care facilities, correctional institutions, mental institutions, nursing homes and facilities, other long-term residential facilities, and shelters for the homeless

- Health care workers who serve high-risk clients

- Foreign-born persons arriving within past 5 years from countries with a high tuberculosis prevalence (eg, most countries in Africa, Asia, and Latin America)

- Medically underserved low-income populations, including high-risk racial or ethnic minority populations, for example African, Hispanic, and Native Americans

Essential components of a tuberculosis prevention and control program. Screening for tuberculosis and tuberculosis infection in high-risk populations. Recommendations of the Advisory Committee for Elimination of Tuberculosis. MMWR 1995;44(RR-11):1–34.

The usual treatment for TB positive women who do not have active disease is isoniazid 300 mg daily for 6 months. This drug generally is considered safe for the fetus in pregnancy. Some exceptions to delaying treatment until the postpartum period include: 1) known recent skin test convertor after a previous negative test; 2) positive skin test result in women exposed to a patient known to have active tuberculosis infection; and 3) HIV-positive women with a positive PPD.

The risk of progression to active disease is highest in the 2 years after seroconversion to positive PPD. For this reason, isoniazid is the recommended medication in women known to have converted within the previous 2 years but with no evidence of active disease. Isoniazid treatment should be started after the first trimester and continued for 9 months (8).

Unfortunately, the time of seroconversion usually is not known. If a chest X-ray is normal, the woman should be treated after pregnancy. Women with HIV infection should receive tuberculosis therapy for 9 months. Women younger than 35 years with an unknown or prolonged (>2 years) duration of PPD positivity should receive isoniazid for 6 months after delivery. Because of concerns about hepatotoxicity, isoniazid prophylaxis is not recommended for unknown or prolonged PPD positivity in the absence of active disease for women older than 35 years. All pregnant women receiving isoniazid also should receive pyridoxine.

Although congenital infection can occur because of either hematogenous spread or fetal aspiration of the bacillus during delivery, most infection comes from postpartum maternal contact. If the mother has active tuberculosis, the child should be separated from her until she is not contagious. If congenital tuberculosis is excluded, isoniazid is given to the infant for 3–4 months after birth. Vaccination with bacillus Calmette–Guérin may be considered.

Influenza

Because pregnant women are more susceptible to the serious aspects of influenza, vaccination is important for them and for those they have contact with, including health care workers. The CDC now recommends that all pregnant women be immunized (10). A flu vaccine given to a pregnant woman not only protects her but also protects her infant from birth to 3–6 months. Pregnant women should receive the inactivated flu vaccine starting in October and November.

The neuraminidase inhibitors zanamivir and oseltamivir have demonstrated efficacy in reducing the duration of influenza symptoms when started within 48 hours of symptom onset. Both are effective against influenza A and B. Oseltamivir also has been approved for chemoprophylaxis to prevent or ameliorate symptoms in women with a significant exposure. However, studies in pregnancy have not been done. Pregnant women should use the medications only if the potential benefit outweighs the potential harm to the fetus.

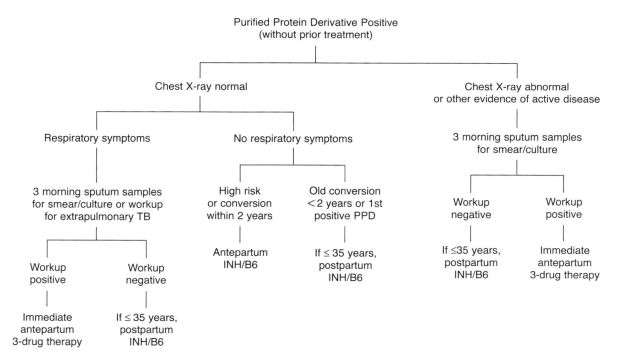

■ FIG. 17. Algorithm for management of pregnancy given a positive purified protein derivative test result. INH indicates isoniazid; PPD, purified protein derivative; TB, tuberculosis. (Reprinted from *Infectious Disease Clinics of North America*, vol 11. Riley L. Pneumonia and tuberculosis, p. 119–233. Copyright 1997, with permission from Elsevier.)

References

1. Selroos O. Sarcoidosis and pregnancy: a review with results of a retrospective study. J Intern Med 1990;227:221–4.

2. Edenborough FP, Stableforth DE, Webb AK, Mackenzie WE, Smith DL. Outcome of pregnancy in women with cystic fibrosis. Thorax 1995;50:170–4.

3. Edenborough FP, Mackenzie WE, Stableforth DE. The outcome of 72 pregnancies in 55 women with cystic fibrosis in the United Kingdom, 1977-1996. BJOG 2000;107:254–61.

4. Olson GL. Cystic fibrosis in pregnancy. Semin Perinatol 1997;21:307–12.

5. Cantwell MF, Shebab ZM, Costello AM, Sands L, Green WE, Ewing EP Jr, et al. Brief report: congenital tuberculosis. N Engl J Med 1994;330:1051–5.

6. Tuberculosis elimination revisited: obstacles, opportunities, and a renewed commitment. Advisory Council for the Elimination of Tuberculosis (ACET). MMWR Recomm Rep 1999;48 (RR-9):1–13.

7. Anderson GD. Tuberculosis in pregnancy. Semin Perinatol 1997;21:328–35.

8. Treatment of tuberculosis. American Thoracic Society; Centers for Disease Control and Prevention; Infectious Diseases Society of America. MMWR Recomm Rep 2003;52 (RR-11):1–77.

9. Montalto NJ. An office-based approach to influenza: clinical diagnosis and laboratory testing. Am Fam Physician 2003;67:111–8.

10. Update: influenza activity—United States, 2003–04 season, and composition of the 2004–05 influenza vaccine. Centers for Disease Control and Prevention. MMWR Morb Mortal Wkly Rep 2004;3:547–52.

LIVER AND ALIMENTARY TRACT DISEASES

Cholestasis of Pregnancy

Intrahepatic cholestasis is the most common liver disorder unique to pregnancy. Patients usually present with pruritus during the third trimester of pregnancy. The normal course of the disorder is mild nocturnal pruritus of the palms and soles that gradually increases and migrates to the trunk with severe, unrelenting, generalized pruritus. The appearance of jaundice is highly variable and is not necessary for diagnosis. Intrahepatic cholestasis tends to recur in subsequent pregnancies and has a higher prevalence in the spring. The disease is common in women of Scandinavian and Chilean ancestry, but over the past 25 years its incidence has decreased in these populations. The disease is more common in close relatives with an autosomal-dominant, sex-limited inheritance (1). Its pathophysiology remains unknown, but seems to be related to increasing estrogen and progesterone associated with pregnancy, especially multiple gestations (2). Its his-

tologic features are indistinguishable from those of other causes of cholestasis (centrilobular cholestasis, canaliculi-containing bile plugs, and bile pigment in hepatocytes).

The diagnosis of intrahepatic cholestasis is confirmed by demonstrating an increase in circulating bile acids (primarily cholic and chenodeoxycholic acids). Levels of cholic acid are significantly higher than those of chenodeoxycholic acid, and thus determination of the former is more sensitive and specific for diagnosis (3). Fasting levels of bile acids 3–4 times the upper limit of normal are considered diagnostic. Ultrasonography of the gallbladder should be performed to rule out obstruction and stones; liver biopsy is rarely indicated. Other diagnostic criteria include mild to moderate increases in alanine aminotransferase and aspartate aminotransferase, but are not diagnostic of the disease. There is no correlation between bile acids, liver function studies, and clinical symptoms. Total bilirubin level usually is elevated less than 5 mg/dL. Impaired enterohepatic circulation of vitamin K may result in decreased production of vitamin K-dependent clotting factors (II, VII, IX, and X), leading to prolongation of prothrombin time in patients with severe and protracted cholestasis of pregnancy. Treatment with vitamin K is recommended to prevent intracranial hemorrhage in the fetus and maternal hemorrhage postpartum (4).

Intrahepatic cholestasis is associated with an increased incidence of prematurity, fetal distress, and late fetal loss (>36 weeks of gestation). Although the extent of these problems remains to be delineated, the incidence of fetal compromise appears to be acute. Fetal testing is of questionable value in predicting fetal demise (5). Because of late, sudden fetal loss, consideration of early delivery after determining fetal lung maturity is recommended by some clinicians (6); others recommend induction of labor at 38 weeks (1). Deposits of bile salts in the placenta and increased levels of bile salt metabolites in amniotic fluid have been described, but how they adversely affect the fetus is unknown (7). Some clinicians have speculated that these deposits are related to an anoxic event. No clinical parameters have been correlated with fetal death in pregnant women with intrahepatic cholestasis.

Taking cornstarch baths or using antihistamines such as diphenhydramine or hydroxyzine may provide symptomatic relief in a few patients. Women with more severe symptoms require systemic therapy. Cholestyramine, phenobarbital, dexamethasone, S-adenosylmethionine, and epomediol have been used with varying success.

Ursodeoxycholic acid originally was introduced as an agent for the treatment of gallstones and is currently the medication of choice for cholestasis. It effectively reduces levels of cholic acids and bile acids while significantly decreasing pruritus. Additionally, small studies suggest that fetal wastage is decreased in patients treated with ursodeoxycholic acid. In most cases, the pruritus resolves in the first 24–48 hours after delivery. Trials for all therapeutic interventions are small and inconsistent, and no consistent recommendations can be made (8).

Acute Fatty Liver of Pregnancy

Until recently, acute fatty liver of pregnancy (AFLP) was associated with a maternal mortality of nearly 90% of cases. Recent reports suggest that most patients survive with proper supportive care and early diagnosis and delivery. Acute fatty liver of pregnancy usually is first seen during the third trimester and is associated with first pregnancies, multiple gestations, and male fetuses. The signs and symptoms of preeclampsia may be found in approximately 20% of patients with AFLP. Recently, the pathophysiology and genetics of AFLP have been elucidated.

The etiology of AFLP is an enzymatic defect in the fetus. Inherited as an autosomal recessive disorder, the fetus has a congenital deficiency of long-chain 3-hydroxy-acyl coenzyme A dehydrogenases (LCHAD) with a 1528G-->C mutation on one or both alleles. Because of this defect, there is an accumulation of straight-chain fatty acids, which results in mitochondrial disruption and, eventually, severe liver dysfunction in the mother. If the infant is normal or a heterozygote, the mother is unaffected.

Pregnancy is associated with increased triglyceride breakdown, with the accumulated fatty acids causing a toxic reaction to hepatocytes (9). One study suggests that 79% of the mothers of infants with this deficiency had either HELLP (hemolysis, elevated liver enzymes, and low platelet count) syndrome or AFLP (10). Current recommendations are that metabolic screening for LCHAD deficiency be performed in individuals affected with AFLP or recurrent HELLP syndrome (11). Chorionic villus sampling has been advocated for families where both partners are known carriers to determine if the fetus is affected.

The clinical course of AFLP begins with nonspecific constitutional symptoms and epigastric or abdominal pain, followed in about a week with jaundice and neurologic symptoms. Serum amylase, creatinine, bilirubin, uric acid, alanine aminotransferase, and aspartate aminotransferase levels are elevated. In contrast to viral hepatitis, liver transaminase levels are only moderately elevated, at 200–500 IU/L (12).

Coagulation abnormalities become evident as the disease progresses. These abnormalities include hypofibrinogenemia, increased fibrin degradation products, thrombocytopenia, and prolonged prothrombin and activated partial thromboplastin times. If the course of the disorder continues to progress, profound hypoglycemia can result from liver failure. Leukocytosis and anemia caused by microangiopathic destruction of red blood cells also are seen. Liver biopsy, with frozen section showing infiltration of hepatocytes with small droplets of fat (demonstrated with oil red O stain), remains the definitive diagnostic study, although this finding also may be present in preeclampsia. Electron microscopy examination reveals mitochondrial disruption.

CT and MRI have been helpful in establishing the diagnosis of AFLP. Differential diagnoses include the following:

- Chemical hepatitis
- Cholangitis
- Hemolytic uremic syndrome
- Thrombotic thrombocytopenia purpura septicemia
- Budd–Chiari syndrome
- Pancreatitis
- Acute hepatitis
- Systematic lupus erythematosus
- HELLP syndrome
- Severe pregnancy-induced hypertension or eclampsia

Treatment of pregnant patients with AFLP is immediate delivery. The route of delivery for women with the condition should depend on the clinical situation. Involvement of multiple organ systems is common. Special attention should be directed to combating infection with broad-spectrum antibiotics and treating coagulation dysfunction, usually with platelets, fresh frozen plasma, cryoprecipitate, and packed red cell transfusion. Use of H_2-receptor antagonists helps reduce the incidence of gastrointestinal bleeding. Although transaminase levels usually normalize promptly after delivery, other liver functions may remain abnormal for days to weeks. Multiple cases of successful liver transplantation have been reported, and transfer to a tertiary-care center with these services available should be considered.

Liver Transplantation

Gonadotropin activity returns soon after liver transplantation; pregnancies have been reported as early as 3 months postsurgery. Normal menstrual function returns in 90% of women by 7 months posttransplantation. It has been suggested that contraception be used for 1–2 years after a transplantation procedure so that stable levels of immunosuppressive drugs are achieved, steroids have been tapered off, and the risk of infections, specifically CMV infection, is lessened (13). As experience increases, certain trends have been noted. Patients treated with cyclosporine have been noted to have more renal dysfunction at conception and a higher incidence of hypertensive problems in pregnancy (preeclampsia and HELLP syndrome). Intrauterine growth restriction is more common and is associated with an increased risk of hypertension and preeclampsia. The risks of spontaneous abortion, stillbirth, and congenital malformations are not increased. Cyclosporine levels are high in breast milk and, therefore, breastfeeding should be discouraged. These patients also have a higher incidence of anemia, SGA infants, and cesarean delivery. Some transplant centers currently recommend tacrolimus (FK 506) as the immunosuppressant agent of choice during pregnancy to prevent hypertension (14). Regardless of the agent chosen, close monitoring of drug levels is recommended during pregnancy because of changing drug distribution and renal clearance. Infants born to mothers on either cyclosporine or tacrolimus may have transient hyperkalemia and increased creatinine levels that decrease after several days. Preterm PROM is also common and is thought to be related to systemic steroids that most patients take daily to prevent rejection. All pregnant patients who have had liver transplantation should be considered high risk, and the disease should be managed in conjunction with transplant teams. The most common cause of maternal mortality was in patients with recurrent hepatitis C (15).

Inflammatory Bowel Disease

The inflammatory bowel diseases, ulcerative colitis and Crohn's disease (regional enteritis), are idiopathic disorders that have their peak incidence during the reproductive years. Ulcerative colitis primarily involves the mucosa in the colon and rectum, whereas Crohn's disease is most commonly found in the terminal ileum and colon. Crohn's disease is transmural, causes fistulas found from mouth to anus, and may involve the perineum. Symptoms of both disorders include cramping pain, diarrhea, hematochezia, and weight loss; in 10% of cases, differentiation between the 2 is impossible. Unlike ulcerative colitis, Crohn's disease tends to run a more subacute and chronic course. Patients with colitis must be evaluated carefully for an infectious etiology before symptoms are ascribed to inflammatory bowel disease. Rectal bleeding is less common in patients with Crohn's disease, and the absence of rectal involvement essentially excludes ulcerative colitis. Extraintestinal manifestations of inflammatory bowel disease include arthritis of the spine; ocular inflammation; aphthous ulcers; hepatitis; and renal involvement with stones, fistula formation, and hydronephrosis.

Reports of pregnancy outcomes in patients with inflammatory bowel disease are conflicting. Important variables are the state of the disease at the beginning of gestation (ie, remission versus active disease) and its clinical course during gestation. Active disease is associated with a slight increase in spontaneous abortion and poor pregnancy outcome. These patients, particularly women with Crohn's disease, should delay conception until their disease is in remission (16). Pregnancy is associated with a 15–30% chance of exacerbation of inflammatory bowel disease. Women with new-onset disease during pregnancy are at increased risk for pregnancy loss. Patients with quiescent disease at conception usually do not have disease reactivation. Controversy exists as to whether flare-ups are more common in the postpartum period.

Treatment of inflammatory bowel disease is not altered greatly by pregnancy and includes oral sulfasalazine, oral or rectal corticosteroids, and occasionally immunosuppression with systemic corticosteroids. Each of these medications may be continued during pregnancy. A new chimeric monoclonal antibody to tissue necrosis factor alpha (TNF-α) given by infusion is being used in severe disease. Preliminary findings suggest that there have been no deleterious effects during pregnancy (17). Surgery may be required to treat fistulas, bowel obstruction, hemorrhage, abscess formation, perforation, or malignancy or when medical management fails. Indications for surgery remain the same for the pregnant patient. Occasionally, patients with active disease, severe dehydration, and perforations may require long periods of total parenteral nutrition.

Pregnancy After Gastrointestinal Bypass

Bariatric surgery is considered the most effective tool to control weight in morbidly obese patients. Newer procedures, specifically laparoscopic gastric banding, are likely to increase the number of patients who desire weight loss. Many of these patients are infertile because of anovulation. After surgery, with weight loss, they may regain ovulatory function and become pregnant. Few long-term studies are available to compare results, but those available suggest that pregnancy outcomes, both maternal and fetal, are generally good (18).

Once the patient becomes pregnant, the gastric bands should be decompressed because of persistent nausea and vomiting. Intragastric band migration during pregnancy has been reported (19). Because of rapid weight loss due to malabsorption after bariatric surgery, it has been suggested that pregnancy be delayed for the first year. Patients who had a pregnancy both before and after bariatric procedures had less weight gain on average (12.7 kg versus 20.4 kg), less gestational diabetes, less macrosomia, and fewer cesarean births than patients with obesity alone (20). Despite concerns of ketosis and fetal outcome, significant IUGR has not been reported. Because of concerns that patients may return to previous hyperphagic behaviors, surgeons recommend 4 high-protein meals daily rather than 6 meals daily. Supplemental vitamins, especially folic acid, should be given because of absorption concerns.

Hyperemesis Gravidarum

Nausea and vomiting of pregnancy affect 70–85% of pregnant women (21). Hyperemesis gravidarum affects 0.5–2% of pregnancies, is the most common indication for hospital admission in the first part of pregnancy, and is second only to preterm labor as the most common reason for hospitalization during pregnancy (22). It appears to be an escalation of severity of nausea and vomiting of pregnancy. Commonly cited criteria for diagnosing hyperemesis gravidarum include persistent vomiting not related to other causes, a measure of acute starvation (usually large ketonuria), and some discrete measure of weight loss, most often at least 5% of prepregnancy weight.

Failure to treat early symptoms increases the likelihood of hospital admission for hyperemesis gravidarum. Recommendations for prevention and treatment include the following (23):

- Taking a multivitamin at the time of conception may decrease the severity of nausea and vomiting of pregnancy.

- Vitamin B_6 or vitamin B_6 plus doxylamine is safe and effective and should be considered first-line pharmacotherapy.

- In patients with hyperemesis gravidarum who also have suppressed TSH levels, treatment of hyperthyroidism should not be undertaken without evidence of intrinsic thyroid disease (including goiter or thyroid autoantibodies).

- Treatment of nausea and vomiting of pregnancy with ginger has shown beneficial effects and can be considered as a nonpharmacologic option.

- In refractory cases of nausea and vomiting of pregnancy, antihistamine H_1 receptor blockers, phenothiazines, and benzamides have been shown to be safe and efficacious in pregnancy.

- Early treatment of nausea and vomiting of pregnancy is recommended to prevent progression to hyperemesis gravidarum.

- Treatment of severe nausea and vomiting of pregnancy or hyperemesis gravidarum with methylprednisolone may be efficacious in refractory cases; however, the risk profile of methylprednisolone suggests it should be a treatment of last resort.

- Intravenous hydration should be used for the patient who cannot tolerate oral liquids for a prolonged period or if clinical signs of dehydration are present. Correction of ketosis and vitamin deficiency should be strongly considered. Dextrose and vitamins, especially thiamine, should be included in the therapy when prolonged vomiting is present.

- Enteral or parenteral nutrition should be initiated for any patient who cannot maintain her weight because of vomiting.

Nausea and vomiting of pregnancy occurs before 9 weeks of gestation in virtually all affected women. If nausea and vomiting first occurs after 9 weeks, other conditions, such as cholelithiasis, should be considered for the differential diagnosis.

References

1. Germain AM, Carvajal JA, Glasinovic JC, Kato CS, Williamson C. Intrahepatic cholestasis of pregnancy: an intriguing pregnancy-specific disorder. J Soc Gynecol Investig 2002;9:10–4.

2. Lammert F, Marschall HU, Glantz A, Matern S. Intrahepatic cholestasis of pregnancy: molecular pathogenesis, diagnosis and management. J Hepatol 2000;33:1012–21.

3. Walker IA, Nelson-Piercy C, Williamson C. Role of bile acid measurement in pregnancy. Ann Clin Biochem 2002;39:105–13.

4. Fagan EA. Intrahepatic cholestasis of pregnancy. Clin Liver Dis 1999;3:603–32.

5. Alsulyman OM, Ouzoumian JG, Ames-Castro M, Goodwin TM. Intrahepatic cholestasis of pregnancy: perinatal outcome associated with expectant management. Am J Obstet Gynecol 1996;175:957–60.

6. Davies MH, da Silva RC, Jones SR, Weaver JB, Elias E. Fetal mortality associated with cholestasis of pregnancy and the potential benefit of therapy with ursodeoxycholic acid. Gut 1995;37:580–4.

7. Mullally BA, Hansen WF. Intrahepatic cholestasis of pregnancy: review of the literature. Obstet Gynecol Surv 2002;57:47–52.

8. Burrows RF, Clavisi O, Burrows E. Interventions for treating cholestasis in pregnancy. The Cochrane Database of Systematic Reviews 2001, Issue 4. Art. No.: CD000493. DOI: 10.1002/14651858.CD000493.

9. Ibdah JA, Yang Z, Bennett MJ. Liver disease in pregnancy and fetal fatty acid oxidation defects. Mol Genet Metabol 2000;71:182–9.

10. Ibdah JA, Bennett MJ, Rinaldo P, Zhao Y, Gibson B, Sims HF, et al. A fetal fatty-acid oxidation disorder as a cause of liver disease in pregnant women. N Engl J Med 1999:340:1723–31.

11. Strauss AW, Bennett MJ, Rinaldo P, Sims HF, O'Brien LK, Zhao Y, et al. Inherited long-chain 3-hydroxyacyl-CoA dehydrogenase deficiency and a fetal-maternal interaction cause maternal liver disease and other pregnancy complications. Semin Perinatol 1999;23:100–12.

12. Treem WR. Mitochondrial fatty acid oxidation and acute fatty liver of pregnancy. Semin Gastrointest Dis 2002;13:55–66.

13. Riely CA. Contraception and pregnancy after liver transplantation. Liver Transpl 2001;7:S74–6.

14. Jain A, Venkataramanan R, Fung JJ, Gartner JC, Lever J, Balan V, et al. Pregnancy after liver transplantation under tacrolimus. Transplantation 1997;64:559–65.

15. Armenti VT, Herrine SK, Radomski JS, Mortiz MJ. Pregnancy after liver transplantation. Liver Transpl 2000;6:671–85.

16. Kane S. Inflammatory bowel disease in pregnancy. Gastroenterol Clin North Am 2003;32:323–40.

17. Katz JA, Lichtenstein GR, Keenan GF, et al. Outcome of pregnancy in women receiving Remicade (infliximab) for the treatment of Crohn's disease or rheumatoid arthritis [abstract]. Gastroenterol 2001;120 suppl:A69.

18. Martin LF, Finigan KM, Nolan TE. Pregnancy after adjustable gastric banding. Obstet Gynecol 2000;95: 927–30.

19. Weiss HG, Nehoda H, Labeck B, Hourmont K, Marth C, Aigner F. Pregnancies after adjustable gastric banding. Obes Surg 2001;11:303–6.

20. Wittgrove AC, Jester L, Wittgrove P, Clark GW. Pregnancy following gastric bypass for morbid obesity. Obes Surg 1998;8:461–4; discussion 465–6.

21. Jewell D, Young G. Interventions for nausea and vomiting in early pregnancy. The Cochrane Database of Systematic Reviews 2003, Issue 4. Art. No.: CD000145. DOI: 10.1002/14651858.CD000145.

22. Gazmararian JA, Petersen R, Jamieson DJ, Schild L, Adams MM. Deshpande AD, et al. Hospitalizations during pregnancy among managed care enrollees. Obstet Gynecol 2002;100:94–100.

23. Nausea and vomiting of pregnancy. ACOG Practice Bulletin No. 52. American College of Obstetricians and Gynecologists. Obstet Gynecol 2004;103:803–14.

NEUROLOGIC DISEASES

Seizure Disorders

Seizure disorders affect between 0.5% and 2% of the population and are the most common neurologic problem in pregnancy. Approximately 75% of these disorders are idiopathic, generally classified as generalized tonic–clonic seizures, partial complex seizures that may or may not become generalized, and absence seizures (petit mal). Controversy exists about the effects of seizure disorders on pregnancy, the effects of pregnancy on seizure disorders, and the antiepileptic drugs used to treat these disorders.

Studies have shown that control of seizure disorders may deteriorate during pregnancy and up to 25% of women with epilepsy will experience an increase in frequency (1). Factors that contribute to increased seizures include lower antiepileptic drug levels. If drug levels are monitored at regular intervals and dosages adjusted accordingly, seizure control can be maintained throughout pregnancy (2). Drug levels may fluctuate in pregnancy owing to a variety of factors. For example, gastrointestinal absorption is reduced and is often erratic as a result of progestational effects on bowel motility. Hepatic microsomal enzyme metabolism of many drugs increases during pregnancy. The large increase in glomerular filtration rate during pregnancy enhances the clearance of drugs that are eliminated by the kidneys. Monitoring free drug levels, which may increase in pregnancy because albumin is decreased, is recommended for phenobarbital, phenytoin, carbamazepine, valproic acid, and primidone. Some experts recommend monthly monitoring of lamotrigine because its clearance is markedly increased in pregnancy. Measuring the serum trough level of antiepileptic drugs has been recommended (3).

The underlying risk of fetal malformations is believed to be increased in women with untreated seizure disorders. Results from one study challenge this notion, documenting a rate of congenital anomalies that was similar among pregnant women with epilepsy but not exposed to antiepileptic drugs during the first trimester of pregnancy (0 of 98) and pregnant women without epilepsy and without exposure to antiepileptic drugs (9 of 508) (4). This study and others also demonstrated that compared to monotherapy, polytherapy with multiple antiepileptic drugs further increases the risk of fetal anomaly (4).

Although evidence that antiepileptic drugs are teratogenic is not conclusive, most studies suggest that all antiepileptic drugs are associated with major congenital malformations at a 2–3-fold higher rate than in the general population (4, 5). Use of the older antiepileptic drugs has been associated with a variety of anomalies, including NTDs associated with valproate; oral clefts and cardiac defects with phenobarbital, carbamazepine, and valproate; and facial and digital dysmorphology with phenytoin and carbamazepine. The teratogenic effects of the newer antiepileptic drugs lamotrigine, gabapentin, topiramate, felbamate, oxcarbazepine, and levetiracetam are not yet defined. Preliminary reports of lamotrigine use by 200 pregnant women suggest that when used as monotherapy, the risk of major malformations may be as low as 2% (5). Gabapentin may be more commonly prescribed, with its low side-effect profile. It is well absorbed, neither protein bound nor metabolized, and is renally excreted.

Although the mechanisms of teratogenesis are unknown, 2 possibilities relate to the higher levels of free radical arene oxide metabolites and antifolate effects. Phenytoin, carbamazepine, and phenobarbital are metabolized to oxidative intermediates, which are inactivated by epoxide hydrolase. In pregnant women treated with antiepileptic drugs, fetuses with lower epoxide hydrolase activity as measured in amniotic fluid had an increased risk of congenital anomalies. Valproate, which is associated with fetal NTDs, inhibits epoxide hydrolase activity. This may explain in part the higher rates of anomalies identified when valproate is added to any other antiepileptic drugs in a polytherapy regimen (1). Lower folic acid levels noted with antiepileptic drug treatment may contribute to the risk of anomalies. Folic acid supplementation of 1–4 mg per day is recommended, though the optimal dosage is unknown.

Preconception consultation with a neurologist is recommended to determine if the patient treated with antiepileptic drugs is a candidate to stop antiepileptic drugs or, if she is on polytherapy, to reduce therapy to a single agent. In the second trimester, consider maternal biochemical testing such as maternal serum alpha-fetoprotein, detailed fetal ultrasonography, and possibly amniocentesis to define risk of anomalies. A general recommendation to stop antiepileptic drug treatment is not appropriate if the risk of seizures is significant because the attendant complications (eg, status epilepticus, hazards of seizures with normal activity, including driving) can have serious effects on both the mother and fetus.

In the third trimester, oral vitamin K supplementation (10 or 20 mg daily) has been advocated by some experts because antiepileptic drugs are associated with a reduction in fetal vitamin K levels. Reduction in vitamin K–dependent coagulation factors may contribute to early hemorrhagic disease of the newborn. This recommendation remains controversial because study results have documented conflicting results as to whether maternal supplementation decreases the risk of early hemorrhagic disease. In any event, parenteral administration of vitamin K to the neonate is recommended at birth.

Myasthenia Gravis

Myasthenia gravis is an autoimmune neuromuscular disorder characterized pathologically by an immunologically mediated reduction of acetylcholine receptors at the neuromuscular junction in skeletal muscle. Clinically, patients note weakness and easy fatigue with repetitive skeletal muscle use. Respiratory muscles may become involved and respiratory difficulties may ensue (myasthenic crisis). Ptosis and diplopia are common presentations. The prevalence is 2–10 per 100,000 people, with women aged 20–30 years affected more often. Its occurrence in pregnancy, then, is not rare. Co-management with a neurologist is a prudent course of action. In pregnancy, the course of myasthenia gravis is unpredictable, although recent studies confirm that in general, most patients experience either no change or improvement in symptoms (6). Relapse may manifest with worsening ptosis, dyspnea, respiratory difficulties, or other signs of skeletal muscle weakness.

Most patients who have myasthenia gravis are treated with an oral anticholinesterase drug such as pyridostigmine, a Category C drug with no known adverse fetal effects. Other treatment options include thymectomy, prednisone, and other immunosuppressive drugs, such as azathioprine, cyclosporine, and, rarely, plasmapheresis. The need for anticholinesterase drugs may increase during labor and delivery. Patients may experience respiratory difficulty or fatigue in the second stage of labor and may benefit from an assisted second stage. In this context, anticholinesterase drugs are best administered parenterally in the form of neostigmine because of poor oral absorption of pyridostigmine during labor. The conversion of an oral to intravenous dose is approximately 60 mg oral pyridostigmine to 0.5 mg intravenous neostigmine.

Consultation with an obstetric anesthesiologist before labor should be considered because of interactions between commonly used anesthetic agents and myasthe-

nia. For example, patients with myasthenia can have prolonged weakness after nondepolarizing muscle relaxants and prolonged duration or increased toxicity from local ester anesthetics (eg, 2-chloroprocaine) metabolized by acetylcholinesterase. These agents should be avoided in patients treated with anticholinesterase agents. For pain control, epidural analgesia should be considered to reduce respiratory requirements and fatigue. Narcotic analgesics (eg, meperidine) may be given, although patients with myasthenia gravis may be more sensitive than others to their respiratory depressant effects. Magnesium sulfate is contraindicated because of its effect on neuromuscular transmission. Aminoglycosides and several other drugs (eg, propranolol, barbiturates) have been noted to potentially exacerbate muscle weakness and should be used with caution (7).

Rarely, cholinergic crisis may occur as a result of overdosage of anticholinesterase drugs. It may be difficult to distinguish a cholinergic crisis and myasthenic crisis because both are characterized by muscle weakness. With cholinergic crisis, treatment with anticholinesterase drugs is discontinued and atropine is recommended, whereas with myasthenic crisis, more intensive treatment is needed. Administration of a very short-acting anticholinesterase agent, such as edrophonium, may differentiate, with improvement in symptoms suggestive of inadequate anticholinesterase therapy and deterioration suggestive of too much therapy.

Transient neonatal myasthenia gravis is likely the result of transplacental passage of maternal antibodies directed against the acetylcholine receptor and may occur in up to 50% of newborns of women with myasthenia gravis (6). Its occurrence has not been associated with either severity of maternal disease or titer of maternal acetylcholine receptor antibodies. Clinical presentation usually occurs within the first week of life, with difficulties in sucking, swallowing, or respiration.

Paraplegia and Quadriplegia

Patients with spinal cord injuries are able to become pregnant and give birth without major complications. In the few published studies, in general, pregnancy complications for patients with quadriplegia or paraplegia do not appear to increase except for urinary tract infections, pressure ulcers, and autonomic hyperreflexia. Urinary tract infections are more common in some patients because of an indwelling catheter. Cesarean deliveries also have been reported at a higher rate.

Patients with traumatic spinal cord injury at T5 vertebra spinal level or higher are at risk for autonomic hyperreflexia syndrome because central regulation of the sympathetic nervous system below the level of the lesion is lost. This syndrome is characterized by acute onset of headache, nasal congestion, upper thorax cutaneous vasodilation, flushing and blotching, hypertension, and reflex bradycardia. Blood pressures can reach malignant levels, leading to myocardial infarction and stroke. Any noxious stimuli to the nervous system below the level of the injury, such as labor, delivery, cervical examinations, and cystitis, have the potential to precipitate this syndrome. Prior to labor and delivery, consultation with an anesthesiologist is recommended. Epidural anesthesia has been advocated and appears to prevent the autonomic hyperreflexia syndrome in labor and delivery (8).

A concern in patients with quadriplegia or paraplegia (T10 injury or higher) is the lack of sensation below the spinal cord injury and the inability to perceive uterine contractions. In the second and third trimester, patients can be taught to palpate for uterine contractions, or if this is not possible, to use a home uterine contraction monitoring device. In the third trimester, examination of the cervix at each visit may be helpful. Cesarean delivery is reserved for obstetric indications. Vaginal delivery should be anticipated with a passive second stage of labor; use of forceps or vacuum extraction may be necessary.

Cerebrovascular Disease

Cerebral infarction and transient ischemic attacks are rare in young women but are increased up to 13-fold in pregnancy and the postpartum period. Risk may be highest in the postpartum period (9). The etiology is unknown but is perhaps related to the hypercoagulable state of pregnancy. Atherosclerosis is responsible for less than 25% of cases during pregnancy. Other etiologies include atrial fibrillation, paradoxical embolism from DVT of the lower extremities, and endocarditis. The diagnosis may be confirmed by MRI and CT scanning. Evaluation should further include electrocardiogram, echocardiogram, thrombophilic assessment, prothrombin and partial thromboplastin time, complete blood count, serum cholesterol and triglyceride, and assessment of carotid arteries. It is not clear whether the benefits of anticoagulation in acute thrombotic stroke and a decrease in the risk of recurrence outweigh the risks of intracerebral hemorrhage (10). The recurrence risk of ischemic or occlusive cerebrovascular disease has been estimated in the 1–2% range for a subsequent pregnancy (11). Vaginal delivery, unless obstetrically contraindicated, is preferable to cesarean birth.

Patients that present with severe acute headaches with or without other neurologic signs, such as mental status changes, seizures, cranial nerve abnormalities, and deficit in motor control of the extremities, are suspect for subarachnoid hemorrhage and intracranial venous thrombosis. Intracranial venous thrombosis is a rare complication, generally diagnosed with MR angiography and CT scanning. Treatment is uncertain and prognosis in general is tenuous. Incidence of subarachnoid hemorrhage (SAH) is 1–5 per 10,000 pregnancies with a mortality rate of 30–40% (12). Hemorrhage typically occurs antepartum, in the latter half of pregnancy, but also can occur postpartum. The 2 major etiologies of SAH are cerebral vascular aneurysms and arteriovenous malformations, with indistinguishable clinical presentations. Initial evaluation generally depends on imaging such as CT and MRI. Cerebral angiography is useful in identifying the site of the lesion. After the initial hemorrhage, recurrent bleeding is a major morbidity that increases mortality with each subsequent bleed. Early neurosurgical intervention has been associated with better maternal and fetal outcomes. Some experts suggest that patients with a surgically corrected aneurysm can undergo labor and vaginal delivery. Delivery recommendations for uncorrected aneurysm or arteriovenous malformations are not well defined. Cesarean delivery has been recommended by some.

Multiple Sclerosis

Multiple sclerosis, the cause of which remains unknown, has no adverse effect on pregnancy, and pregnancy has no detrimental effect on multiple sclerosis. Clinically, symptoms include diplopia, transient blindness or eye pain (optic neuritis), weakness, spasticity, ataxia, tremor, dysarthria, and bladder dysfunction. No specific cure is available.

Treatment includes medication (eg, corticosteroids) to diminish severity of an acute flare, medications to address specific symptoms (eg, amitriptyline for neurogenic pain), and newer agents to reduce the risk of recurrence. Currently, these newer agents include interferons β-1a and β-1b and glatiramer. Experience with these medications is insufficient to detail their risk to pregnancy or the fetus, but anecdotal reports suggest that the risk is small. During pregnancy, the rate of relapse decreases, with the greatest reduction in the third trimester. Conversely, relapse increases 2-fold in the first 3–6 months postpartum.

The course of disease is unpredictable, though certain factors, such as progressive disease from onset, motor and cerebellar signs, and an abnormal result of MRI of the head, are associated with a poor prognosis, whereas complete recovery after the initial attack, dominant sensory symptoms, and absence of recurrence after 5 years are associated with a favorable prognosis.

References

1. Liporace J, D'Abreu A. Epilepsy and women's health: family planning, bone health, menopause, and menstrual-related seizures. Mayo Clin Proc 2003;78:497–506.

2. Pennell PB. Antiepileptic drug pharmacokinetics during pregnancy and lactation. Neurology 2003;61(suppl 2): S35–42.

3. Schoenenberger RA, Tanasijevic MJ, Jha A, Bates DW. Appropriateness of antiepileptic drug level monitoring. JAMA 1995;274:1622–6.

4. Holmes LB, Harvey EA, Coull BA, Huntington KB, Khoshbin S, Hayes AM, Ryan LM. The teratogenicity of anticonvulsant drugs. N Engl J Med 2001;344:1132–8.

5. Pennell PB. The importance of monotherapy in pregnancy. Neurology 2003;60 (suppl);S31–8.

6. Batocchi AP, Majolini L, Evoli A, Lino MM, Minisci C, Tonali P. Course and treatment of myasthenia gravis during pregnancy. Neurology 1999;52:447–52.

7. Branch DW, Porter TF. Autoimmune disease. In: James DK, Steer PJ, Weiner CP, Gonik B, editors. High risk pregnancy: management options. 2nd ed. London: Saunders; 1999. p. 853–84.

8. Hambly PR, Martin B. Anaesthesia for chronic spinal cord lesions. Anaesthesia 1998;53:273–89.

9. Kittner SJ, Stern BJ, Feeser BR, Hebel R, Nagey DA, Buchholz DW, et al. Pregnancy and the risk of stroke. N Engl J Med 1996;335:768–74.

10. Moonis M, Fisher M. Considering the role of heparin and low-molecular-weight heparins in acute ischemic stroke. Stroke 2002;33:1927–33.

11. Lamy C, Hamon JB, Coste J, Mas JL. Ischemic stroke in young women: risk of recurrence during subsequent pregnancies. French Study Group on Stroke in Pregnancy. Neurology 2000;55:269–74.

12. Fox MW, Harms RW, Davis DH. Selected neurologic complications of pregnancy. Mayo Clin Proc 1990;65:1595–618.

DIABETES MELLITUS

Preexisting Diabetes

Preexisting diabetes complicates approximately 0.1–0.3% of pregnancies in the United States. Perinatal mortality associated with diabetes has declined from approximately 65% before the discovery of insulin to well below 5% at present. The most significant remaining cause of fetal death among women with diabetes is congenital malformation. The dramatic improvement in survival rates has resulted in part from general advances in perinatal care but particularly from the development of a team approach to the management of diabetes, which stresses maintaining excellent glycemic control during pregnancy.

PRECONCEPTIONAL CARE

The incidence of congenital anomalies is 4-fold higher among infants of women with diabetes than among the general population. Anomalies of the cardiac, renal, vertebral, and central nervous systems arise during the first 8 weeks of gestation, at a time when it is unusual for patients to seek prenatal care. Studies have demonstrated a strong correlation between elevated levels of glucose and ketone bodies (as well as other metabolic aberrations) in the embryonic and preembryonic milieu and the likelihood of malformations. Furthermore, a number of case reviews have demonstrated a reduction in the rate of malformations when improved metabolic control is insti-

tuted before or during very early pregnancy. Therefore, the management and counseling of diabetic women of reproductive age should begin before conception (1). In fact, every medical visit for a female with diabetes should be considered a preconception visit.

Ideally, metabolic control should be at optimal levels before conception. Many authorities suggest delaying conception until glycosylated hemoglobin levels have remained in the normal or near-normal range for at least 3 months. A thorough history, physical examination, and laboratory evaluation should be undertaken to determine the presence or absence of vascular disease and other potentially complicating factors. Appropriate contraceptive advice should be given so that a woman with diabetes can plan her pregnancy. Women with diabetes, like other women considering pregnancy, should be counseled to ingest at least 400 mg of folic acid daily before conception and in early pregnancy to lower the likelihood of NTDs in their offspring. Preconceptional care of women with diabetes is cost-effective in terms of preventing many of the complications of diabetes during pregnancy.

SELF-MONITORING OF BLOOD GLUCOSE

Self-monitoring of blood glucose, along with intensive therapy, has made maintenance of near-normal glycemia a therapeutic reality for pregnant women with diabetes. Patients are instructed to monitor their ambient glucose levels frequently throughout the day by using reagent strips impregnated with glucose oxidase and a portable reflectance meter or similar system. Some diabetes care centers suggest fasting and preprandial measurements; others use fasting and 1- or 2-hour postprandial testing. In a randomized trial of women with severe gestational diabetes, as well as 2 descriptive studies of pregnancies in women with preexisting diabetes, postprandial glucose measurements were more predictive than preprandial monitoring of certain adverse outcomes among infants of mothers with diabetes (2–4). Target glucose values are fasting levels of 60–90 mg/dL and 1-hour postprandial values below 130–140 mg/dL or 2-hour postprandial values below 120 mg/dL. All patients and their families should be instructed in the use of glucagon to treat severe hypoglycemia.

INSULIN, ORAL AGENTS, AND DIET THERAPY

In most pregnant women with diabetes, the condition can be managed successfully with an insulin regimen consisting of multiple injections of mixtures of short-acting and intermediate-acting insulin timed to maintain blood glucose in the desired range. The second-generation oral agent glyburide has been shown not to cross the placenta at term and has been demonstrated to be similarly effective to insulin in treating gestational diabetes in a single randomized trial, but little information is available regarding the use of oral antidiabetes agents in early to mid-pregnancy for treating preexisting diabetes.

Metformin is increasingly useful in treating insulin resistance syndrome, enhancing the likelihood of conception. A number of case series have been published to describe its use at various times in pregnancy. Because this agent can cross the placenta (5) and acts as an insulin sensitizer in addition to suppressing hepatic insulin production, it might be expected to enhance the effects of fetal hyperinsulinemia. Because of this theoretic possibility and a lack of well-controlled animal or human studies, women with diabetes who conceive while taking metformin should be switched to insulin during pregnancy.

Diet is critical to successful regulation of maternal diabetes. Most diets include 30–35 kcal/kg of ideal body weight, with a high protein intake (90–125 g) and the addition of snacks between meals. The protein content may need to be reduced when diabetic nephropathy is present. Flexibility in the diet regimen is necessary to suit the patient's preferences and activity schedule.

Fetal Surveillance

Early ultrasound examination to confirm the gestational age of the fetus is suggested for women with diabetes mellitus. In an attempt to detect NTDs and other anomalies, a determination of maternal serum alpha-fetoprotein levels and other serum markers should be offered at 16–20 weeks in association with an ultrasound study at 18–20 weeks. Because maternal serum alpha-fetoprotein values may be lower in diabetic pregnancies, interpretations may need to be altered accordingly. Repeated ultrasound examinations at monthly intervals between 28 weeks of gestation and term are useful in establishing the pattern of fetal growth and changes in amniotic fluid volume.

Programs of fetal surveillance are initiated in the third trimester, when the risk of fetal death appears to be greatest. The severity of the diabetes and the presence of other complicating factors (eg, nephropathy, hypertension, fetal growth disturbance, poor or undocumented metabolic control) should determine the need for and frequency of fetal testing. Antenatal testing should be performed at least weekly and more often if complicating factors are present. The primary benefit of normal test results is reassurance for the physician and the patient that the pregnancy can continue, thus allowing further fetal maturation. For women with severe vascular disease, testing is often initiated at the time of potential extrauterine viability, whereas surveillance may be delayed until as late as 35 weeks of gestation when the diabetes is well controlled and the pregnancy is otherwise uncomplicated. The nonstress test, oxytocin challenge test, nipple stimulation test, biophysical profile, and maternal assessment of fetal activity are all accepted methods of fetal evaluation.

Timing and Route of Delivery

Improved fetal surveillance and better metabolic management of diabetes have reduced the likelihood of unexplained fetal death in late pregnancy. As a result, scheduling elective preterm delivery for patients with diabetes is no longer routine, although the rate of elective intervention at 38 weeks or beyond continues to be higher than the rate for women without diabetes complications. Before elective delivery, amniocentesis should be performed to document fetal pulmonary maturity in patients with poor or undocumented metabolic control or those at less than 39 weeks of gestation by accurate dating. Problems such as hypertension, nephropathy, or altered fetal growth may necessitate early delivery as soon as fetal maturity can be documented. Occasionally, evidence of fetal or maternal compromise may dictate delivery before fetal lung maturity.

Diabetes is not an indication for cesarean delivery, but its complications may be. For example, because of the increased likelihood of shoulder dystocia in the vaginal delivery of large infants of women with diabetes, recommendations have been made for elective cesarean delivery when fetal weight exceeds predetermined limits. Some authorities suggest a fetal weight threshold of 4,000 g; others recommend 4,500 g because the predictive accuracies of various methods of estimating fetal weight are less than optimal (6). A decision analytic model predicted that a policy of elective cesarean section for women with diabetes with an ultrasound estimated fetal weight above either 4,000 g or 4,500 g resulted in similar numbers of cesarean deliveries (443–489) and similar total costs (under $1,000,000) needed to prevent 1 permanent brachial plexus injury (7). These results were much more favorable than those generated using similar policies for pregnant women without diabetes.

Gestational Diabetes

Gestational diabetes has been defined as glucose intolerance of varying severity diagnosed during pregnancy by glucose tolerance testing. Women with gestational diabetes should undergo a 75-g, 2-hour oral glucose tolerance test within 1 or 2 months after delivery to determine whether they have type 1 or type 2 diabetes, prediabetes (impaired fasting glucose or impaired glucose tolerance), or normal glycemia (see Table 13). If the test shows impaired glucose tolerance or impaired fasting glucose, diabetes testing should be repeated annually. If the postpartum glucose tolerance test is normal, then glycemia should be reassessed at least every 3 years (8). Within 10–20 years after delivery, approximately one half of women who had gestational diabetes will develop type 2 diabetes. Among certain ethnic groups, women with gestational diabetes develop type 2 diabetes at an accelerated rate: up to 50% of Hispanic women will develop the disease within 5 years.

The clinical significance of gestational diabetes continues to be challenged. The risk of complications such as fetal macrosomia, traumatic or operative delivery, neonatal hypoglycemia, and jaundice are all increased in such pregnancies. Recent evidence suggests that childhood

TABLE 13. Diagnostic Criteria for Diabetes in the Nonpregnant State

| | Prediabetes | | |
Diabetes	Impaired Fasting Glucose	Impaired Glucose Tolerance	Normal
Fasting plasma glucose ≥126 mg/dL 2-h OGTT plasma glucose ≥200 mg/dL	Fasting plasma glucose ≥100 and <126 mg/dL	75-g, 2-hour OGTT plasma glucose ≥140 and <200 mg/dL	Fasting plasma glucose <100 mg/dL 75-g, 2-h OGTT plasma glucose <140 mg/dL

OGTT indicates oral glucose tolerance test.

Adapted from The Expert Committee on the Diagnosis and Classification of Diabetes Mellitus. Follow-up report on the diagnosis of diabetes mellitus. Diabetes Care 2003;26:3160–7.

and adult obesity, as well as diabetes, may be increased among offspring of mothers with gestational diabetes.

SCREENING AND DIAGNOSIS

There has not been a well-controlled study to demonstrate the benefits of universal screening for gestational diabetes. The American College of Obstetricians and Gynecologists and the American Diabetes Association recommendations for screening for gestational diabetes are similar (8, 9). Traditional risk factors (family history, previous macrosomic infant, poor obstetric history, glycosuria) identify only 40–60% of cases of gestational diabetes. Certain factors, such as age younger than 25 years, normal body weight, no first-degree family history of diabetes, and not being a member of a high-risk ethnic group, place women at lower risk for gestational diabetes. Therefore, routine screening may not be cost-effective in these women. Patients who manifest all of these characteristics may be candidates for selective screening based on obstetric risk factors.

A 50-g, 1-hour oral glucose challenge test has been suggested for screening for diabetes. This test usually is performed at 24–28 weeks of gestation, although performing the test earlier may be worthwhile when strong risk factors such as a previous history of gestational diabetes are present. A 3-hour oral glucose tolerance test should be performed when the screening test value exceeds a predetermined limit. When a threshold of 140 mg/dL is used, 14% of individuals will meet the criteria for the 3-hour glucose tolerance test. With a threshold of 130 mg/dL, an additional 10% of cases of gestational diabetes will be identified, but 23% of patients will be required to undergo the 3-hour diagnostic test.

Normal values for the glucose tolerance test differ from those used in nonpregnant women. Table 14 lists two conversions of the original O'Sullivan criteria. Any 2 values meeting or exceeding the threshold confirm the diagnosis of gestational diabetes. A number of studies have demonstrated excess morbidity even when only the lower set of thresholds is exceeded. In 1998, the Fourth International Workshop Conference on Gestational Diabetes recommended using the lower of the 2 sets of thresholds, which is the Carpenter conversion (10). In all likelihood, the relationship between maternal glucose levels and fetal outcome is a continuum, and the choice of diagnostic criteria is relatively arbitrary.

TREATMENT

Women with gestational diabetes should be counseled about appropriate diet. The use of oral hypoglycemic agents has been considered contraindicated in pregnancy because the earlier agents, whose mechanism of action is

TABLE 14. Detection of Gestational Diabetes

Test	Plasma Glucose Level (mg/dL)*
50-g, 1-h screen	130 or 140
O'Sullivan criteria	
NDDG conversion: 100-g oral glucose tolerance test	
Fasting	105
1 h	190
2 h	165
3 h	145
Carpenter conversion: 100-g oral glucose tolerance test	
Fasting	95
1 h	180
2 h	155
3 h	140

NDDG indicates National Diabetes Data Group.

*Result is upper limit of normal.

Data from Carpenter MW, Coustan DR. Criteria for screening tests for gestational diabetes. Am J Obstet Gynecol 1982;144:768–73; National Diabetes Data Group. Classification and diagnosis of diabetes mellitus and other categories of glucose intolerance. Diabetes 1979;28:1039–57.

to stimulate pancreatic insulin production and release, cross the placenta. There was concern that they could stimulate the fetal pancreas, exacerbating the problem of fetal hyperinsulinemia. A recent randomized trial demonstrated no significant difference in neonatal outcome between women with severe gestational diabetes treated with glyburide, a second-generation sulfonylurea, and those treated with insulin (11). A previous study used isolated single cotyledons in vitro to demonstrate that very little glyburide was transferred across the human placenta (12). Such findings suggest that it may become acceptable to treat gestational diabetes with specific oral agents, which would be more comfortable for patients than insulin injections.

The most important intervention in gestational diabetes is surveillance of maternal blood glucose levels during the third trimester. Circulating glucose should be monitored in the fasting state and postprandially at least every week. Some clinicians prefer to use daily self-monitoring of blood glucose, as described for women with preexisting diabetes.

The thresholds for initiating insulin therapy are somewhat arbitrary. The potential for perinatal mortality is probably increased, and insulin therapy should be instituted when the goals for metabolic control during pregnancy in women with preexisting diabetes are exceeded (fasting levels of 60–90 mg/dL and 1-hour postprandial values below 130–140 mg/dL or 2-hour postprandial values below 120 mg/dL). Even lower thresholds may be required to reduce the likelihood of macrosomia.

For women with gestational diabetes who are receiving insulin or have hypertension, a history of stillbirth, or other risk factors, fetal evaluation should be instituted in a fashion similar to that described for women with preexisting diabetes. If glucose levels remain in the desired range throughout pregnancy and other complications are absent, the potential for perinatal mortality is probably not increased. Nevertheless, daily determinations of fetal movement may provide reassurance to the pregnant woman and the clinician and allow the pregnancy to proceed to term. A randomized trial of induction of labor at 38 weeks versus expectant management revealed similar rates of cesarean delivery (13); however, the number of infants with macrosomia increased with expectant management. There was no statistically significant impact on shoulder dystocia. As with preexisting diabetes, ultrasound evaluation may be used to help identify macrosomia.

References

1. Kitzmiller JL, Buchanan TA, Kjos S, Combs CA, Ratner RE. Pre-conception care of diabetes, congenital malformations, and spontaneous abortions. Diabetes Care 1996;19: 514–41.

2. Combs CA, Gunderson E, Kitzmiller JL, Gavin LA, Main EK. Relationship of fetal macrosomia to maternal postprandial glucose control during pregnancy. Diabetes Care 1992; 15:1251–7.

3. de Veciana M, Major CA, Morgan MA, Asrat T, Toohey JS, Lien JM, et al. Postprandial versus preprandial blood glucose monitoring in women with gestational diabetes mellitus requiring insulin therapy. N Engl J Med 1995;333: 1237–41.

4. Jovanovic-Peterson L, Peterson CM, Reed GF, Metzger BE, Mills JL, Knopp RH, et al. Maternal postprandial glucose levels and infant birth weight: the Diabetes in Early Pregnancy Study. National Institute of Child Health and Human Development—Diabetes in Early Pregnancy Study. Am J Obstet Gynecol 1991;164:103–11.

5. Hague WM, Davoren PM, McIntyre DR, Noms R, Xiaonian X, Charles B. Metformin crosses the placenta: a modulator for fetal insulin resistance? BMJ web site http://bmj.bmjjournals.com/cgi/content/full/327/7420/880 (4 Dec 2003).

6. American College of Obstetricians and Gynecologists. Fetal macrosomia. ACOG Practice Bulletin 22. Washington, DC: ACOG; 2000.

7. Rouse DJ, Owen J, Goldenberg RL, Cliver SP. The effectiveness and costs of elective cesarean delivery for fetal macrosomia diagnosed by ultrasound. JAMA 1996;276: 1480–6.

8. Gestational diabetes mellitus. American Diabetes Association. Diabetes Care 2004;27 suppl 1:S88–90.

9. Gestational diabetes. ACOG Practice Bulletin No. 30. American College of Obstetricians and Gynecologists. Obstet Gynecol 2001;98:525–38.

10. Metzger BE, Coustan DR. Summary and recommendations of the Fourth International Workshop-Conference on Gestational Diabetes Mellitus. The Organizing Committee. Diabetes Care 1998;21 suppl 2:B161–7.

11. Langer O, Conway DL, Berkus MD, Xenakis EM, Gonzales O. A comparison of glyburide and insulin in women with gestational diabetes mellitus. N Engl J Med 2000;343:1134–8.

12. Elliott BD, Langer O, Schenker S, Johnson RF. Insignificant transfer of glyburide occurs across the human placenta. Am J Obstet Gynecol 1991;165;807–12.

13. Kjos SL, Henry OA, Montoro M, Buchanan TA, Mestman JH. Insulin-requiring diabetes in pregnancy: a randomized trial of active induction of labor and expectant management. Am J Obstet Gynecol 1993;169:611–5.

THYROID DISEASES

Clinical Physiology

Thyroid hormones, thyroxine (T_4) and triiodothyronine (T_3), act in target tissues principally by binding to nuclear receptors, which induce specific changes in gene expression. These actions include a critical role in fetal central nervous system development. T_4 is the main product of the thyroid gland, providing a stable hormonal reservoir for extrathyroidal conversion to T_3. Pituitary TSH is the principal regulator of thyroid growth and hormone production. Thyroid-stimulating hormone stimulates thyroid cells by binding to a membrane receptor, which acts via the cyclic adenosine monophosphate second messenger system. Thyroid-stimulating immunoglobulins that bind this same receptor are the cause of hyperthyroid Graves' disease. Rarely, an inherited mutation of the TSH receptor can cause it to bind and be activated by hCG; this can cause familial gestational thyrotoxicosis in which hyperthyroidism develops during pregnancy and resolves after delivery.

At the end of the first trimester of pregnancy, levels of serum TSH are subnormal in 18% of normal women. The timing of this occurrence coincides with peak serum hCG concentrations, which acts as a thyroid stimulator because of the molecular similarity between hCG and TSH. This suggests a likely physiologic role for hCG in stimulating thyroidal hormone production in early pregnancy. The stimulatory effects of hCG are magnified in patients with hyperemesis gravidarum.

Fetal thyroid development begins late in the first trimester and is independent of the mother. Trans-placental passage of maternal thyroid hormones is minimal, but these hormones are likely important for fetal brain development before the appearance of the fetal thyroid gland. Maternal immunoglobulins causing autoimmune thyroid diseases cross the placenta and occasionally can cause transient thyroid dysfunction in the fetus and neonate—transient hyperthyroidism when the mother has Graves' disease and transient hypothyroidism when the mother has autoimmune thyroiditis. The fetus also is exposed to the drugs commonly used to treat hyperthyroidism.

Hypothyroidism

Overt hypothyroidism occurs in 2% of women. Mild hypothyroidism, also called subclinical or mild hypothyroidism, is evidenced only by an elevated serum TSH level. Transient hypothyroidism affects approximately 5% of postpartum women.

CAUSES

The principal cause of hypothyroidism is autoimmune (Hashimoto's) thyroiditis. Although there is a familial predisposition, the specific genetic and environmental factors that trigger this condition are unknown. Autoimmune thyroiditis is present in approximately 7% of women of childbearing age. Many of these women have mild hypothyroidism associated with mild or no symptoms. These women with decreased thyroid reserve are also at high risk of progressing to overt hypothyroidism, particularly during pregnancy, when the metabolic clearance of the thyroid hormones is accelerated. Progressive gland failure is particularly likely if women with mild hypothyroidism also have antithyroid antibodies. Patients with underlying autoimmune thyroiditis usually have a diffuse, firm, and painless goiter; however, the gland may be nonpalpable in the atrophic variant of the disease.

Hypothyroidism also occurs frequently after surgical or radioactive iodine therapy for hyperthyroidism. Thyroid gland irradiation in the course of treatment for head and neck tumors also can cause hypothyroidism. All patients who have received these therapies should be monitored yearly with a serum TSH measurement for the possible development of hypothyroidism. Transient thyroid gland inflammation causes spontaneously resolving hypothyroidism in postpartum thyroiditis and subacute thyroiditis. Hypothyroidism is rarely the result of pituitary or hypothalamic diseases causing TSH deficiency.

CLINICAL FEATURES

Recent studies have shown the negative effect on fetal outcome of undiagnosed or inadequately treated hypothyroidism during pregnancy. There are clear relationships between elevated maternal TSH and both fetal mortality and subsequent childhood neuropsychologic development. In one study, serum TSH in stored serum samples from 9,403 women with singleton pregnancies was found to be elevated (>6 mU/L) in 2% of cases. The fetal death rate was higher in those pregnancies than in the women with a normal TSH (3.8% versus 0.9%, odds ratio 4.4, 95% confidence interval 1.9–9.5) (1). In a related study, 62 women with elevated serum TSH levels were retrospectively identified from among 25,216 pregnant women whose sera had been stored (2). When the 7–9-year-old children of these women were compared with those of 124 matched euthyroid women, their full-scale IQ scores averaged 4 points lower ($P = .06$). Fifteen percent had IQ scores of 85 or less, whereas only 5% of the children born to euthyroid mothers did. The children of the 48 mothers whose hypothyroidism was not treated during pregnancy had IQ scores that were 7 points lower on average than the children of euthyroid control mothers ($P = .005$). Furthermore, there was an inverse correlation between severity of the mothers' hypothyroidism and their offsprings' IQ (3).

DIAGNOSIS

Overt primary hypothyroidism is characterized by a low serum free T_4 or free T_4 index and an elevated serum TSH. During pregnancy, the serum total T_4 level may remain normal due to the increased level of T_4-binding globulin; accurate diagnosis of primary hypothyroidism can be ensured by serum TSH measurement. Autoimmune thyroiditis can be confirmed by the presence of serum antithyroid peroxidase antibodies. For unclear reasons, several studies have shown that circulating antithyroid antibodies may be associated with habitual abortion, even when thyroid gland function is normal.

Because there is an apparent increase in the rate of thyroid hormone degradation during pregnancy, women with diminished thyroid gland reserve may develop hypothyroidism or progress from mild to overt hypothyroidism during gestation.

THERAPY

Levothyroxine is the treatment of choice for hypothyroidism. Its conversion to T_3 provides a stable hormonal milieu. Levothyroxine is well absorbed, unless there is co-administration of medications that include ferrous sulfate, calcium carbonate, cholestyramine, aluminum hydroxide, and sucralfate. Levothyroxine should be taken at least 4 hours apart from these medications, and should probably be taken on an empty stomach. The levothyroxine dose requirement is weight related (approximately 1.6 mg/kg) and should be adjusted to maintain the serum TSH within the lower one half of the reference range, eg, 0.5–2.0 mU/L. In approximately three quarters of pregnant women, the levothyroxine dose requirement is increased by 25–100% (4). This is probably due both to an increased T_4 requirement to occupy the larger circulating TBG pool and to acceleration of the T_4 clearance rate. This can occur during early, middle, or late pregnancy. Consequently, serum TSH should be reassessed at least every trimester of pregnancy. Postpartum, the prepregnancy levothyroxine dose usually can be resumed. All hypothyroid women with childbearing potential should be prospectively instructed to continue their thyroxine and contact the physician managing their thyroid condition when they become pregnant. Serum TSH should be assessed immediately to ensure that a possible increased dose requirement is met.

Treatment of mild hypothyroidism is justified in pregnancy because thyroid hormone deficiency has been associated with increased fetal loss and subtly impaired subsequent childhood neuropsychologic development, as described previously.

Administration of excessive levothyroxine doses should be avoided. Even mild T_4 excess, which is recognizable solely by a suppressed serum TSH, has been associated with cortical bone loss and atrial fibrillation. Initially, a low levothyroxine dose should be used (eg, 0.025 mg/kg/d) in women with known or suspected ischemic heart disease, which can be exacerbated by levothyroxine therapy.

Hyperthyroidism

The treatment of thyroid disease in pregnancy is straightforward: achieve and maintain maternal euthyroidism. Uncontrolled thyrotoxicosis is associated with high rates of fetal loss and possible malformations.

Less commonly, hyperthyroidism may be due to autonomously functioning benign thyroid neoplasia: toxic adenoma and toxic multinodular goiter. Transient thyrotoxicosis also results from the unregulated glandular release of thyroid hormone in subacute (painful) thyroiditis and in postpartum (painless, silent, or lymphocytic) thyroiditis. Rarely, thyroid gland overactivity is caused by a choriocarcinoma that secretes hCG or a pituitary adenoma that secretes TSH. Ovarian teratomas (struma ovarii) can produce thyroid hormones ectopically and

may cause hyperthyroidism if this tissue is stimulated in Graves' disease or contains an autonomously function neoplasm. Thyrotoxicosis is also caused by the iatrogenic prescription or factitious ingestion of T_4 or T_3, the latter often occurring in patients with eating disorders. Recently, a rare form of familial gestational thyrotoxicosis has been described in which a germline mutation of the TSH receptor renders it responsive to hCG with resulting recurrent hyperthyroidism whenever an affected woman becomes pregnant (5).

CLINICAL FEATURES

The symptoms and signs of hyperthyroidism in pregnancy are similar to the nonpregnant state. Weight may increase or decrease. Thyrotoxicosis may present with vomiting and may be confused with hyperemesis gravidarum. On examination, tachycardia, lid lag, tremor, proximal muscle weakness, and warm, moist skin are often present. Goiter is present in most younger women with Graves' disease.

DIAGNOSIS

Most thyrotoxic patients have elevated total and free T_4 and T_3 concentrations. However, as discussed above, high serum total T_4 or T_3 levels are not pathognomonic of hyperthyroidism. In all of the common forms of thyrotoxicosis, the serum TSH concentration is undetectable or very low in sensitive assays (ie, ones with detection limits of 0.1 mU/L). Consequently, serum TSH measurement is an extremely accurate way to exclude the diagnosis of hyperthyroidism. Patients with a low TSH concentration despite normal free T_4 and T_3 concentrations are said to have subclinical hyperthyroidism.

It is essential to differentiate accurately among the causes of hyperthyroidism because distinct forms of treatment often are indicated. Although the radioiodine uptake and scan are useful in the differential diagnosis of chemically established hyperthyroidism in the nonpregnant patient, radioisotopic studies are contraindicated during pregnancy. In patients with Graves' disease, serum immunoglobulins that mimic TSH-mediated adenylate cyclase activation (thyroid-stimulating immunoglobulins) or compete with TSH for receptor binding (thyroid-binding inhibitory immunoglobulins) can be detected, but seldom are required for diagnosis. High levels of maternal thyroid-stimulating immunoglobulins do predict a greater likelihood of neonatal hyperthyroidism in pregnant women with Graves' disease, including those who may themselves be euthyroid after previous thyroid ablation therapy.

THERAPY

The treatment of choice for pregnant women with hyperthyroid Graves' disease is antithyroid medication, either propylthiouracil or methimazole. Propylthiouracil also partially inhibits conversion of extrathyroidal T_4 to T_3 (6). Methimazole has a longer half-life and can be administered in a single daily dose. The notion that propylthiouracil crosses the placenta less readily than methimazole has been questioned recently. Although methimazole has been anecdotally associated with a congenital scalp anomaly, aplasia cutis, as well as more severe fetal anomalies, it also has been used widely and safely in pregnant women. The lowest dose of drug required to maintain the free T_4 concentration at the upper limit of normal should be used. Euthyroidism typically is restored in 3–10 weeks. As pregnancy progresses, the activity of Graves' disease often wanes, and the antithyroid dosage can be reduced or discontinued. Although continued antithyroid medication is effective in controlling hyperthyroidism, remissions are sustained in less than one half of patients after a course of drug therapy. Relapses are particularly common in the postpartum period.

All patients should be cautioned about the drug's minor side effects (eg, fever, rash, arthralgias), which are infrequent (5%), and particularly about major drug toxicities (eg, hepatitis, vasculitis, agranulocytosis), which are rare (0.2–0.5%). If a remission is achieved, lifelong monitoring is warranted. Long-term follow-up studies have documented that children exposed to antithyroid drugs in utero grow and develop normally. Concurrent levothyroxine therapy will not protect the fetus from hypothyroidism because levothyroxine crosses the placenta poorly. Following birth, antithyroid drugs are safe to use in lactation. Approximately 2% of fetuses may experience hypothyroidism as a result of propylthiouracil therapy, which may lead to the development of goiter. Fetal management during pregnancy should include serial ultrasonography to ensure adequate weight gain and targeted ultrasonography in the late third trimester to detect evidence of fetal goiter. Expert newborn care is essential.

In nonpregnant patients who have been treated with radioactive iodine, the radioiodine will have been excreted or will have decayed within 3 months. However, pregnancy probably should be avoided for 4–6 months after radioiodine therapy until most patients have become euthyroid or are taking T_4 replacement therapy.

Beta-adrenergic blocking agents are useful adjunctive therapy for control of sympathomimetic symptoms in hyperthyroid patients. Neonatal bradycardia and hypoglycemia can occur when these agents are used at the time of delivery. Beta blockers are usually the sole treatment for patients with spontaneously resolving hyperthyroidism caused by thyroiditis. Patients with subacute thyroiditis also are treated with aspirin or other nonsteroidal antiinflammatory drugs for relief of thyroid pain. In 20% of patients, a 2–8-week course of antenatal corticosteroids is required. Thyroid surgery is indicated only in thyrotoxic pregnant women who have a major side effect from an antithyroid drug or who do not follow instructions for therapy.

Neonatal thyrotoxicosis secondary to the transplacental passage of antibodies occurs only in about 1% of mothers with Graves' disease. Neonates with Graves' disease present with failure to thrive, irritability, tachycardia, goiter, heart failure, and craniosynostosis. If the mother received antithyroid medication during the pregnancy, the child may not become hyperthyroid until 7–10 days postpartum. If neonatal thyrotoxicosis is diagnosed by finding elevated serum thyroid hormones, suppressed serum TSH, and positive TSH-receptor antibodies, antithyroid drug therapy should be continued for 6–8 weeks, until the passively transferred antibodies have been cleared from the infant's circulation.

Some women with hyperemesis gravidarum develop concomitant mild biochemical hyperthyroidism. This phenomenon is thought to result from the extremely high serum levels of hCG that are often observed in hyperemesis. Serum free T_4 levels correlate with serum hCG concentrations as well as the severity of nausea and vomiting. Although more than half of patients with so-called "gestational thyrotoxicosis" have suppressed serum TSH levels and elevated free T_4 levels, they rarely display the clinical features of hyperthyroidism, including goiter and eye findings. In general, the hyperthyroidism resolves without specific therapy as the hyperemesis wanes, usually by 20 weeks of gestation. If it persists beyond this point, the patient probably has true thyrotoxicosis due to mild Graves' disease and should be treated with antithyroid drugs.

Complicated thyrotoxicosis, sometimes called *thyroid storm*, is a medical emergency that is typically triggered by infection or other systemic illness in a thyrotoxic patient. The condition is manifested by fever, tachycardia, agitation or psychosis, tremor, and, sometimes, abdominal pain, vomiting, and dehydration. Prompt identification and intensive care are mandatory for such patients. It is almost always seen in untreated or noncompliant patients.

Postpartum Thyroid Disease

A spectrum of autoimmune thyroid dysfunction occurs during the postpartum period in approximately 5–10% of women (7). The classical sequence of events is transient hyperthyroidism followed by transient hypothyroidism, with the onset 1–8 months after delivery and each phase lasting 2–12 weeks. Other common patterns include transient hyperthyroidism (due to either Graves' disease or transient hyperthyroidism with low radioiodine uptake) or transient hypothyroidism alone. When patients present with postpartum hyperthyroidism, it may be difficult to distinguish postpartum thyroiditis from recurrent or new-onset Graves' disease. The thyroid uptake of radioiodine is an important diagnostic tool because it is elevated in Graves' disease and low in postpartum thyroiditis. Although this test is contraindicated in women who are breastfeeding, it can be performed safely with iodine-123 or technetium-99m pertechnetate if breastfeeding is suspended for several days until radioactivity above the background level is no longer detectable in breast milk.

The presence of orbital involvement, a ratio of serum T_3 to serum T_4 concentration greater than 20, or serum anti-TSH receptor antibodies also favors the diagnosis of Graves' disease.

Because 25% of women with type 1 diabetes develop postpartum thyroiditis (8), assessment of this patient population during the postpartum period should be considered. Women with previous episodes of postpartum thyroiditis are likely to have recurrences after subsequent pregnancies.

Postpartum thyroiditis is relatively common, occurring in 5–10% of pregnancies. The resultant thyroid dysfunction is usually not evident at the time of the routine postpartum assessment; the majority of cases will develop within 3 to 6 months of delivery. Although depression has been reported to occur more frequently in the patients with postpartum thyroid dysfunction, more recent literature suggests that the association is less certain (9).

Thyroid Nodules and Cancer

In the pregnant woman discovered to have a thyroid nodule, fine-needle aspiration biopsy is the test of choice; radionuclide thyroid scanning is contraindicated. If the biopsy is benign or suspicious, T_4 suppression therapy should be initiated. In the case of a suspicious nodule, surgery can be performed after delivery if the nodule failed to shrink. If the patient clearly has thyroid carcinoma, 2 options can be considered: 1) thyroid surgery in the second trimester; or 2) T_4 suppression therapy and close observation for tumor growth followed by postpartum surgery (10). The latter would be particularly reasonable for papillary tumors, which typically have an indolent growth pattern.

References

1. Allan WC, Haddow JE, Palomaki GE, Williams JR, Mitchell ML, Hermos RJ, et al. Maternal thyroid deficiency and pregnancy complications: implications for population screening. J Med Screen 2000;7:127–30.

2. Haddow JE, Palomaki GE, Allan WC, Williams JR, Knight GJ, Gagnon J, et al. Maternal thyroid deficiency during pregnancy and subsequent neuropsychological development of the child. N Engl J Med 1999;341:549–55.

3. Klein RZ, Sargent JD, Larsen PR, Waisbren SE, Haddow JE, Mitchell ML. Relation of severity of maternal hypothyroidism to cognitive development of offspring. J Med Screen 2001;8:18–20.

4. Mandel SJ, Larsen PR, Seely EW, Brent GA. Increased need for thyroxine during pregnancy in women with primary hypothyroidism. N Engl J Med 1990;323:91–96.

5. Arafah BM. Increased need for thyroxine in women with hypothyroidism during estrogen therapy. N Engl J Med 2001;344:1743–9.

6. Rodien P, Bremont C, Sanson ML, Parma J, Van Sande J, Costagliola S, et al. Familial gestational hyperthyroidism caused by a mutant thyrotropin receptor hypersensitive to human chorionic gonadotropin. N Engl J Med 1998; 339:1823–6.

7. Mandel SJ, Cooper DS. The use of antithyroid drugs in pregnancy and lactation. J Clin Endocrinol Metab 2001; 86:2354–9.

8. Browne-Martin K, Emerson CH. Postpartum thyroid dysfunction. Clin Obstet Gynecol 1997;40:90–101.

9. Alvarez-Marfany M, Roman SH, Drexler AJ, Robertson C, Stagnaro-Green A. Long-term prospective study of postpartum thyroid dysfunction in women with insulin dependent diabetes mellitus. J Clin Endocrinol Metab 1994;79:10–6.

10. Lucas A, Pizarro E, Granada ML, Salinas I, Foz M, Sanmarti A. Postpartum thyroiditis: epidemiology and clinical evolution in a nonselected population. Thyroid 2000; 10:71–7.

11. Moosa M, Mazzaferri EL. Outcome of differentiated thyroid cancer diagnosed in pregnant women. J Clin Endocrinol Metab 1997;82:2862–6.

HEMATOLOGIC DISORDERS

Anemia in pregnant women has been defined as hemoglobin levels of less than 11 g/dL in the first and third trimesters and less than 10.5 g/dL in the second trimester (Fig. 18). Although anemia is somewhat more common among indigent pregnant women, it by no means is restricted to them. The frequency of anemia during pregnancy varies considerably, depending primarily on whether supplemental iron is taken during pregnancy. In several studies, women who took iron supplements had a mean hemoglobin concentration that was 1 g/dL greater than that of women not taking supplements.

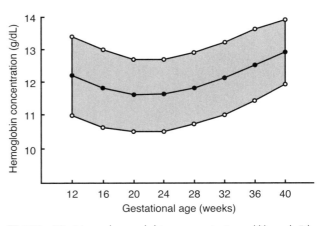

■ **FIG. 18.** Mean hemoglobin concentrations (*) and 5th and 95th percentiles (o) for healthy pregnant women taking iron supplements. (Centers for Disease Control and Prevention. CDC criteria for anemia in children and childbearing-aged women. MMWR Morb Mortal Wkly Rep 1989;38:400–4.)

The modest fall in hemoglobin levels observed in healthy pregnant women who are not deficient in iron or folate is caused by a greater expansion of plasma volume relative to the increase in hemoglobin mass and erythrocyte volume. The disproportion between the rates at which plasma and erythrocytes are added to the maternal circulation is usually greatest during the second trimester. The term *physiologic anemia*, long used to describe this process, is an oxymoron and should be discarded. Late in pregnancy, plasma expansion essentially ceases while hemoglobin mass continues to increase; thus hemoglobin concentration increases.

The initial evaluation of a woman with moderate anemia includes hemoglobin electrophoresis and red cell indices to ensure adequate hemoglobin identification. It also should include hematocrit, examination of peripheral blood smear, and measurement of levels of serum iron or ferritin or both.

Any disorder that causes anemia in women of childbearing age may complicate pregnancy. A classification based primarily on etiology and including most of the common causes of anemia in pregnant women is shown in Box 14.

Iron Deficiency Anemia

The 2 most common causes of anemia during pregnancy and the puerperium are iron deficiency and acute blood loss. The iron requirements of pregnancy are considerable. In a typical gestation with a single fetus, the maternal need for iron induced by pregnancy averages close to 1,000 mg: approximately 300 mg for the fetus and placenta and approximately 500 mg for the expansion of maternal hemoglobin mass. Another 200 mg is shed

through the gut, urine, and skin. This total amount considerably exceeds the iron stores of most women.

Moderate iron deficiency anemia during pregnancy (for example, a hemoglobin concentration of 9 g/dL) usually is not accompanied by obvious morphologic changes in erythrocytes. With this degree of anemia from iron deficiency, however, serum ferritin levels are lower than normal. In general, normal ferritin levels (Table 15) exclude iron deficiency, but decreased values do not confirm it (1). The serum iron-binding capacity is elevated, but by itself this is of little diagnostic value because it also is elevated during normal pregnancy in the absence of iron deficiency. Most clinicians consider a ratio of less than 15% for serum iron/iron-binding capacity to indicate iron deficiency anemia.

The objectives of treatment are correction of the deficit in hemoglobin mass and, eventually, restitution of iron stores. Taking into account the amount of iron absorption from the gastrointestinal tract, the clinician can accomplish both of these objectives with orally administered simple iron compounds—ferrous sulfate, fumarate, or gluconate—that provide a daily dose of about 200 mg of elemental iron (ie, 325 mg of ferrous sulfate three times daily or iron compounds in combination with prenatal vitamins) (Table 16). (The Institute of Medicine recommends 20 mg/d for pregnancy women, double the recommended dosage for nonpregnant women.) There is no need to prescribe ascorbic acid or fruit juices or to withhold food to enhance iron absorption nor is there any advantage from delayed-release or sustained-release medications. To replenish iron stores, oral therapy should be continued for 3 months or so after the anemia has been corrected. After 7–10 days of therapy with an iron compound, reticulocytosis can be seen and hemoglobin may increase by at least 1 g per week in patients with severe anemia.

BOX 14

Causes of Anemia During Pregnancy

Acquired
- Iron deficiency
- Anemia caused by acute blood loss
- Megaloblastic anemia
- Acquired hemolytic anemia
- Anemia of inflammation or malignancy
- Aplastic or hypoplastic anemia

Hereditary
- α- and β-thalassemias
- Sickle cell hemoglobinopathies
- Other hemoglobinopathies
- Hereditary hemolytic anemias

TABLE 15. Normal Iron Indices During Pregnancy

Index	Normal Value
Plasma iron	40–175 µg/dL
Plasma total iron-binding capacity	216–400 µg/dL
Transferrin saturation	16–60%
Serum ferritin	>10 µg/dL

TABLE 16. Oral Iron Supplementation

Preparation	Elemental Iron (mg)
Ferous sulfate 300 mg	60
Ferous gluconate 300 mg	34
Feosol, elixir 5 mL	45

In select cases—for example, patients with malabsorption syndromes or those with severe anemia (Hgb <8.5g/dL) who will not take iron therapy—there is a role for parenteral iron therapy (2, 3). The required dose of iron dextran needed to correct anemia and replenish iron stores is calculated using the following formula:

$$\text{Iron dextran (mL)} = (14 - \text{patient's Hgb}) \times (\text{wt in kg}) \times (0.0476) + \text{wt in kg}/5 \text{ [maximum 14]}$$

Anaphylaxis is a risk with intravenous iron dextran administration; therefore, a test dose should be administered first. The maximum rate of the full dose is 1 mL/min.

Subcutaneous erythropoietin has been administered successfully to correct iron deficiency anemia in pregnancy (4–6). In patients with significant anemia who had failed treatment to correct anemia with oral iron therapy alone, the addition of erythropoietin to oral iron therapy resulted in correction of anemia within 2 weeks in 73% of patients.

Despite the fact that iron deficiency anemia is the most common nutritional deficiency in the world, the maternal and perinatal complications associated with anemia have not been extensively studied (7–9). Severe anemia has been associated with increased low birth weight babies, induction rates, operative vaginal and cesarean deliveries, and prolonged labor (10).

Anemia Associated With Chronic Diseases

Anemia may be associated with chronic disease states, such as inflammatory bowel disease, chronic renal failure, and systemic lupus erythematosus. The etiology of such anemia may result from both decreased production and increased destruction of erythrocytes. The treatment of chronic anemia in pregnancy may be difficult, and treatment response may vary. Besides iron and folic acid, human recombinant erythropoietin has been used for the treatment of these anemias in pregnant women, especially those associated with chronic renal failure. Hypertension is a potentially worrisome side effect.

Sickle Cell Hemoglobinopathies

Hemoglobin S results from a single β-chain substitution of glutamic acid by valine because of a substitution of A for T at codon 6 of the β-globin gene. Sickle cell anemia (SS disease), sickle cell–hemoglobin C disease (SC disease), and sickle cell–β-thalassemia disease (S-β-thalassemia disease) are the most common of the sickle hemoglobinopathies.

The inheritance of the gene for S hemoglobin from each parent results in sickle cell anemia (SS disease). Although pregnancy outcomes have been improving, complications from sickle hemoglobin diseases are still significant (11, 12). This is especially true of women with hemoglobin SS disease, in whom anemia often becomes more intense, vasoocclusive episodes with severe pain—so-called *sickle cell crises*—usually become more frequent, and infections and pulmonary complications are more common. In addition to excessive maternal mortality, more than one third of pregnancies end in abortion, stillbirth, or neonatal death (Table 17).

The management of pregnant women with sickle cell hemoglobinopathies includes close observation with careful evaluation of all symptoms, physical findings, and laboratory studies. One rather common danger is that symptomatic women may categorically be considered to be suffering from sickle cell crisis. As a result, ectopic pregnancy, cholecystitis, or other serious obstetric or medical problems that cause pain, anemia, or both may be overlooked.

Intense sequestration of sickled erythrocytes with infarction in various organs may develop acutely, especially late in pregnancy, during labor and delivery, and early in the puerperium. When partial exchange transfusion is employed, the goal of therapy is to maintain Hgb A above 50% and the hematocrit above 25%.

Acute chest syndrome is characterized by pain, fever, cough, and pulmonary infiltrates (13, 14). It also may result in significant illness and even death in women with sickle cell disease. The exact etiology of this syndrome is unclear, but it has been reported to be associated with infection, microvascular occlusion from sickle hemoglobin, and fat embolism. The treatment for this syndrome basically is supportive.

Special circumstances during pregnancy appreciably increase morbidity among these women. Bacteriuria is common and urinary tract infections, including acute pyelonephritis, are increased substantially. Bacteriuria eradication is important to prevent most symptomatic infections. Pneumonia, especially caused by *Streptococcus pneumoniae*, is common, and polyvalent pneumococcal vaccine is recommended for these women. Because of substantial perinatal mortality and IUGR, careful fetal surveillance is mandatory, as is the use of other methods of antepartum assessment.

Sickle Cell Trait

About 8% of African Americans are heterozygous for the sickle cell gene. Sickle cell trait should not be considered a deterrent to pregnancy on the basis of increased risk to the mother. The risk of urinary tract infection is twice as high. Conflicting data exist regarding an association (increased or decreased) risk with pregnancy-induced hypertension (15). It appears that sickle cell trait does not unfavorably influence the frequency of abortion, perinatal mortality, or low birth weight.

The probability of a serious sickle cell hemoglobinopathy in offspring of women with sickle cell trait is 1 in 4 whenever the father carries a gene for an abnormal hemoglobin or for β-thalassemia. Prenatal diagnosis of sickle cell disease is available.

TABLE 17. Pregnancy Outcomes Reported Since 1956 for Women with Sickle Cell Anemia and Hemoglobin Sickle Cell Disease

Type of Disease	Number and Rate				
	Women	Pregnancies	Maternal Deaths (per 100,000)	Spontaneous Abortions (per 100)	Perinatal Deaths (per 1,000)
Sickle cell anemia (SS)	1,144	2,145	~2,500	20	~180
Sickle cell–hemoglobin C (SC) disease	293	740	~2,300	16	~75

Adapted from Hematological disorders. In: Cunningham FG, Gant NF, Leveno KJ, Gilstrap LC III, Hauth JC, Wenstrom KD. Williams obstetrics. 21st ed. New York (NY): McGraw-Hill; 2001. p. 1317.

Megaloblastic Anemia

Although uncommon in pregnancy, megaloblastic anemia can occur as a result of folic acid anemia. The sequence of changes that result from folate deficiency is unaltered by pregnancy. The earliest biochemical evidence is low plasma concentrations of folic acid. The earliest morphologic evidence is usually hypersegmentation of neutrophils. Macrocytes usually are seen on peripheral smear. As anemia becomes more intense, an occasional nucleated erythrocyte appears in the peripheral blood. As maternal folate deficiency and, in turn the anemia, become more severe, thrombocytopenia, leucopenia, or both may develop.

Treatment of pregnancy-induced megaloblastic anemia should include folic acid, a nutritious diet, and iron. As little as 1 mg of folic acid administered orally once daily produces a striking hematologic response. By 4–7 days after treatment is begun, the reticulocyte count is increased appreciably, and leucopenia and thrombocytopenia are promptly corrected. Severe megaloblastic anemia during pregnancy typically is accompanied by an appreciably smaller blood volume than in a normal pregnancy, but soon after folic acid therapy has been started, the blood volume usually increases considerably and may intensify the anemia transiently. Folic acid requirements increase as gestation advances, and anemia may develop in the setting of folic acid deficiency. Pregnancies with multiple gestation should be supplemented with 1 mg of folic acid daily. Several drugs, including phenytoin, primidone, para-aminosalicylic acid, and sulfasalazine may decrease serum folate concentrations and cause deficiency.

Of note, oral contraceptives also may impair folate metabolism, and dihydrofolate reductase inhibitors (eg, methotrexate, trimethoprim) can interfere with folic acid utilization.

Thrombocytopenia

GESTATIONAL THROMBOCYTOPENIA

Gestational thrombocytopenia occurs in 5% of pregnancies and typically is not associated with maternal, fetal, or neonatal sequelae (16). The lower limit of normal platelet counts in pregnancy has been reported to be 106–120 × 10^9/L. However, it is well recognized that platelet counts can drop much lower than this range, with a lower threshold of gestational thrombocytopenia being 70 × 10^9/L. Gestational thrombocytopenia is characterized by mild asymptomatic thrombocytopenia in a patient without any history of thrombocytopenia (other than in a prior pregnancy), typically occurring in the third trimester without any fetal thrombocytopenia and with spontaneous resolution (17). Recurrent gestational thrombocytopenia has been reported in 18% of pregnancies. (See Box 15 on differential diagnosis.)

At delivery, routine obstetric management for the patient and fetus/neonate is recommended. Women with platelet counts at 50–100 × 10^9/L can safely have a regional anesthetic. Although severe thrombocytopenia rarely has been reported in the setting of presumed gestational thrombocytopenia, fortunately fetal intracranial hemorrhage is not a feature of this disease.

BOX 15

Differential Diagnosis of Thrombocytopenia

Preeclampsia and preeclampsia-related syndrome

Autoimmune thrombocytopenia from lupus, drugs, antiphospholipid antibody, human immunodeficiency virus disease, or idiopathic etiology

Thrombotic thrombocytopenic purpura or hemolytic uremic syndrome

Disseminated intravascular coagulation

Bone marrow disease

Hypersplenism

Congenital platelet disorders

Spurious thrombocytopenia from ethylene diaminetetraacetic acid

IDIOPATHIC THROMBOCYTOPENIC PURPURA

Idiopathic thrombocytopenic purpura (ITP, also called isoimmune thrombocytopenic purpura) is an autoimmune disorder in which antiplatelet antibodies of the reticuloendothelial system, namely IgG antibodies, initiate a process of platelet destruction (18). The principal site of antibody production is the maternal spleen and secondarily the bone marrow. Platelet destruction results in maternal thrombocytopenia. In addition, antiplatelet IgG antibodies can cross the placenta to cause fetal thrombocytopenia. When new-onset thrombocytopenia is discovered in pregnancy, the diagnosis of ITP often is made as a diagnosis of exclusion once other causes of thrombocytopenia are ruled out (see Box 15). Criteria for ITP include normal blood count, except for thrombocytopenia, blood smear showing an increased percentage of large platelets, normal coagulation studies, bone marrow with increased size and number of megalokaryocytes, and lack of other cause of thrombocytopenia.

Fortunately, the risk of severe thrombocytopenia (platelet count $< 50 \times 10^9$/L) occurs in approximately 10% of cases, but the risk of serious morbidity, namely intracranial hemorrhage, occurs in less than 1% of cases. In fact, an estimated rate of 2 per 100,000 births has been suggested for intracranial hemorrhage due to ITP. The presence of chronic ITP and antiplatelet antibodies place a fetus at risk for thrombocytopenia. Fetuses at highest risk for morbidity are those whose siblings have experienced serious morbidity (intracranial hemorrhage). Given the rarity of sequelae from fetal thrombocytopenia from ITP, routine obstetric management in most cases of either new onset ITP or chronic ITP is appropriate (17, 19–21). In select cases of ITP, a more aggressive approach to the management of labor and delivery may be indicated (prior affected sibling with severe thrombocytopenia and intracranial hemorrhage) and may include cordocentesis to determine the fetal platelet count. If significant thrombocytopenia (platelet count $< 50 \times 10^9$/L) is noted at cordocentesis, options include in utero transfusion of platelets and cesarean delivery. Thus, considerable attention has been directed to identifying fetuses with potentially dangerous thrombocytopenia. Unfortunately, the correlation between fetal and maternal platelet counts is not strong. There also is little correlation of maternal IgG circulating platelet antibody, platelet-associated antibody, and fetal platelet count.

The management of thrombocytopenia associated with ITP depends on the patient's experience with ITP and the presence of other relevant medical conditions, the severity and setting of the thrombocytopenia, and gestational age at which it occurs. Early on in pregnancy, treatment of thrombocytopenia should occur if the maternal platelet count is in the 30×10^9/L – 50×10^9/L range, or if the patient is symptomatic. Initial treatment should consist of steroid administration (1 mg/kg of prednisone per day). Other options for severe thrombocytopenia include intravenous gamma globulin (IVIG) with regimens ranging from 400 mg/kg/day for 3 days to higher dose IVIG (for example, 1 g/kg/day). Rh immune globulin (WinRho) is another option for ITP for patients who are Rhesus positive (22). One of the side effects of Rh immune globulin therapy is mild anemia.

Splenectomy should be reserved for the most refractory cases. Although splenectomy initially will dramatically improve the thrombocytopenia, thrombocytopenia can still occur in patients with chronic ITP. Other pregnancy-associated risks include risk of fetal death and preterm labor.

At delivery, the principal maternal risk is hemorrhage. A maternal platelet count of $50–100 \times 10^9$/L is considered safe for vaginal or cesarean delivery. For neuraxial anesthesia, a platelet count of 80×10^9/L is considered adequate for catheter placement (23). For immediate treatment of thrombocytopenia for delivery, platelet transfusion is an option. For severe thrombocytopenia, if platelet transfusion is considered necessary, it should be done just before surgery, preferably with single donor platelets. Postpartum, medications associated with an increased risk of bleeding (nonsteroidal antiinflammatory agents, for example) should be avoided.

Because thrombocytopenia can occur in neonates born of mothers with ITP, serial platelet counts in the newborn are required. Neonatal thrombocytopenia is correlated with prior maternal splenectomy, maternal platelet count less than 50×10^9/L, and neonatal thrombocytopenia in a sibling. For severe thrombocytopenia (typically in the range of $< 20 \times 10^9$/L) requiring immediate correction, platelet transfusion is indicated.

THROMBOTIC THROMBOCYTOPENIC PURPURA AND HEMOLYTIC UREMIC SYNDROME

Thrombotic thrombocytopenic purpura (TTP) and hemolytic uremic syndrome are thrombotic microangiopathic diseases in which intravascular platelet aggregation causes transient ischemia (24). They are characterized by thrombocytopenia and hemolytic anemia and frequently can cause multisystem organ failure. The conditions occur in 1/25,000 pregnancies. Typically, TTP has 5 distinguishing features: fever, hemolytic anemia, thrombocytopenia, neurologic symptoms, and renal abnormalities. Elevations in blood urea nitrogen (BUN) and creatinine are rarely greater than 100 mg/dL and 3 mg/dL, respectively. Typically, hemolytic uremic syndrome has more renal impairment and less neurologic involvement than TTP. Typically, TTP occurs in women in their 20s and 30s; hemolytic uremic syndrome is primarily a disease of children. A characteristic differentiating feature of TTP and hemolytic uremic syndrome is antecedent gastrointestinal illness, which is common with hemolytic uremic syndrome and rare with TTP. Renal failure and hypertension often occur early with TTP and are severe, while they are less common and occur later with TTP. Thrombocytopenia and bleeding are more severe in TTP. Neurologic manifestations are unusual with hemolytic uremic syndrome.

The treatment for TTP and hemolytic uremic syndrome is plasmapheresis. Patients with TTP have a progressive deteriorating course, and the disease is fatal (almost 90% of cases) unless treated. Both conditions can occur during and following a normal pregnancy or occur following preeclampsia. Unlike preeclampsia, TTP and hemolytic uremic syndrome do not typically resolve with only delivery.

Von Willebrand's Disease

Von Willebrand's disease (vWD) is the most common inherited bleeding disorder, affecting up to 1% of the population. The disease occurs because of qualitative abnormalities, quantitative abnormalities, or both of von Willebrand's factor (vWF) (25). Circulating as a series of multimers, vWF plays an important role in primary hemostasis by binding to both platelets and the endothelium, forming an adhesive bridge. It also acts as a carrier protein for factor VIII. Four types of vWD have been identified (Box 16).

Consistent with the rise of the majority of the circulating clotting factors, levels of vWF rise during the second and third trimesters of pregnancy to 2–3 times the baseline. Treatment is not needed during pregnancy in the majority of women with vWD. However, plasma levels of factor VIII and vWF fall quickly after delivery, and excessive bleeding may occur at this time. Diminished factor VIII levels appear to be the most important deter-

minant of excess bleeding at delivery. Factor VIII levels should be at or above 50% for a cesarean delivery. (See Box 17 for management considerations.) Regarding peripartum management, for patients who respond to desmopressin (DDAVP), administer DDAVP immediately postpartum and 12 hours later; follow factor levels as an outpatient. Consider oral contraception to manage menorrhagia associated with the disease. (See Fig. 19 for care of nonresponders.)

Desmopressin is a synthetic analog of antidiuretic hormone and increases vWF and factor VIII levels. It also promotes the release of vWF from endothelial cell storage sites and potentially enhances hemostasis in patients with platelet function defects. Desmopressin can be administered intravenously, by subcutaneous injection,

---

BOX 16

Types of von Willebrand's Disease

According to the 1993 International Society of Thrombosis and Haemostasis classification, there are 4 types of vWD:

- Type 1 vWD: Most common (70–80%); decreased synthesis or excess proteolytic degradation, normal multimers; vWFAg is reduced 20–50%. (R/Type 3 het)

- Type 2 vWD: Four subtypes (mutations resulting in qualitative alterations in vWF function)

- Type 3 vWD: Severe form of disease (absence or near absence of vWF), autosomal recessive

- Acquired vWD: Usually @ monoclonal gammaglobulinopathies or lymphoproliferative disorders. Mechanism: Ig-vWF complex with clearance; selective absorption of vWF to malignant cells

VWD indicates von Willebrand's disease; vWF, von Willebrand's factor.

BOX 17

Management of von Willebrand's Disease During Pregnancy

First trimester:

  Identify variant of vWD.
  Identify response to DDAVP.
  Obtain baseline vWF: Ag, vWF activity, factor VIII level.
  Check hepatitis B status.

Second trimester:

  Administer hepatitis B vaccine series if nonimmune.
  Plan for anesthesia consultation.
  Test response to DDAVP.

Third trimester:

  Monitor FVIII, vWF: Ag levels, vWF activity.
  Review birth plan: epidural, dose/ timing of DDAVP (and/or factor VIII concentrate, Humate-P).
  Obtain test response to DDAVP.

At 38 weeks of gestation:

  Assay vWF levels.
  If vWF level is less than 50 IU/dL, start DDAVP for known responders, or replacement therapy for others.

In labor:

  Invasive fetal monitoring can be used, but consideration should be given about the potential for injury to an affected fetus.
  Treatment of vWD may be required after delivery, and during the first 2–4 weeks postpartum.
  Elective neonatal procedures should be withheld until the infant's vWD and factor VIII status have been determined.

DDAVP indicates desmopressin; vWD, von Willebrand's disease; vWF, von Willebrand's factor.

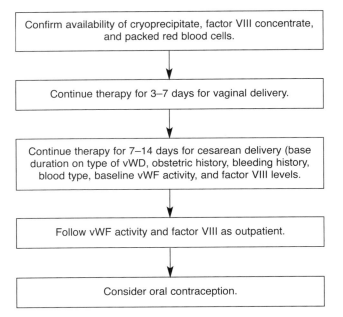

FIG. 19. Management algorithm for patients with von Willebrand's disease (vWD) who do not respond to desmopressin (DDAVP). vWF indicates von Willebrand's factor.

or by intranasal spray. Desmopressin is suitable for patients with Type I, Type IIA, and Type IIN, while it is not helpful in Type IIB and Type III. When given intravenously for prophylaxis before invasive procedures or for acute bleeding episodes, a dose of 0.3 μg/kg (maximum 20 μg) is diluted in 50 mL of normal saline and infused over 20–30 minutes; the same dose is given with subcutaneous therapy. An increase in vWF and factor VIII levels is expected at approximately 30–60 minutes after the infusion, and the response persists for 6–12 hours. A repeat dose may be given at 8–12 hours; subsequent doses are often switched to once daily doses.

Intranasal administration is an excellent choice for milder bleeding cases. The usual dose is 300 μg for adults. The vWF levels achieved with 300 μg of intranasal spray (DDAVP) are approximately equivalent to that seen with an intravenous dose of 0.2 μg/kg. Side effects of desmopressin include facial flushing, headache, and tingling. Hypertension or hypotension is rare. Thrombosis is rare. Tachyphylaxis will occur after repeated administration. Water retention and consequent hyponatremia can occur. Avoid the concomitant use of ibuprofen (26). Other treatment options include factor VIII concentrate, recombinant factor VIIa, and cryoprecipitate.

References

1. Alper BS, Kimber R, Reddy AK. Using ferritin levels to determine iron-deficiency anemia in pregnancy. J Fam Practice 2000;49:829–32.

2. Bashiri A, Burstein E, Sheiner E, Mazor M. Anemia during pregnancy and treatment with intravenous iron: review of the literature. Eur J Obstet Gynecol Reprod Biol 2003;110:2–7.

3. Komolafe JO, Kuti O, Ijadunola KT, Ogunniyi SO. A comparative study between intramuscular iron dextran and oral ferrous sulphate in the treatment of iron deficiency anaemia in pregnancy. J Obstet Gynaecol 2003;23:628–31.

4. Scott LL, Ramin SM, Richey M, Hanson J, Gilstrap LC 3rd. Erythropoietin use in pregnancy: two cases and a review of the literature. Am J Perinatol 1995;12:22–4.

5. Sifakis S, Angelakis E, Vardaki E, Koumantaki Y, Matalliotakis I, Koumantakis E. Erythropoietin in the treatment of iron deficiency anemia during pregnancy. Gynecol Obstet Invest 2001:51:150–6.

6. Thorp M, Pulliam J. Use of recombinant erythropoietin in a pregnant renal transplant recipient. Am J Nephrol 1998;18:448–51.

7. Cogswell ME, Parvanta I, Ickes L, Yip R, Brittenham GM. Iron supplementation during pregnancy, anemia, and birth weight: a randomized controlled trial. Am J Clin Nutr 2003;78:773–81.

8. Mungen E. Iron supplementation in pregnancy. J Perinat Med 2003;31:420–6.

9. Erdem A, Erdem M, Arslan M, Yazici G, Eskandari R, Himmetoglu O. The effect of maternal anemia and iron deficiency on fetal erythropoiesis: comparison between serum erythropoietin, hemoglobin and ferritin levels in mothers and newborns. J Matern Fetal Neonatal Med 2002;11:329–32.

10. Malhotra M, Sharma JB, Batra S, Sharma S, Murthy NS, Arora R. Maternal and perinatal outcome in varying degrees of anemia. Int J Gynaecol Obstet 2002;79:93–100.

11. Rust OA, Perry KG Jr. Pregnancy complicated by sickle hemoglobinopathy. Clin Obstet Gynecol 1995;38:472–84.

12. Smith JA, Espeland M, Bellevue R, Bonds D, Brown AK, Koshy M. Pregnancy in sickle cell disease: experience of the Cooperative Study of Sickle Cell Disease. Obstet Gynecol 1996;87:199–204.

13. Stuart MJ, Setty BN. Sickle cell acute chest syndrome: pathogenesis and rationale for treatment. Blood 1999;94:1555–60.

14. Kress JP, Pohlman AS, Hall JB. Determination of hemoglobin saturation in patients with acute sickle chest syndrome: a comparison of arterial blood gases and pulse oximetry. Chest 1999;115:1316–20.

15. Stamilio DM, Sehdev HM, Macones GA. Pregnant women with the sickle cell trait are not at increased risk for developing preeclampsia. Am J Perinatol 2003;20:41–8.

16. Rouse DJ, Owen J, Goldenberg RL. Routine maternal platelet count: an assessment of a technologically driven screening practice. Am J Obstet Gynecol 1998;179:573–6.

17. George JN, Woolf SH, Raskob GE, Wasser JS, Aledort LM, Ballem PJ, et al. Idiopathic thrombocytopenic purpura: a practice guideline developed by explicit methods for the American Society of Hematology. Blood 1996;88:3–40.

18. Cines DB, Blanchette VS. Immune thrombocytopenic purpura. N Engl J Med 2002;346:995–1008.

19. Silver RM, Branch DW, Scott JR. Maternal thrombocytopenia in pregnancy: time for a reassessment. Am J Obstet Gynecol 1995;173:479–82.

20. Gill KK, Kelton JG. Management of idiopathic thrombocytopenic purpura in pregnancy. Semin Hematol 2000;37:275–89.

21. Payne SD, Resnik R, Moore TR, Hedriana HL, Kelly TF. Maternal characteristics and risk of severe neonatal thrombocytopenia and intracranial hemorrhage in pregnancies complicated by autoimmune thrombocytopenia. Am J Obstet Gynecol 1997;177:149–55.

22. Michel M, Novoa MV, Bussel JB. Intravenous anti-D as a treatment for immune thrombocytopenic purpura (ITP) during pregnancy. Br J Haematol 2003;123:142–6.

23. Webert KE, Mittal R, Sigouin C, Heddle NM, Kelton JG. A retrospective 11-year analysis of obstetric patients with idiopathic thrombocytopenic purpura. Blood 2003;102:4306–11.

24. Esplin MS, Branch DW. Diagnosis and management of thrombotic microangiopathies during pregnancy. Clin Obstet Gynecol 1999;42:360–7.

25. Rodeghiero F. von Willebrand disease: still an intriguing disorder in the era of molecular medicine. Haemophilia 2002;8:292–300.

26. Garcia EB, Ruitenberg A, Madretsma GS, Hintzen RQ. Hyponatraemic coma induced by desmopressin and ibuprofen in a woman with von Willebrand's disease. Haemophilia 2003;9:232–4.

RENAL DISEASE

Over the past 3 decades, improved understanding of the interplay between pregnancy and renal disease, as well as recognition of the importance of hypertension and increased ability to control it, has led to a realization that pregnancy may be successfully accomplished in most, though not all, women with renal disease.

The most obvious changes seen during pregnancy, the increase in the size of the kidney and dilation of the ureters, have been recognized for years. The cause of these changes has been debated; however, it is generally held that both the direct compression of the ureters by the enlarging, dextrorotated uterus and ovarian vein plexuses and the effect of increased progesterone levels on the smooth muscles of the ureter play a role. This may rarely lead to symptomatic hydronephrosis (0.2% of pregnancies), with about 7% of cases necessitating placement of a stent due to failure of analgesics and conservative therapy.

In recent years, it is the advances in understanding of the functional changes that have been most notable. The functional increase is characterized by an increase in renal plasma flow, which peaks in the second trimester at 60–80% above nonpregnant levels and then falls back to 50% above nonpregnant levels in the third trimester. The glomerular filtration rate increases to 30% above prepregnancy levels in the first trimester, peaks at 50% above

prepregnancy levels in the second trimester, and maintains this increase through the third trimester. Endothelial-derived relaxing factor (EDRF), which is nitric oxide (NO), has been demonstrated to be the most likely primary mediator of this dramatic alteration in renal hyperfiltration (1). In a series of experiments that evaluated the role of nitric oxide in a rat model, investigators observed that inhibition of NO synthetase altered renal hemodynamics in pregnant rats, increasing renal resistance in vivo and increasing myogenic reactivity in vitro to levels comparable to nonpregnant controls (2). These studies also showed that back-up mechanisms appear to exist, with vasodilatory prostaglandins likely playing a fail-safe role when the NO-EDRF system is suppressed. Further work revealed that endothelin, which normally acts as a vasoconstrictor, is the mediator of low vascular tone in pregnant rats via some combination of the mechanisms of stimulation of an endothelin B subtype, tonic stimulation of NO-EDRF, or a feedback inhibition of endothelin production. Finally, these investigators showed that relaxin plays a role in gestational alterations in renal function by increasing glomerular filtration rate and decreasing osmolality (3–5). Relaxin is a hormone produced by the corpus luteum. Its production is increased dramatically by hCG. Although all of these observations are in rat models and cannot necessarily be translated verbatim to humans, they have stimulated further research and helped increase our appreciation of the complexity of gestational renal hemodynamics, with the hope that a more complete understanding of the normal physiology will allow us to better understand and treat pathologic derangements of that system.

The effect of pregnancy on renal disease and vice versa depends on the degree of renal insufficiency and the etiology. It is important to consider both renal disease secondary to systemic diseases and primary renal disease. In general, the impact of renal insufficiency on pregnancy is related to the serum creatinine. In women with minimal renal insufficiency (serum creatinine <1.4 mg/dL), fetal mortality is only mildly increased, and the underlying disease is not irreversibly worsened. However, as the serum creatinine rises, so does the risk to the mother and fetus (Table 18) (6). When the preconception serum creatinine is 2.0 mg/dL or higher, the risk of a rapid decline to end-stage renal disease is 33%. The risks of prematurity and growth restriction also increase as creatinine levels increase.

The next important factor to influence pregnancy outcome in women with renal disease is the presence of preconceptional hypertension. Although even controlled hypertension is associated with a higher incidence of preeclampsia and preterm delivery, it is uncontrolled hypertension that is predictive of poor maternal and fetal outcomes. For this reason, control of hypertension is one of the most important aspects of care. Angiotensin-converting enzyme inhibitors, among the most widely prescribed antihypertensive medications in this population, are contraindicated in pregnancy because they are associated with oligohydramnios leading to pulmonary

TABLE 18. Pregnancy's Effect on Renal Disease

Creatinine Level	Effect
≥1.4 mg/dL	Cesarean birth rate increases to more than 50%
1.4–2.5 mg/dL	Rates of prematurity increase to approximately 55% Rates of intrauterine growth restriction increase to approximately 30%
≥2.0 mg/dL	Decline in renal function accelerates
1.4–2.0 mg/dL	Risk of accelerated decline is approximately 2%
≥2.0 mg/dL	Risk of rapid decline is 33%
≥2.5 mg/dL	Rates of prematurity increase to 70% Rates of intrauterine growth restriction increase to 55%

hypoplasia. Fortunately, ACE inhibitors do not appear to be teratogenic. Consequently, women may remain on this therapy until pregnancy is diagnosed, allowing them the benefits of the medication's renoprotective effect.

During pregnancy, the therapies most commonly used for hypertension in patients with renal disease include α-methyldopa, labetalol, and calcium channel blockers. Among calcium channel blockers, nifedipine is the most widely studied in pregnancy, although usually in the role of a tocolytic. However, in patients with nephropathy outside of pregnancy, diltiazem is the calcium channel blocker that is most effective in decreasing proteinuria and preserving renal function (7). This led one group to retrospectively compare pregnancies in women with renal disease who were treated with diltiazem to those not requiring therapy (8). Although they showed a lower rate of IUGR, improved blood pressure control, and less proteinuria in the diltiazem-treated group, the small size of the trial (only 4 treated patients compared to 3 controls) did not allow for statistically significant conclusions. Nonetheless, by reminding us of the findings outside of pregnancy, it suggests that diltiazem is an appropriate alternative to ACE inhibitors and possibly the optimal choice.

Another aspect of chronic renal disease that may cause difficulty is a nephrotic level of proteinuria. In these cases, massive protein loss may lead to hypoalbuminemia and significant body edema. In extreme cases, this edema may be very uncomfortable, and small doses of diuretics may be administered. Whether the degree of proteinuria is itself a prognostic indicator for pregnancy outcome is still an open question. Several authors have suggested that proteinuria is not an independent marker for outcome (6); others believe that it is (9).

Primary Renal Disease

Primary renal disease is divided into glomerulonephritis (eg, membranoproliferative glomerulonephritis, IgA nephropathy, focal glomerulosclerosis, congenital nephrosis) and chronic tubulointerstitial disease (eg, reflux, adult polycystic kidney disease, chronic obstruction). The evidence that pregnancy outcomes vary significantly based on individual disease is lacking, and the outcomes between the two large categories, glomerulonephritis and tubulointerstitial diseases, have not been shown to be clearly different. Indeed, a single-center study of women with renal disease included 46 pregnancies in 38 women with a variety of primary renal diseases and reported that 98% of pregnancies were associated with a healthy infant without severe handicap 2 years after delivery.

Diabetic Nephropathy

Although women with diabetic nephropathy were once considered to require more pessimistic counseling, recent studies have suggested that with close attention to glycemic control, pregnancy does not pose an unreasonable risk of an accelerated decline in renal function. Two studies of women with type 1 diabetes and diabetic nephropathy found no evidence that pregnancy had a deleterious effect on renal function during follow-up of 3–16 years (10, 11). Another study of 11 women with type 1 diabetes did show accelerated progression of nephropathy after pregnancy (12). In a randomized trial of tight control in type 1 diabetes, all women who became pregnant were treated intensively. No difference was found in progression of albuminuria between those who did and those who did not become pregnant (13).

Yet it is clear that, as with other nephropathies, prepregnancy renal function is predictive of obstetric outcome. A series of 72 pregnancies in 58 women demonstrated that a high serum creatinine was associated with preterm delivery prior to 32 weeks of gestation, very low birth weight, and neonatal hypoglycemia (14). These findings were independent of total urinary protein excretion or glycemic control. A study that evaluated the influence of proteinuria found that it was of some prognostic value, with patients with less than 1 g proteinuria prior to 20 weeks of gestation having a substantially lower risk of pregnancy complications and long-term deterioration in renal function (15). The investigators suggested this was most likely due to this group representing a cohort of women with microalbuminuria in whom pregnancy exacerbated protein excretion, resulting in the diagnosis of nephropathy. Overall though, pregnancy outcomes in women with diabetic nephropathy appear similar to outcomes in women with other nephropathies.

Lupus Nephritis

Although many women with lupus do not have renal involvement, those who do may become exceptionally ill during pregnancy and have perinatal morbidity and mortality exceeding those of other nephropathies. A recent review of the risks of pregnancy in women with lupus nephritis pointed out the most critical determinants of outcome were quiescence of disease for at least 6 months prior to conception and the presence of antiphospholipid antibodies (14). For instance, in a representative study, fetal loss was noted in 83% of patients with antiphospholipid antibodies compared to 13% in whom no antibodies were detected (16). Investigators noted that proteinuria and hypertension were also independent predictors of adverse fetal outcome.

Renal Dialysis

Although most women on dialysis have irregular or absent menses, pregnancy can occur and be maintained while on dialysis. In 1 study, 1.5% of women of reproductive age on dialysis became pregnant over a 2-year period. In another, 7.3% of married women younger than 50 years became pregnant during long-term dialysis. The lack of regular menstruation is problematic because gestation is frequently quite advanced by the time pregnancy is recognized. Early studies were somewhat pessimistic, but recent literature has reported that successful pregnancy occurs in more than 50% of women. In 1 center, of 18 pregnancies in 15 women, 10 were successful (17). Another single-center study of 17 pregnancies reported success in 12 cases, and in this report, success was more common in women undergoing hemodialysis (13, or 78.6%) than continuous ambulatory peritoneal dialysis (6, or 33.3%). However, the U.S. Registry for Pregnancy in Dialysis Patients found that although conception rates in peritoneal dialysis patients were just under half that in hemodialysis patients, the outcomes in the 2 groups were the same (18). Infant survival was 46.4% in the hemodialysis group and 47.6% in the peritoneal dialysis group. In the subgroup of women undergoing intensive hemodialysis (≥ 20 hours/week), survival may be as high as 85%. The data from the registry also found that prematurity and IUGR were common complications, with 84% of fetuses delivered preterm (mean gestational age of 32.9 weeks) and 28% small for gestational age. The obstetric management of these patients is not substantially altered with the exception of taking great care to avoid magnesium toxicity if magnesium sulfate is chosen as a tocolytic. Also, indomethacin should be used cautiously because it may have an effect on any residual renal function a patient may have, increasing their need for dialysis. As with any chronic medical conditions that pose a high risk of stillbirth and IUGR, patients should be followed with early fetal surveillance. With regard to the route of delivery, cesarean births are reserved for routine obstetric indications (18). For patients undergoing peritoneal dialysis who must deliver by cesarean birth, the abdomen should be drained preoperatively and the surgery performed extraperitoneally, if possible. Peritoneal dialysis may be resumed 24 hours postoperatively, but if transperitoneal cesarean delivery is required and leakage occurs, hemodialysis should be substituted for 2 weeks.

The goals of dialysis during pregnancy do not differ substantially from goals in the nonpregnant state; however, certain modifications are necessary. The minimum goal for dialysis is to maintain the BUN below 80 mg/dL, and a BUN below 50–60 mg/dL is much preferred. To limit hypotension and decreased uterine perfusion, the volume of exchanges must be limited. In most pregnant women on hemodialysis, exchanges occur daily or 6 of 7 days per week by the start of the third trimester. Increasing the number of hours of hemodialysis to 20 or more results in a decreased rate of prematurity and improved infant survival. Women on dialysis often are anemic and may require transfusions. In order to maintain the hematocrit and reduce the need for transfusion, erythropoietin has been used in pregnancy for a number of conditions, including renal anemia, and appears to be well tolerated. It may increase the hematocrit to more than 30% in most patients. It is important to note that because dialysis increases removal of water-soluble vitamins, pregnant women should be given supplements. In particular, it is recommended that folic acid be increased 4-fold.

Renal Transplantation

When conception occurs after renal transplantation and the pregnancy continues past the first trimester, the outcome is successful more than 90% of the time. It has been shown that the graft undergoes the same functional and anatomic changes seen in the normal kidney in relation to its preconceptional function. Three case–control studies that have looked at the question of whether pregnancy is detrimental to the graft have found no evidence of negative consequences; another study suggested an adverse affect. The disparate findings between these studies have not been adequately explained. It appears that the risk of deterioration of function is highest in cases in which there is preexisting chronic rejection, proteinuria, or decreased renal function (serum creatinine ≥ 2.5 mg/dL).

Overall, graft rejection is noted in 9% of patients during pregnancy and up to 15% if a 3-month postpartum interval is included. Serial assessment of renal function is appropriate to monitor for graft rejection, and the onset of fever, oliguria, renal enlargement, or tenderness should prompt an evaluation for rejection. The onset or exacerbation of hypertension should be treated aggressively and the diagnosis of preeclampsia must be considered. A review of more than 3,300 pregnancies in transplant patients provides useful guidelines for counseling patients. These pregnancies were complicated by hypertension or preeclampsia, or both, in 30% of cases. Another common maternal complication is urinary tract infection, which is seen in 40% of cases. For this reason, monthly urine cultures are appropriate to screen for asymptomatic bacteriuria. Also, anemia may occur more often and with greater severity in these women. Erythropoietin is helpful in increasing the hematocrit. As might be expected, fetal survival and maternal course were better for women whose serum creatinine was less than or equal to 1.4 mg/dL. Nonetheless, even though fetal survival was

96% with serum creatinine less than or equal to 1.4 mg/dL, it was still 75% in the group with moderate renal insufficiency.

The chief perinatal risk is prematurity, which is seen in about 40% of women. Preterm births are the primary cause of low birth weight infants, with a birth weight of less than 2,500 g seen in almost 50% of patients and a birth weight of less than 1,500 g in approximately 15% of patients.

Although many series report high cesarean delivery rates, women with transplants are candidates for vaginal delivery because the graft does not obstruct labor, and renal function is not affected by the mode of delivery. Considering these issues, it has been suggested that the best candidates for pregnancy are those who meet the following criteria:

- Good health and at least 2 years posttransplantation
- No (or minimal) proteinuria
- No hypertension
- No evidence of graft rejection
- No pelvic caliceal distention on a recent intravenous pyelogram
- Stable renal function
- On maintenance immunosuppression

The mainstay of immunosuppression during pregnancy for renal transplants has become cyclosporine, although some patients may be on azathioprine or prednisone. Cyclosporine does not appear to be teratogenic or directly harmful to the fetus, but it has been associated with an increased risk of low birth weight (49.5%) and very low birth weight infants (17.8%) compared to women taking only azathioprine and prednisone (39.1% and 7.7%, respectively). However, those observations may be explained by a higher incidence of pregestational hypertension, a higher mean creatinine, and shorter mean interval from transplant to pregnancy in the cyclosporine group. Cyclosporine levels have been reported both to increase and to decrease in pregnancy. Given the difficulty in predicting how levels will be affected in any given patient, levels should be checked frequently.

Azathioprine is another commonly used immunosuppressant. Although it readily crosses the placenta, the fetal liver lacks the enzyme required for conversion to the active form. Consequently, the fetus is relatively protected from the drug. Although listed as a category D drug, it has been widely used in pregnancy and found to be relatively safe with teratogenicity suggested in only 1 small study of 48 patients, 5 of whom had anomalies.

Prednisone is also a mainstay of therapy, particularly when an acute rejection occurs. It does cross the placenta efficiently, with the fetal concentration approximately one tenth of the maternal. Although there have been reports of adrenal insufficiency and thymic hypoplasia in infants of women on high doses of prednisone during pregnancy, the risk is quite small when the dose is less than or equal to 15 mg/day. Most reports have not suggested prednisone is a teratogen; however, 4 large epidemiologic studies have associated the use of corticosteroids in the first trimester with nonsyndromic orofacial clefts. Although this risk should be discussed with a patient, this association should not lead one to withhold prednisone when it is the appropriate therapy.

There are other, newer immunosuppressants for which only limited data on use during pregnancy are available. A review of 100 pregnancies in women on tacrolimus reported a 70% live birth rate, although 2 of those neonates subsequently died (19). One third of the neonates had a complication, with the most frequent being hypoxia, hyperkalemia, and renal dysfunction. Of the 100 pregnancies, 26 had preconception exposure and 45 had first-trimester exposure. The investigators reported that 4 fetuses (5.6% of the 71 deliveries) had fetal anomalies, slightly higher than the rate in the general population but similar to the incidence of anomalies in transplant patients on other immunosuppressants. However, all 4 of these fetuses had both preconception and first-trimester exposure. Although the investigators did not discuss this in detail, this would mean that nearly 10% of fetuses exposed in the first trimester had anomalies. There was no consistent pattern in the anomalies noted, but with the limited data available, tacrolimus should be used only with caution in the first trimester.

The use of mycophenolate mofetil outside of pregnancy has increased dramatically over the past decade. The annual report of the Organ Procurement and Transplantation Network in the United States showed use of mycophenolate mofetil after renal transplantation increased from 11.9% in 1995 to 79.6% in 2000 (20). Mycophenolate mofetil is embryotoxic and teratogenic in animals, and for this reason, women generally have been switched to other immunosuppressants when they were attempting to conceive or were found to be pregnant. Until recently, concerns regarding human teratogenicity had not been borne out. A few infants had been born to women treated with mycophenolate mofetil without apparent ill effect (21). But the report of an infant girl born to a woman taking mycophenolate mofetil, tacrolimus, and prednisone noted the possible teratogenic effect of hypoplastic nails and short fifth fingers (22). More recently, a case was reported of a woman who received mycophenolate mofetil, tacrolimus, and prednisone through 13 weeks of gestation, when her pregnancy was diagnosed (23). Her mycophenolate mofetil was then replaced by azathioprine for the remainder of the pregnancy. At 22 weeks of gestation, the pregnancy was terminated due to multiple congenital anomalies that were similar to those described in animals exposed to mycophenolate mofetil. These 2 reports, particularly the latter, suggest that mycophenolate mofetil is likely teratogenic in humans and should be avoided during pregnancy, at least during organogenesis.

Observations were reported on 7 pregnancies in women using 0KT3, an immunoglobulin G that crosses the placenta. Of the 5 surviving infants, all were reported to be doing well initially.

Urolithiasis

The incidence of urinary calculi complicating pregnancy has been quoted to range from 1:1,500 to 1:244 (24). Although stones will, more likely than not, pass spontaneously, pregnancy complicates the diagnosis and treatment of stones. In women presenting with unilateral colicky pain, the diagnosis of nephrolithiasis or ureterolithiasis must be considered. Urinalysis is helpful when it reveals microscopic hematuria, but definitive diagnosis requires imaging studies. The main modality used in pregnancy is ultrasonography. Ultrasound examination will allow for assessment of the dilation of the upper urinary tract and can detect the stone directly; however, the sensitivity of ultrasonography for stone detection is only about 85%. When ultrasound examination fails to reveal a stone, but clinical suspicion is high, several options are available. Both an abdominal X-ray and a "single-shot" intravenous pyelogram (IVP) have been suggested as reasonable steps. Some have suggested using a radioisotope nephrogram, which exposes the patient to one tenth (or less) the radiation dose of an IVP. However, although a nephrogram may diagnose an obstruction, it will convey less additional information than an IVP. Perhaps the best choice is a helical CT scan, with a sensitivity of about 95% to detect a stone.

Once the diagnosis is made, initial therapy consists of hydration and analgesics. About 80% of stones up to 4 mm will pass spontaneously. Pain should be managed with narcotics. A urine culture also should be obtained with appropriate antibiotic administration if a urinary tract infection is diagnosed. For patients who do not have spontaneous stone passage, the traditional interventional therapy during pregnancy is placement of internal stents. Stents can be placed blindly, but a great deal of success has been achieved with ultrasound guidance. Stents will provide symptomatic relief, but they can cause complications themselves. Stent encrustation may occur on long-indwelling stents, and stent migration has been reported (more common with a double–J than pigtail). In cases of a stone in the distal ureter, ureteroscopy with stone extraction by mini-basket or disintegration by ultrasonography has been used successfully. More recently, the use of uteroscopy with laser lithotripsy during pregnancy has been reported with encouraging results. Finally, the traditional therapy of nephrostomy is available in pregnancy, but the inconvenience and associated risk of infection make it a less desirable option.

References

1. Conrad KP, Gandley RE, Ogawa T, Nakanishi S, Danielson LA. Endothelin mediates renal vasodilation and hyperfiltration during pregnancy in chronically instrumented conscious rats. Am J Physiol 1999;276:F767–76.

2. Gandley RE, Conrad KP, McLaughlin MK. Endothelin and nitric oxide mediate reduced myogenic reactivity of small renal arteries from pregnant rats. Am J Physiol Regul Integr Comp Physiol 2001;280:R1–7.

3. Danielson LA, Kercher LJ, Conrad KP. Impact of gender and endothelin on renal vasodilation and hyperfiltration induced by relaxin in conscious rats. Am J Physiol Regul Integr Comp Physiol 2000;279:R1298–304.

4. Danielson LA, Sherwood OD, Conrad KP. Relaxin is a potent renal vasodilator in conscious rats. J Clin Invest 1999;103:525–33.

5. Novak J, Danielson LA, Kerchner LJ, Sherwood OD, Ramirez RJ, Moalli PA, et al. Relaxin is essential for renal vasodilation during pregnancy in conscious rats. J Clin Invest 2001;107:1469–75.

6. Jones DC, Hayslett JP. Outcome of pregnancy in women with moderate or severe renal insufficiency [published erratum appears in N Engl J Med 1997;336:789]. N Engl J Med 1996;335:226–32.

7. Griffin KA, Picken MM, Bakris GL, Bidani AK. Class differences in the effects of calcium channel blockers in the rat remnant kidney model. Kidney Int 1999;55:1849–60.

8. Khandelwal M, Kumanova M, Gaughan JP, Reece EA. Role of diltiazem in pregnant women with chronic renal disease. J Matern Fetal Neonatal Med 2002;12:408–12.

9. Hemmelder MH, de Zeeuw D, Fidler V, de Jong PE. Proteinuria: a risk factor for pregnancy-related renal function decline in primary glomerular disease? Am J Kidney Dis 1995;26:187–92.

10. Miodovnik M, Rosenn BM, Khoury JC, Grigsby JL, Siddiqi TA. Does pregnancy increase the risk for development and progression of diabetic nephropathy? Am J Obstet Gynecol 1996;174:1180–9; discussion 1189–91.

11. Rossing K, Jacobsen P, Hommel E, Mathiesen E, Svenningsen A, Rossing P, et al. Pregnancy and progression of diabetic nephropathy. Diabetologia 2002;45:36–41.

12. Purdy LP, Hantsch CE, Molitch ME, Metzger BE, Phelps RL, Dooley SL, et al. Effect of pregnancy on renal function in patients with moderate-to-severe diabetic renal insufficiency. Diabetes Care 1996;19:1067–74.

13. Diabetes Control and Complications Trial Research Group. Effect of pregnancy on microvascular complications in the diabetes control and complications trial. Diabetes Control and Complications Trial Research Group. Diabetes Care 2000;23:1084–91.

14. Khoury JC, Miodovnik M, LeMasters G, Sibai B. Pregnancy outcome and progression of diabetic nephropathy. What's next? J Matern Fetal Neonatal Med 2002;11:238–44.

15. Gordon M, Landon MB, Samuels P, Hissrich S, Gabbe SG. Perinatal outcome and long-term follow-up associated with modern management of diabetic nephropathy. Obstet Gynecol 1996;87:401–9.

16. Moroni G, Quaglini S, Banfi G, Caloni M, Finazzi S, Ambroso G, et al. Pregnancy in lupus nephritis. Am J Kidney Dis 2002;40:713–20.

17. Chao AS, Huang JY, Lien R, Kung FT, Chen PJ, Hsieh PC. Pregnancy in women who undergo long-term hemodialysis. Am J Obstet Gynecol 2002;187:152–6.

18. Hou S. Conception and pregnancy in peritoneal dialysis patients. Perit Dial Int 2001;21 suppl 3:S290–4.

19. Kainz A, Harabacz I, Cowlrick IS, Gadgil SD, Hagiwara D. Review of the course and outcome of 100 pregnancies in 84 women treated with tacrolimus. Transplantation 2000;70:1718–21.

20. Organ Procurement and Transplantation Network and the Scientific Registry of Transplant Recipients. The 2003 OPTN/SRTR Annual Report. Available at http://www.optn.org/data/annualReport.asp. Retrieved October 8, 2004.

21. Hou S. Pregnancy in renal transplant recipients. Adv Ren Replace Ther 2003;10:40–7.

22. Pergola PE, Kancharla A, Riley DJ. Kidney transplantation during the first trimester of pregnancy: immunosuppression with mycophenolate mofetil, tacrolimus, and prednisone. Transplantation 2001;71:994–7.

23. Le Ray C, Coulomb A, Elefant E, Frydman R, Audibert F. Mycophenolate mofetil in pregnancy after renal transplantation: a case of major fetal malformations. Obstet Gynecol 2004;103:1091–4.

24. Lewis DF, Robichaux AG 3rd, Jaekle RK, Marcum NG, Stedman CM. Urolithiasis in pregnancy. Diagnosis, management and pregnancy outcome. J Reprod Med 2003; 48:28–32.

DERMATOLOGIC DISEASE

Physiologic changes in the skin during gestation may result in hyperpigmentation, hirsutism, increased sebum production, or hair loss. Although some of these conditions are believed to result from alterations in the hormonal milieu of pregnancy, for most skin changes, little information is available on the precise causes. Furthermore, many dermatologic conditions, such as eczema, may appear during pregnancy but are not specific to pregnancy. Some conditions, such as papular dermatitis of pregnancy, are no longer recognized as separate entities. About 20% of pregnant women will complain of "itching" during pregnancy, but less than 10% of these will prove to have a diagnosable entity.

Conditions Specific to Pregnancy

At present there appears to be agreement that the following conditions are specific to pregnancy:

- Polymorphic eruption of pregnancy (also known as pruritic urticarial papules and plaque of pregnancy)
- Pruritic folliculitis
- Prurigo of pregnancy
- Pemphigoid gestationis (also known as herpes gestationis)
- Intrahepatic cholestasis of pregnancy

A variety of laboratory abnormalities, especially hormonal, have been reported with some of these entities. Two hundred women with dermatoses in pregnancy were studied with analyses of serum direct immunofluorescence, direct immunofluorescence in biopsies, serum analyses of IgE, IgM, BhCG, estradiol, cortisol, androgens, sex hormone binding globulin, and liver function tests. When these tests produced abnormal results, serum bile acid levels were analyzed. All these determinations were comparable to pregnant patients without dermatoses except for suppressed cortisol levels in cases of polymorphic eruption of pregnancy and abnormal liver function test results and bile acid levels in obstetric cholestasis. Their immunofluorescence findings were uniformly positive in pemphigoid gestationis (plus complement C3 deposition). Immunofluorescence studies were negative in 90% of polymorphic eruption of pregnancy cases and in all cases of pruritic folliculitis.

Histologic studies also appear not to be helpful in separating these conditions because similar microscopic findings are described in polymorphic eruption of pregnancy, pruritic folliculitis, and pemphigoid gestationis. Prurigo is histologically described as showing an upper dermal perivascular infiltrate of monocytes and obstetric cholestasis as showing only acanthosis, hyperkeratosis, and the effects of excoriation. Immunofluorescence and C3 studies are useful in identifying the lesions of pemphigoid gestationis. In the absence of clear laboratory test results, the diagnosis will depend on clinical observation in most instances.

POLYMORPHIC ERUPTION OF PREGNANCY

With an incidence of 1 in 200 pregnancies, polymorphic eruption of pregnancy is the most common pregnancy-related dermatosis. Pruritus is the major symptom and can be severe. The lesions of polymorphic eruption of pregnancy typically begin on the abdomen with sparing of the umbilicus and initially consist of 1–2-mm erythematous papules surrounded by pale halos that coalesce into urticarial plaques (Figs. 20 and 21). In contrast to herpes gestationis, face, palms, soles, and the periumbilical area usually are not affected.

The etiology and pathogenesis are unknown. Affected women are more commonly primigravida with prominent striae and have an increased incidence of twins, triplets, or hydramnios, each associated with greater abdominal and uterine distention. It has been hypothesized that increased skin tension results in skin damage, which manifests as striae; this may play a role in the etiology of polymorphic eruption of pregnancy. One study demonstrated male DNA in these lesions occurring in 50% of mothers with male fetuses (1). No male DNA was found in unaffected mothers with male or female fetuses. The investigators speculated that with better laboratory techniques than those available to them, more male DNA might have been found in affected mothers bearing male fetuses. The ratio of male to female fetuses in women affected by polymorphic eruption of pregnancy is about 2 to 1. Further study is necessary to corroborate these findings.

Most cases (75%) occur in the third trimester, and the condition rarely develops postpartum. Polymorphic eruption of pregnancy does not appear to recur with subsequent pregnancies or with use of hormonal contraception.

Therapy with topical steroids generally is successful in most women but some require systemic therapy. Moderately potent topical steroids have been reported to be effective. Antipruritic agents such as antihistamines are helpful as well. Because late pregnancy use can result in suppression of the fetal adrenals, a warning must be given to those who will care for the newborn. Rarely, early delivery has been used for maternal relief. Some observations indicate that symptoms worsen immediately postpartum but decline within 2 weeks. This condition is not associated with an elevated risk for adverse fetal or maternal outcome.

PEMPHIGOID GESTATIONIS

Pemphigoid gestationis (formerly known as herpes gestationis) is a rare, pruritic, autoimmune, bullous disease of the skin that occurs principally during pregnancy. The reported incidence of pemphigoid gestationis is 1 in 1,700–50,000 pregnancies. The onset of the disease is usually during the second and third trimesters and occasionally may occur immediately postpartum. Clinically, the patient presents with very pruritic lesions that initially closely resemble those of polymorphic eruption of pregnancy. Later, when bullae and vesicles develop, they then may closely resemble dermatitis herpetiformis or

bullous pemphigoid (Fig. 22). Bullae result from IgG binding to the cutaneous basement membrane by attaching to the bullous pemphigoid antigen 2.

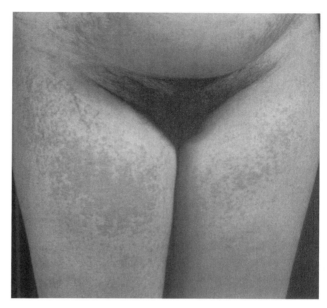

■ **FIG. 21.** Pruritic urticarial papules and plaques of pregnancy. Papular urticaria-like lesions also are present on the upper thighs. (Diseases in pregnancy. In: Fitzpatrick TB, Johnson RA, Wolff K, Polano MK, Surmond D. Color atlas and synopsis of clinical dermatology, common and serious diseases. 3rd ed. New York (NY): McGraw-Hill Companies; 1997. p. 417. Copyright McGraw-Hill Companies.)

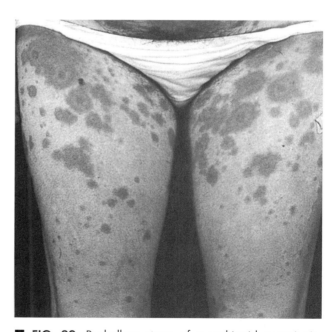

■ **FIG. 22.** Pre-bullous stage of pemphigoid gestationis, showing typical annular urticated plaques. (Parish LC, Brenner S, Ramos-e-Silva M. Women's dermatology from infancy to maturity. New York (NY): Parthenon Publishing; 2001. Fig. 6, p. 404.)

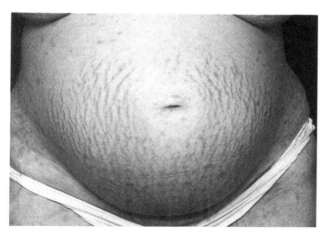

■ **FIG. 20.** Early polymorphic eruption showing typical periumbilical sparing. (Parish LC, Brenner S, Ramos-e-Silva M. Women's dermatology from infancy to maturity. New York (NY): Parthenon Publishing; 2001. Fig. 9, p. 408.)

Exacerbations are common during the postpartum period. The etiology of pemphigoid gestationis is unknown, but a genetic predisposition is suggested. Clinical presentation, together with a perilesional skin biopsy displaying complement and IgG deposition along the basement membrane between epidermis and dermis, establishes the diagnosis.

The condition may recur with subsequent pregnancies and may be associated with an increased incidence of IUGR, prematurity, and stillbirth, although these risks of fetal complications are debated. Fetal concern is heightened by the belief of some investigators that the primary immunologic event (it is strongly related to HLA-DR3 and HLA-DR4) actually takes place in the placenta and the maternal skin lesions are a secondary event. Therefore, increased fetal surveillance is recommended during the third trimester, but no specific requirements have been defined.

Treatment is aimed at controlling pruritus and reducing the formation of new vesicles. Colloidal oatmeal baths and topical emollients sometimes provide sufficient relief. In mild cases, treatment would next progress to the use of topical steroids. Systemic corticosteroids are often required for maternal comfort. Transient neonatal herpes gestationis (neonatal pemphigoid gestationis) has been reported in some cases. Rarely, the infant may show lesions of the skin that are similar to those of the mother. Neonatal disease usually is mild and spontaneously resolves within a short period.

The disease may worsen and require more vigorous therapy in the postpartum period in up to 75% of patients. The patient also should be advised that the disease may return with the use of hormonal contraception (25%) and during subsequent pregnancies and may be more severe. Subsequent pregnancies with a different paternal genetic contribution are still subject to recurrence of pemphigoid gestationis. Several reports warn that other autoimmune diseases, particularly Graves' disease and Hashimoto's, may occur in such women.

PRURIGO OF PREGNANCY

Papular dermatitis of pregnancy is perhaps a "catch all" diagnosis when other conditions have been excluded. It may include Nurse's disease. It is characterized by small, pruritic, erythematous, papular, or nodular lesions limited to the extensor surfaces of the extremities and resembling insect bites. The abdomen may be affected. The disease may begin at any time during gestation and may recur in subsequent pregnancies. The incidence of the disease is 1 in 300 pregnancies.

In the past, the entity was believed to be associated with increased fetal risk and abnormal biochemical findings, such as elevated hCG and diminished cortisol levels. Subsequent reports have not substantiated those findings, and fetal risk is no longer described. Liver function tests are normal and bile acid levels are not increased.

Histologic studies are nonspecific. Many patients give a personal or family history of atopy and about half have elevated serum IgE. These findings suggest that this entity is actually a pregnancy-enhanced manifestation of atopic dermatitis.

Treatment is usually topical with the use of mild emollients, midpotency corticosteroids, or oral antihistamines. The lesions resolve after delivery.

PRURITIC FOLLICULITIS OF PREGNANCY

The lesions of pruritic folliculitis of pregnancy (formerly known as PUPP) are erythematous papules with a more generalized distribution than prurigo of pregnancy but mainly on the chest and back. About 80% of cases appear in the third trimester. The lesions are suggestive of cystic acne seen in women taking steroids. Not all lesions are pruritic to the same degree; overall, symptoms are relatively mild.

The entity is easily confused with polymorphic eruption of pregnancy and with prurigo of pregnancy and may be underreported. Hormone levels, liver function tests, and immunofluorescence studies of biopsies show no abnormalities. Histologic studies are nonspecific. Most reports regarding maternal and fetal effects show no serious problems; one study has suggested IUGR may be associated.

Treatment may not be required. If therapy is needed, topicals, including moderately potent corticosteroids, are used. Ultraviolet B therapy has been described with reported success.

Coincidental Dermatoses

The following conditions are noted in pregnancy but are not specific diseases of pregnancy.

PIGMENTED NEVI AND HYPERPIGMENTATION

During pregnancy, melanogenesis increases. Thus any existing nevi may grow and darken, and new ones may appear. No treatment is required, but surveillance is prudent. Generalized hyperpigmentation can be found in most pregnancies. Darkening of the areolae, linea nigra, umbilicus, vulva, and perianal skin may occur as early as the first trimester. Chloasma, hyperpigmentation of the face, usually affects the areas over the malar eminences, cheeks, and forehead. It is a cosmetic problem for some women, who should be warned that exposure to direct sunlight will intensify the pigmentation both during pregnancy and later.

Useful treatments for the condition include chemical peels and bleaching agents. Treatment with such agents should always be combined with use of sunscreens that block ultraviolet A and B light. Some of the more common bleaching agents include hydroxyquinone 2% or 4% and azelaic acid, which work by blocking the conversion of dopa to melanin by enzymatic inhibition of tyrosinase, and can be combined with a keratolytic (all-trans retinoic acid, known as *tretinoin*). Use of tretinoin in pregnancy is absolutely contraindicated as an oral preparation, but topical tretinoin is readily metabolized by the skin. Its use, however, is strongly discouraged unless the benefits to mother outweigh the fetal risks. It generally is not used for cosmetic reasons in pregnancy. Chemical peeling also may be used; it involves the use of a topical agent that exfoliates skin, revealing organized repairing skin. Postinflammatory hyperpigmentation may result.

HAIR CHANGES

Telogen effluvium, or hair loss after a shift of anagen follicles to telogens, often is seen during the postpartum period. Generally the hair regrows completely in 3–6 months. Drug therapy is seldom helpful; reassurance is the best approach. Alopecia areata may either occur or improve during pregnancy. Intralesional corticosteroids may be helpful.

Mild degrees of hirsutism are common during pregnancy and primarily affect the face and extremities. During pregnancy, the proportion of hair in the anagen (growing) phase is increased, although elevated androgen levels from placental sources may contribute to hirsutism. Mild hirsutism rarely requires therapy. Excessive hirsutism with virilism warrants investigation for an androgen-secreting tumor. Hyperreactio luteinalis (gestational ovarian thecalutein cysts), which is manifested by bilateral enlarged cystic ovaries and elevated androgen levels, also can cause hair growth; the ovarian cysts do not require surgical therapy, and involute following pregnancy.

ACNE

The sweat and sebaceous glands are especially active during pregnancy, probably as a result of increased progesterone secretion. Acne may worsen during pregnancy but usually improves as a result of increased production of sex hormone binding globulin. Good skin hygiene should be encouraged. Topical therapy may be used, but tetracycline should not be prescribed. Isotretinoin, an effective medication used to treat cystic acne, is a potent teratogen. The teratogenic risk is so serious that the manufacturer recommends that women of reproductive age initiate a secure form of contraception 1 month before starting therapy and continue that contraception for 1 month after stopping isotretinoin use. Additionally, all women of reproductive age should have a negative pregnancy test result within the week before taking the first dose of isotretinoin. Tretinoin is teratogenic (delayed bone development) in animal fetuses in doses 500–1,000 times the human dose, but with doses used for human treatment and the rapid metabolism by the skin, it is considered pregnancy risk category C; use is condoned only if the maternal benefits outweigh fetal risks. It is suggested that even exposure to tretinoin during the first trimester does not pose a significant risk to the fetus (2). Salicylic acid preparations may be used in pregnancy; however, safety data are limited. Their use in lactation is not advocated, because of the potential for bleeding disorders in neonates (3). (See Table 19 for a list of medications for dermatologic conditions and risks of use in pregnancy.)

TABLE 19. Medications for Dermatologic Conditions and Risks of Use in Pregnancy

Medication	Pregnancy Risk Category	Comment
Adapalene	C	Topical retinoid
Benzoyl peroxide	C	Antibacterial and comedolytic
Clindamycin, topical or oral	B	
Cholestyramine	C	Prevents vitamin absorption
Erythromycin topical or oral	B	Use ethylsuccinate, base, or lactiobionate; not estolate
Isotretinoin	X	Known teratogen
Metronidazole	B	Contraindicated in first trimester; disulfiram reaction
Ursodeoxycholic acid	B	Reduced cholesterol content of bile; not for use in first trimester
Steroids, topical	C	Use of super potent and potent topical steroids can suppress maternal and fetal adrenals, cause fetal abnormalities; use of lower potency (intermediate and mild) drugs is preferable

PSORIASIS

Psoriasis seldom arises de novo during gestation. The effect of pregnancy on preexisting psoriasis is unpredictable. Generalized lesions often improve, whereas localized lesions, particularly those of inverse psoriasis (also called seborrheic psoriasis), may become aggravated. Postpartum exacerbation of psoriasis frequently occurs. Psoriasis itself has no known deleterious effect upon the fetus, but fetal effects must be considered before prescribing any dermatologic treatments.

PYOGENIC GRANULOMA

Pyogenic granuloma is a misnomer; a bacterial cause for the condition has not been demonstrated. This disorder is relatively common and affects both men and women. The clinical description is that of a bright red, or blue and black, vascular nodule microscopically composed of proliferating capillaries and stromal edema. The lesion resembles those associated with some forms of melanoma and must be distinguished from that as well as other malignancies. Pressure on the lesion does not cause blanching, and it is easily traumatized, causing bleeding. During pregnancy these lesions may become very large and prominent. When they occur in pregnancy on the gingiva, they are referred to as telangiectatic epulis. Pyogenic granulomas may involute spontaneously, but if persistent, they should be biopsied and then treated by removal or local destruction.

References

1. Aractingi S, Berkane N, Bertheau P, Le Goue C, Dausset J, Uzan S, et al. Fetal DNA in skin of polymorphic eruptions of pregnancy. Lancet 1998;352:1898–901.

2. Jick SS, Terris BZ, Jick H. First trimester topical tretinoin and congenital disorders. Lancet. 1993;341:1181–2.

3. Akhavan A, Bershad S. Topical acne drugs: review of clinical properties, systemic exposure, and safety. Am J Clin Dermatol 2003;4:473–92.

IMMUNOLOGIC DISORDERS

The immunologic disorders affecting pregnancy may be classified as either autoimmune or alloimmune. Autoimmune diseases likely to be encountered by the obstetrician are rheumatoid arthritis, systemic lupus erythematosus, antiphospholipid syndrome, systemic sclerosis, myasthenia gravis, and herpes gestationis. Other rare autoimmune diseases less likely to be encountered include Sjögren's syndrome, ankylosing spondylitis, and mixed connective tissue disease. Alloimmune disorders are the result of an immune response to antigens of different individuals of the same species. Alloimmune diseases of significant obstetric consequence include hematologic alloimmunization and alloimmune thrombocytopenia.

Rheumatoid Arthritis

Rheumatoid arthritis (RA) is a chronic debilitating disease characterized by symmetrical polyarthritis of the small joints of the hands and feet. Most individuals affected by RA are women; the female-to-male ratio ranges from 2 to 1 to 4 to 1. Frequently its onset is during childbearing years. Overall, RA affects about 1% of the adult population and complicates pregnancy in approximately 1 in 1,000 to 1 in 2,000 cases. Although the etiology of RA is unknown, it is probably secondary to environmental exposure upon an underlying genetic predisposition. The HLA-DRB 1 genotypes are associated with RA, but it remains controversial whether there is an association with disease incidence, severity, or both. Rheumatoid arthritis does not appear to have adverse effects on pregnancy. In comparison, pregnancy appears to favorably affect the symptoms of RA because in the majority of women, RA dramatically improves during pregnancy. However, 10% of pregnant women may experience worsening of their symptoms. This worsening of symptoms continues during breastfeeding. A relapse of RA is observed within 6 months after delivery in approximately 90% of women (1).

Goals of therapy should include reduction of inflammation and pain and preservation of joint function. Given that RA usually improves during pregnancy, analgesics and antiinflammatory agents are first-line therapy. The primary therapeutic agents during pregnancy are acetaminophen for simple analgesia and aspirin and other NSAIDs for antiinflammatory action. Contraindications for use of NSAIDs include late pregnancy (>37 weeks of gestation), aspirin-induced asthma, congestive heart failure, and renal dysfunction. Corticosteroids may be used short term, either during initiation of therapy or during acute exacerbations, or chronically in low doses. The risk of neonatal adrenal suppression after maternal treatment with hydrocortisone or prednisolone is very low, probably secondary to the placental metabolism of these corticosteroids. Intraarticular steroids also may be used during pregnancy.

Other medications that can be used with caution by pregnant women with RA include hydroxychloroquine, sulfasalazine, gold salts, cyclosporine, and D-penicillamine. Methotrexate and cyclophosphamide should be avoided in pregnancy because of their potential mutagenic and teratogenic effects. Nonpharmacologic therapy, including rest, appropriate use of heat and cold, assistive devices, and physical therapy, also are important components of caring for pregnant women with RA.

Systemic Lupus Erythematosus

Systemic lupus erythematosus (SLE) is an idiopathic chronic inflammatory disease that affects multiple organ systems. It occurs predominantly in women; the female-to-male ratio during the reproductive years is 9 to 1. Its prevalence is approximately 1–2 in 1,000 in the general population and 1 in 2,000 to 3,000 pregnancies (2). The prevalence of SLE is greater among minority women, including African-American, Hispanic, Asian, and Native-American women, than among white women. Patients may present with vague constitutional symptoms, with fatigue being the most common. Weight loss, fever, arthralgia, myalgias, and a malar (butterfly) rash or other cutaneous symptoms occur in 80% or more of patients. Fertility does not appear to be affected by SLE. A genetic predisposition is suggested by the observations that SLE occurs in 5–12% of relatives of patients with SLE; furthermore, the concordance among monozygotic twins is greater than 50%, and human leukocyte antigens B8, DR3, and DR2 occur more frequently in individuals with SLE.

The diagnosis of SLE is suspected by the clinical presentation and confirmed by the presence of circulation autoantibodies (Box 18). In 1997, the American College of Rheumatology revised the criteria for the diagnosis of SLE (Box 19).

Clinically obvious renal disease occurs in 50% of patients with SLE. Proteinuria is the most common presentation and usually worsens in pregnancy. Four basic histologic and clinical categories of lupus nephropathy exist. Diffuse proliferative glomerulonephritis is the most common and most severe lesion. Hypertension, moderate to heavy proteinuria, nephritic syndrome, hematuria, pyuria, casts, hypocomplementemia, and circulation immune complexes often are seen at the same time. Focal proliferative glomerulonephritis, membranous glomerulonephritis, and mesangial nephritis are progressively less severe.

The effects of SLE on pregnancy outcome are related to the presence of hypertension, renal impairment, or antiphospholipid syndrome. If none of these are present, chances of a normal pregnancy outcome are good. The presence and degree of renal impairment and hypertension antedating pregnancy is related to the frequency of superimposed preeclampsia. Overall, 20–30% of pregnant women with SLE have complications of pregnancy-induced hypertension.

Whether pregnancy predisposes women to increased SLE disease flares remains controversial. Flares may be related to disease activity at the outset of pregnancy. The rate of disease flare is lower if the disease is under good control for at least 6 months before conception. Approximately 15–60% of women with SLE have an exacerbation during pregnancy or the postpartum period.

BOX 18

Systemic Lupus Erythematosus Antibodies

Antinuclear antibody (ANA): Initial screening test

Anti-double-stranded DNA (anti-dsDNA): Most specific for systemic lupus erythematosus, found in 80–90% of untreated patients, may be related to disease activity

Anti-single-stranded DNA (anti-ssDNA): Less specific

Anti-Sm antigen (Sm)

Antinuclear ribonucleoprotein (nRNP): Mixed connective tissue disease

Anti-Ro/SSA: Specific for Sjögren's syndrome and systemic lupus erythematosus; associated with nephritis, associated with neonatal lupus

Anti-La/SSB: Associated with neonatal lupus

Anticardiolipin: Vascular thromboses; recurrent pregnancy loss

BOX 19

Revised Criteria for Classification of Systemic Lupus Erythematosus

To be classified as having systemic lupus erythematosus, an individual must have at least 4 of the following 11 criteria simultaneously or serially:

- Malar rash
- Discoid rash
- Photosensitivity
- Oral ulcers
- Arthritis (nonerosive arthritis involving 2 or more peripheral joints)
- Serositis (pleuritis or pericarditis)
- Renal disorders (proteinuria > 0.5 g/d or 3+ if quantitation not performed, or cellular casts)
- Neurologic disorders (seizures or psychosis, or other central or peripheral neuropsychiatric syndrome)
- Hematologic disorders (hemolytic anemia, leukopenia, lymphopenia, or thrombocytopenia)
- Immunologic disorders (Anti-DNA, or Anti-Sm, or positive findings of antiphospholipid antibodies: an abnormal serum level of IgG or IgM anticardiolipin antibodies; lupus anticoagulant; or false-positive serologic test for syphilis)
- Antinuclear antibody

Tan EM, Cohen AS, Fries JF, Masi AT, McShane DJ, Rothfield NF, et al. The 1982 revised criteria for the classification of systemic lupus erythematosus. Arthritis Rheum 1982;25:1271–7.

Hochberg MC. Updating the American College of Rheumatology revised criteria for the classification of systemic lupus erythematosus [letter]. Arthritis Rheum 1997;40:1725.

Most SLE exacerbations during pregnancy are treated with low to moderate doses of corticosteroids, which may be given for 4–6 weeks. There is no evidence that prophylactic corticosteroids will prevent SLE disease flares. Distinguishing between an exacerbation of SLE involving active nephritis and preeclampsia may be difficult because each may present with proteinuria, hypertension, and evidence of multiorgan dysfunction. Elevated levels of anti-double-stranded DNA, low levels of classical pathway complement components, and active urinary sediment with cellular casts and hematuria suggest a lupus flare over preeclampsia. In addition to hypertensive flare, other manifestations of worsening SLE include cerebritis, carditis, nephritis, and pneumonitis.

Neonatal lupus erythematosus (NLE) is a rare condition of the fetus and neonate. It is characterized by dermatologic, cardiac, or hematologic abnormalities. It results from maternal IgG autoantibodies that cross the placenta and cause tissue damage. The lesions appear within the first several weeks after delivery and may last up to 6 months.

The cardiac lesion associated with NLE is congenital complete heart block from fibrosis and disruption of the conduction system. The usual clinical presentation is fixed fetal bradycardia in the range of 60–80 beats per minute detected between 16 and 25 weeks of gestation in a structurally normal heart. Ultrasound evaluation shows atrioventricular dissociation. Hydrops fetalis and even fetal death may occur.

The diagnosis of NLE is confirmed by testing for autoantibodies, especially anti-Ro/SSA and anti-La/SSB. Among all mothers with SLE, the risk of having a fetus or neonate with NLE is less than 5%. Among mothers with SLE and anti-Ro/SSA, the risk of skin lesions that are dermatologic manifestations of NLE is approximately 15%. The risk of congenital heart block is 1–5%. The recurrence risk is 25% for dermatologic manifestations and 10% for congenital heart block.

Optimally, women should receive preconception counseling and a thorough discussion of potential maternal and fetal risks during pregnancy (see Box 20). Pregnant patients should be seen at least every 2 weeks and instructed to be alert to the signs and symptoms of preeclampsia. After 18–20 weeks of gestation, ultrasonography should be performed every 4–6 weeks to assess fetal growth.

Similar to the goals of therapy for rheumatoid arthritis, therapy for SLE should include reduction of inflammation and pain and preservation of joint and organ function. Therefore, drugs most frequently used are analgesics such as acetaminophen and NSAIDs. More severe cases require the use of antimalarials, corticosteroids, and cytotoxic agents. Antimalarials, specifically hydroxychloroquine, appear to be safe for the fetus. A small, randomized study of hydroxychloroquine found beneficial effects without an increase in congenital, neuroophthalmologic, or auditory abnormalities at 1.5–3 years of age

---

BOX 20

Preconception Counseling of Women With Systemic Lupus Erythematosus

Discussion about potential risks:
- Pregnancy loss
- Preterm delivery
- Pregnancy-induced hypertension
- Intrauterine growth restriction

Laboratory evaluation:
- Complete blood count
- Urinalysis
- Serum creatinine
- 24-hour urine collection for creatinine clearance and total protein
- Antiphospholipid antibodies
- Anti-RO, anti-La

---

(3). Antimalarials are not effective in the treatment of fever, SLE nephritis, or neurologic or hematologic disease manifestations. Corticosteroids are another acceptable alternative therapy for treatment for SLE during pregnancy, but they are used only as necessary to treat symptoms of SLE. Systemic corticosteroids are indicated for life-threatening symptoms of SLE such as nephritis or neurologic or hematologic manifestations. Stress-dose steroids (hydrocortisone, 100 mg every 6–8 hours) should be given during labor or at the time of cesarean delivery to all patients who have been treated with steroids within the year. Other medications used to treat SLE, such as azathioprine, methotrexate, and cyclophosphamide, are best avoided during pregnancy.

Antiphospholipid Syndrome

Antiphospholipid syndrome is an autoimmune condition characterized by the production of moderate to high levels of antiphospholipid antibodies and certain clinical features. Clinical manifestations of the syndrome include pregnancy loss (fetal death or recurrent pregnancy loss) and arterial or venous thrombosis (see "Deep Vein Thrombosis"). Autoimmune thrombocytopenia, a false-positive test for syphilis, livedo reticularis, and other features also may be seen. The confirmatory antiphospholipid autoantibody studies include 2 well-characterized antibodies: lupus anticoagulant and anticardiolipin antibody. Antiphospholipid antibodies are found in as many as 50% of patients with SLE but also may occur in patients without overt lupus. Furthermore, antiphospholipid antibodies of the IgG and IgM classes have been reported to be present in 1.8% and 4%, respectively, of otherwise healthy pregnant women. A diagnosis of antiphospholipid syndrome requires that the patient have at least 1 clinical feature of the syndrome along with moderate to high levels of either IgG or IgM anticardiolipin antibodies or the presence of lupus anticoagulant (see Box 11).

TESTING

Testing for both lupus anticoagulant and anticardiolipin antibodies should be done when the diagnosis of antiphospholipid syndrome is considered. Indications for testing are shown in Box 21. The following tests are used for initial testing, verification of results, and confirmation of specific phospholipid specificity:

- Combination of 2 phospholipid-dependent clotting assays (ie, aPTT, dilute Russell viper venom time, or kaolin clotting time)
- Mixing of the patient's plasma with an equal volume of normal plasma to differentiate between the presence of a circulating inhibitor such as lupus anticoagulant and the presence of a clotting factor deficiency
- Enzyme-linked immunosorbent assay (ELISA) using purified cardiolipin as the antigen

---

BOX 21

Indications for Testing for Antiphospholipid Antibodies

Recurrent spontaneous abortion (3 or more spontaneous abortions with no more than 1 live birth)

Unexplained second- or third-trimester fetal death

Severe early-onset preeclampsia (<34 weeks of gestation)

Unexplained venous or arterial thrombosis

Unexplained stroke

Unexplained transient ischemic attack or amaurosis fugax

Systemic lupus erythematosus or other connective tissue disease

Autoimmune thrombocytopenia

Autoimmune hemolytic anemia

Livedo reticularis

Chorea gravidarum

False-positive serologic test for syphilis

Unexplained prolongation in clotting assay

Unexplained severe intrauterine growth restriction

Reprinted from Maternal-fetal medicine: principles and practice. 5th ed. Lockwood CJ, Silver RM. Thrombophilias in pregnancy. Creasy RK, Resnik R, Iams J, editors. p. 1005–21. Copyright 2004, with permission from Elsevier.

Sporadic miscarriage or fetal death infrequently is caused by antiphospholipid antibodies. Testing for antiphospholipid antibodies to screen for pregnancy loss or complications is unwarranted. The importance of identifying the syndrome is not in its prevalence but in the fact that it is a potentially treatable cause of pregnancy loss.

MATERNAL RISKS

Maternal risks include thrombosis and stroke, preeclampsia, postpartum syndrome, and catastrophic antiphospholipid syndrome. Venous thrombosis accounts for approximately 65–70% of events. The single most common site involved is the lower extremities. Arterial thrombosis also has been associated with antiphospholipid antibodies and appears to be a predisposing factor in a modest percentage of cases of stroke. In addition to both arterial and venous thrombosis, antiphospholipid antibodies are associated with transient ischemic attacks and amaurosis fugax. Well over half of thrombotic episodes occur in relation to pregnancy or during the use of combination oral contraceptives. Two prospective studies in pregnant women with the syndrome showed a rate of thrombosis and stroke of 5% and 12%, respectively (4, 5). Heparin thromboprophylaxis or anticoagulation therapy, given during pregnancy and continued for 6 weeks postpartum, is recommended for women with well-characterized antiphospholipid syndrome.

The high incidence (20–50%) of preeclampsia in patients with the syndrome contributes to a high rate of preterm birth. The rate of preeclampsia does not appear to be markedly reduced by treatment with either low-dose aspirin or heparin. Patients with severe, early-onset preeclampsia at less than 34 weeks of gestation have an increased rate of antiphospholipid antibodies (11–17%) and should be tested for antiphospholipid antibodies.

During the immediate postpartum period, complications that may represent an autoimmune exacerbation may occur. These may include fever, pulmonary infiltrates, pleural effusions, thrombosis, and cardiomyopathy. Renal insufficiency and pulmonary hypertension also may accompany this syndrome.

Catastrophic antiphospholipid syndrome, in which there is rapid clinical deterioration associated with an accelerated coagulation vasculopathy, occurs rarely. Patients have high titers of antiphospholipid antibodies and a rapid, deteriorating course of malignant hypertension, pulmonary hypertension, renal insufficiency, widespread thrombosis, and disseminated intravascular coagulopathy. The associated mortality is high, thus the condition should be considered an emergency.

FETAL RISKS

The fetal risks of antiphospholipid syndrome include death and IUGR. Fetal death (death of the conceptus after 10–12 weeks of gestation) appears to be more specific for pregnancy loss related to antiphospholipid antibody than for early embryonic loss. Recurrent first-trimester pregnancy loss is fairly common, affecting approximately 1% of the population. Its link to the syndrome, however, must be carefully assessed. Only patients with moderate to high levels of IgG or IgM anticardiolipin or lupus anticoagulant or both should be considered to have the syndrome.

Antiphospholipid antibodies may be associated with fetal growth impairment. Even with treatment, the rate of fetal growth impairment among liveborn infants approaches 30%. Fetal distress also appears to be more common in pregnancies complicated by antiphospholipid syndrome. Treatment has not been shown to decrease the rate of these complications.

MANAGEMENT

Preconceptional counseling in women with antiphospholipid syndrome should cover the potential maternal and fetal risks, including thrombosis, stroke, preeclampsia, fetal loss, fetal growth impairment, and the need for preterm delivery. Patients should undergo baseline studies assessing the presence of anemia, thrombocytopenia, and underlying renal disease (complete blood count, urinalysis, serum creatinine, and 24-hour urine for creatinine clearance and total protein).

During pregnancy, women with antiphospholipid syndrome may be seen by a physician at least every 2 weeks in the first and second trimesters and weekly thereafter. These patients should be educated about the signs and symptoms of thrombosis, thromboembolism, transient ischemic attacks, amaurosis fugax, and preeclampsia. Serial antiphospholipid antibody determinations are not useful in terms of establishing prognosis or managing therapy. Maternal surveillance for the development of hypertension and proteinuria is crucial. The fetus can be assessed for IUGR with ultrasonography starting at 18–20 weeks of gestation. Heparin thromboprophylaxis should be considered in all women with the syndrome.

Heparin and low-dose aspirin have become the most widely accepted method to prevent fetal loss in women with the syndrome. The optimal dose of heparin needed to achieve good fetal outcome without excessive exposure to osteoporotic risks associated with heparin is uncertain. Average dosages of 17,000–25,000 U of heparin per day have been used in case series. Heparin therapy, however, is not benign. Heparin-induced osteoporosis and fracture may occur in 1–2% of women receiving treatment during pregnancy. Supplemental calcium and vitamin D should be given daily, and axial skeleton weight-bearing exercise should be encouraged. Heparin may be associated with an uncommon idiosyncratic thrombocytopenia known as heparin-induced thrombocytopenia. This complication is immune mediated, and onset usually is 3–15 days after initiation of treatment. Heparin-induced thrombocytopenia may occur in up to 5% of patients. Although most cases are mild and have a benign course, there is also a severe, life-threatening form of the condition. Low-molecular-weight heparin is associated with a lower frequency of heparin-induced thrombocytopenia.

The use of high-dose intravenous immunoglobulin has generated interest because of anecdotal reports of successful pregnancy outcomes in women with antiphospholipid syndrome. However, intravenous immunoglobulin is extremely expensive, and the only randomized study found that the combination of intravenous immunoglobulin and heparin did not improve pregnancy outcome compared with heparin use alone.

Prompt recognition of the signs and symptoms is essential in cases of postpartum syndrome or catastrophic antiphospholipid syndrome. Medical therapies must be individualized, but certain guidelines are useful. First, markedly elevated blood pressure levels should be controlled with antihypertensive medication. Second, anticoagulation with intravenous heparin should be started as long as there is no contraindication. Third, inflammatory conditions should be treated with methylprednisolone. Finally, if catastrophic antiphospholipid syndrome is suspected, treatment with plasmapheresis should be considered.

Systemic Sclerosis

Systemic sclerosis, also known as scleroderma, is characterized by localized or diffuse fibrosis of connective tissue and a progressive obliterative vasculopathy. In the localized form, the disease usually is limited to the skin in the hands and is associated with Raynaud's phenomenon. Systemic sclerosis can be either limited (80%) or diffuse (20%). Patients with early (duration <5 years) diffuse scleroderma are at particularly high risk for developing renal crisis, a condition that may be lethal. Patients in scleroderma renal crisis usually present with thrombocytopenia and daily increases in serum creatinine. Women with moderate to severe renal disease and hypertension also have a substantial risk for developing preeclampsia. Neonatal involvement with skin sclerosis has been reported.

Pregnancy probably is safest among patients with scleroderma without obvious renal, cardiac, or pulmonary disease. Patients with diffuse scleroderma should take a cautious and considered approach to pregnancy. Special attention should be directed to the assessment of renal, cardiac, and pulmonary involvement. Unfortunately, there is no satisfactory treatment for scleroderma. Oral vasodilators for the prevention and treatment of Raynaud's phenomenon may be used. Systemic corticosteroids may be continued. Pregnant women with scleroderma should be seen frequently by their obstetricians, with close observation for preeclampsia and IUGR.

Sjögren's Syndrome

Sjögren's syndrome is a rare autoimmune disorder characterized by the sicca syndrome, including dryness of the eyes (keratoconjunctivitis sicca), mouth (xerostomia), and other mucosal surfaces. Histologically, predominantly lymphocytic infiltrates of the exocrine glands, primarily the lacrimal and salivary glands, are seen. There is a female predominance, with 90% of cases occurring in women between ages 40 and 60 years. Several autoantibodies are associated with Sjögren's syndrome, including anti-SSA/Ro, anti-SSB/La, ANAs, and RF. Treatment is based on symptoms and includes oral and ocular topicals. Low-dose corticosteroids may decrease inflammation of the conjunctival surface. An increase in fetal loss and congenital heart block has been reported in pregnant women with Sjögren's syndrome (6).

Ankylosing Spondylitis

Ankylosing spondylitis (AS) is a chronic inflammatory condition predominantly involving the spine. It is characterized by progressive, ascending stiffening and limitation of back motion and chest expansion. Often, spinal involvement begins at the level of the sacroiliac joints. Radiographically, the presence of a "bamboo spine" is a manifestation of advanced AS. Peripheral arthritis and uveitis are additional clinical manifestations. This is a rare autoimmune condition characterized by a male predominance.

During pregnancy, AS has been reported to worsen in a third of patients, improve in a third, and remain stable in the remaining third (7). An improvement in AS was reported in women with associated uveitis and carrying a female fetus. Sixty percent of women experienced postpartum flares within 6 months following delivery. General anesthesia is potentially difficult in these individuals because of ankylosis of the cervical spine and temporomandibular joints. Moreover, regional anesthesia also may prove difficult because of calcification and ankylosis of the vertebral column. Consultation with an anesthesiologist early in pregnancy is recommended. Treatment for AS is similar to RA.

Mixed Connective Tissue Disease

Mixed connective tissue disease should be considered in an individual who presents with a heterogeneous clinical presentation and does not fit into a definite criteria for another connective tissue disease. The disease is characterized by overlap of different features of different rheumatologic diseases, including RA, SLE, scleroderma, and polymyositis. Antibodies to ribonucleoprotein often are positive. Pregnancy outcome in women with mixed connective tissue disease is similar to those with SLE.

References

1. Ostensen M. Sex hormones and pregnancy in rheumatoid arthritis and systemic lupus erythematosus. Ann N Y Acad Sci 1999;876;131–43; discussion 144.

2. Yasmeen S, Wilkins EE, Field NT, Sheikh RA, Gilbert WM. Pregnancy outcomes in women with systemic lupus erythematosus. J Matern Fetal Med 2001;10:91–6.

3. Levy RA, Vilela VS, Cataldo MJ, Ramos RC, Duarte JL, Tura BR, et al. Hydroxychloroquine (HCQ) in lupus pregnancy: double-blind and placebo-controlled study. Lupus 2001;10;401–4.

4. Branch DW, Silver RM, Blackwell JL, Beading JC, Scott JR. Outcome of treated pregnancies in women with antiphospholipid syndrome: an update of the Utah experience. Obstet Gynecol 1992;80:614–20.

5. Lima F, Khamashta MA, Buchanan NM, Korslake S, Hunt BJ, Hughes GR. A study of sixty pregnancies in patients with the antiphospholipid syndrome. Clin Exp Rheumatol 1996;14:131–6.

6. Julkunen H, Kaaja R, Kurki P, Palosuo T, Friman C. Fetal outcome in women with primary Sjogren's syndrome. A retrospective case-control study. Clin Exp Rheumatol 1995;13:65–71.

7. Ostensen M, Ostensen H. Ankylosing spondylitis—the female aspect. J Rheumatol 1998;25:120–4.

INFECTION

Hepatitis A

Hepatitis A virus (HAV) is caused by a picornavirus and accounts for approximately 50% of all cases of hepatitis in the United States. Approximately 30% of women have serologic evidence of prior infection and are therefore immune. The incidence of acute hepatitis A during pregnancy is less than 1 in 1,000. Hepatitis A infection is acquired primarily by the fecal–oral route, either by person-to-person contact or ingestion of contaminated food or water. Most U.S. cases of hepatitis A result from person-to-person transmission during communitywide outbreaks (1). Children have asymptomatic or unrecognized infections and therefore play an important role in HAV transmission by serving as a source of infection for others (2). Postexposure prophylaxis with immune globulin is indicated for household or other intimate contacts of a person with serologically (IgM anti-HAV) confirmed hepatitis A. Inactivated hepatitis A vaccines are recommended for children older than 2 years in communities where hepatitis A is endemic and among persons traveling to a developing country. Although not studied during pregnancy, the theoretical risk of vaccination to the developing fetus is low.

The usual clinical manifestations of hepatitis A include fever, malaise, anorexia, nausea, abdominal discomfort, dark urine, and jaundice. Symptoms occur in more than 70% of infected adults. The diagnosis is confirmed by identifying IgM-specific antibody in the serum.

Serious complications of hepatitis A are uncommon. A chronic carrier state does not exist, and perinatal transmission of the virus does not occur.

Hepatitis B

Hepatitis B is caused by a small DNA virus and accounts for 40% of all cases of hepatitis in the United States. Acute hepatitis B occurs in 1–2 of 1,000 pregnancies, and chronic hepatitis B occurs in 5–15 of 1,000 pregnancies.

Hepatitis B virus (HBV) is transmitted efficiently by percutaneous or mucous membrane exposure to infectious body fluids. Sexual transmission among adults accounts for most HBV infections in the United States. In the 1990s, transmission among heterosexual partners accounted for 40% of infections, and transmission among men who have sex with men accounted for another 15% of infections. The most common risk factors include having multiple sex partners or a recent history of an STD. Pregnant women who test negative for hepatitis B surface antigen (HbsAg), seek STD treatment, and have not previously been vaccinated should receive hepatitis B vaccine because pregnancy is not a contraindication to vaccination (3).

In adults, only 50% of HBV infections are symptomatic, and about 1% of cases result in acute liver failure and death. In the acute stage of HBV infection, the diagnosis is confirmed by identification of HBsAg and IgM antibody to the core antigen. The presence of hepatitis B envelope antigen (HBeAg) indicates an exceptionally high viral inoculum and active virus replication. No specific therapy is available for women with acute HBV infection. Risk of chronic infection is associated with age at infection: about 90% of infected infants, 60% of children older than 5 years, and 2–6% of adults become chronically infected. Chronic HBV infection is characterized by the persistence of HBsAg in the liver and serum. An estimated 1.25 million people are chronically infected with HBV. Among persons with chronic HBV infection, the risk of death from cirrhosis or hepatocellular carcinoma is 15–20%. Antiviral agents (ie, alpha-interferon or lamivudine) are available for treatment of women with chronic hepatitis B.

Most cases (>90%) of perinatal transmission of HBV occur as a consequence of intrapartum exposure of the infant to maternal blood and genital tract secretions. The remaining cases result from hematogenous transplacental dissemination, breastfeeding, and close postnatal contact between the infant and the infected parent.

Immunoprophylaxis is the principal means of preventing HBV infection in adults and neonates. All pregnant women should be tested for HBsAg, and those who are seronegative should be vaccinated. Two recombinant vaccines are available. Before vaccination, individuals who have been exposed to HBV recently should initially receive passive immunization with hepatitis B immune globulin and simultaneously undergo the vaccination series. Hepatitis B immune globulin should be administered as soon as possible after exposure.

The CDC recommends that all neonates be vaccinated for hepatitis B (4). However, infants delivered to seropositive mothers also need to receive passive immunization with hepatitis B immune globulin.

Hepatitis C

Hepatitis C virus (HCV) is the primary cause of the type of hepatitis previously known as non-A, non-B hepatitis. It is the most common chronic bloodborne infection in the United States; an estimated 2.7 million people are chronically infected, most between ages 40 and 59 years. Persons with acute HCV infection are either asymptomatic or have a mild clinical illness. The diagnosis of HCV infection can be made by detecting either anti-HCV (EIA plus a supplemental antibody test—ie, recombinant immunoblot assay [RIBA]) or HCV RNA [by reverse transcription–polymerase chain reaction]). Chronic infection is common (75–85%), and 60–70% of infected persons have evidence of active liver disease (elevated transaminases). Although antibodies are produced, no protective antibody response has been identified after HCV infection. Antiviral therapy includes alpha interferon alone or in combination with oral ribavirin for a duration of 6–12 months (3).

Hepatitis C is most efficiently transmitted by direct percutaneous exposure to infected blood (eg, sharing needles). The current risk of transfusion-associated hepatitis C is less than 1 per million units transfused. Although less efficient, perinatal and sexual exposures (1.5% prevalence in susceptible long-term spouses) can result in transmission. Perinatal transmission appears to be low (~6%). This is more likely to occur in women with high titers of HCV-RNA or who are coinfected with HIV (5). Because immune globulin does not protect against infection, postexposure prophylaxis for exposed women and immunoprophylaxis for the neonate are not available. There is no available vaccine against HCV.

Hepatitis D and E

Hepatitis D is a defective single-stranded RNA virus that requires the helper function of HBV to replicate. Hepatitis D requires HBV for synthesis of envelope protein composed of HBsAg, which is used to encapsulate the HDV genome. The modes of HDV transmission are similar to those for HBV, with percutaneous exposures the most efficient. Sexual transmission of HDV is less efficient than HBV.

Acute HDV infection may occur as a coinfection with acute HBV. Coinfection is usually self-limiting and rarely leads to chronic hepatitis. Hepatitis D also may develop as a superinfection in a patient who is a chronic carrier of HBV. Approximately 20–25% of chronic HBV carriers eventually become coinfected with HDV. In contrast to coinfection, superinfection leads to chronic hepatitis in almost 80% of patients. Of patients with chronic infection, 70–80% ultimately develop cirrhosis and portal hypertension, and approximately 25% die of hepatic failure.

The diagnosis of hepatitis D can be confirmed by detection of HDV antigen in hepatic tissue or serum and identification of IgM- or IgG-specific antibody. Patients with chronic hepatitis D usually have persistent HDV antigenemia and viremia. Hepatic damage may continue despite the presence of antibody.

Perinatal transmission of HDV is rare. Fortunately the measures used to prevent intrapartum transmission of HBV are almost uniformly effective in preventing transmission of HDV.

Hepatitis E results from fecal–oral transmission of a nonenveloped RNA virus. The epidemiologic features of hepatitis E are similar to those of hepatitis A. Hepatitis E is rare in the United States but is endemic in several developing nations, notably those in Asia, Africa, the Middle East, Central America, and Mexico. It can be diagnosed by identifying HEV–specific IgM and IgG antibody and HEV RNA. Hepatitis E usually is self-limiting and does not result in a chronic carrier state. Fulminant hepatic failure is more common in pregnant women, with an incidence approaching 15% (6). Perinatal transmission does not occur.

Rubella

Rubella is a viral illness caused by a togavirus. It causes a mild febrile rash in adults and children. The most serious consequences of rubella result from infection during the first trimester of pregnancy. Rubella infection can affect all organs in the developing fetus and cause miscarriage, fetal death, and congenital anomalies. Up to 90% of infants born to mothers infected during the first 11 weeks of gestation will develop a pattern of birth defects called congenital rubella syndrome (CRS); the rate of CRS for infants born to women infected during the first 20 weeks of pregnancy is 20%. Infants infected with rubella late in gestation do not exhibit clinical manifestations of CRS but can shed virus.

Although rubella may be confirmed by culture of the virus from nasopharyngeal secretions (throat swabs), serologic tests usually are of more practical value in clinical practice. Enzyme immunoassays specific for IgM and IgG are widely available and relatively easy to perform. Direct identification of virus with reverse transcription–polymerase chain reaction testing also is available.

The number of cases of rubella and CRS have declined 99% since the licensure of the rubella virus vaccine in 1969. CRS now disproportionately affects infants born to foreign-born women. During 1997–1999, 21 of 26 (81%) infants reported with CRS were Hispanic, and 24 of 26 (92%) were born to foreign-born mothers. In recent outbreaks, most cases occurred in persons from Mexico and Central America (7).

Ideally, all women of reproductive age should have a serologic test to confirm their immunity to rubella before they consider pregnancy. Susceptible women should be vaccinated and advised to continue contraception for 3 months. There are no reports of congenital rubella resulting from vaccination, and the maximum theoretical risk is estimated to be no more than 1.6%. For the pregnant patient whose immunologic status is unknown, a rubella serologic screen should be obtained at the time of the first prenatal appointment. Susceptible patients should be targeted for vaccination in the immediate postpartum period.

Cytomegalovirus

Cytomegalovirus infection is caused by a double-stranded DNA herpesvirus. The incidence of primary CMV infection in pregnant women in the United States varies from 1% to 3%. Approximately 50–85% of adults have serologic evidence of previous CMV infection by age 40 years. The virus has been shown to spread in households and among young children in day care centers through infected bodily fluids; simple hand washing with soap and water is effective in removing the virus from the hands. Infection also may be transmitted by sexual contact and blood transfusion. Most CMV infections in adults are subclinical. Symptomatic patients typically present with a mononucleosislike illness.

Cytomegalovirus remains an important cause of congenital viral infection in the United States. The morbidity of CMV congenital infection appears to be almost exclusively associated with *primary* CMV infection during pregnancy. Even in this case, two thirds of the infants will not become infected, and only 10–15% of the remaining third will have symptoms at the time of birth. Neonatal symptoms suggesting generalized infection range from moderate enlargement of the liver and spleen (with jaundice) to fatal illness. Of those neonates, 80–90% will have complications within the first few years of life that may include hearing loss, vision impairment, and varying degrees of mental retardation. After recurrent maternal CMV, only 10% of infants become infected, usually without symptoms at birth, but subsequently may have varying degrees of hearing and mental or coordination problems.

There appears to be little risk of CMV-related complications for women who have been infected at least 6 months prior to conception. For this group, which makes up 50–80% of the women of childbearing age, the rate of newborn CMV infection is 1%, and these infants appear to have no significant illness or abnormalities. The virus also can be transmitted to the infant at delivery from contact with genital secretions or later in infancy through breast milk. However, these infections usually result in little or no clinical illness in the infant.

Maternal CMV infection can be diagnosed by culturing the virus from urine or from genital tract secretions. More commonly, the diagnosis is confirmed by serologic tests. If antibody tests of paired serum samples drawn 2 weeks apart show a 4-fold rise in IgG antibody or a significant level of IgM antibody, meaning equal to at least 30% of the IgG value, or virus is cultured from a urine or throat specimen, the findings indicate that an active CMV infection is present.

Diagnosis of fetal CMV infection should be suspected when ultrasound examination demonstrates fetal anomalies such as abdominal and liver calcifications, echogenic bowel, hepatosplenomegaly, periventricular calcifications, ventriculomegaly, hydrops, and ascites (8). Confirmation of fetal infection is best determined by detection of CMV in amniotic fluid by culture or polymerase chain reaction.

At present, no safe antiviral agent is effective in treating maternal CMV infection or in preventing congenital infection. Routine screening of asymptomatic pregnant women for CMV infection is not indicated.

Toxoplasmosis

Toxoplasmosis is caused by infection with the protozoan parasite *Toxoplasma gondii*. In the United States, an estimated 23% of adolescents and adults have laboratory evidence of infection with *T gondii*. Although these infections usually are either asymptomatic or associated with self-limited symptoms (eg, fever, malaise, and lymphadenopathy), infection in immunosuppressed persons can be severe. In addition, infections in pregnant women can cause serious health problems in the fetus if the parasites are transmitted and cause severe sequelae in the infant (eg, mental retardation, blindness, and epilepsy). Although congenital toxoplasmosis is not a nationally reportable disease and no national data are available regarding its occurrence, extrapolation from regional studies indicates that an estimated 400–4,000 cases occur in the United States each year (9).

Toxoplasma can be transmitted to humans by 3 principal routes: a) ingestion of raw or inadequately cooked infected meat; b) ingestion of oocysts, an environmentally resistant form of the organism that cats pass in their feces, with exposure of humans occurring through exposure to cat litter or soil (eg, from gardening or from unwashed fruits or vegetables); and c) a newly infected pregnant woman passing the infection to her fetus.

Toxoplasma infection can be prevented in large part by: a) cooking meat to a safe temperature; b) peeling or thoroughly washing fruits and vegetables before eating; c) cleaning cooking surfaces and utensils after they have contacted raw meat, poultry, seafood, or unwashed fruits or vegetables; d) pregnant women avoiding changing cat litter or, if no one else is available to change the cat litter, using gloves, then washing hands thoroughly; and e) not feeding raw or undercooked meat to cats and keeping cats inside to prevent acquisition of *Toxoplasma* by eating infected prey.

Congenital toxoplasmosis can occur if the mother develops a primary infection during pregnancy. Approximately one third of infants born to mothers with primary infection will be affected. The frequency of fetal infection is higher when maternal infection occurs in the third trimester (60–65%) than when it occurs in the first trimester (15–20%). However, the severity of infection is greater when the mother is infected during the first trimester.

Approximately one third of infected neonates have evidence of clinical disease at birth. The characteristic triad of congenital toxoplasmosis is intracerebral calcification, chorioretinitis, and hydrocephalus. Other findings may include anemia, jaundice, splenomegaly, generalized lymphadenopathy, seizures, microcephaly, mental retardation, and hearing impairment.

The diagnosis of toxoplasmosis in adults and children may be confirmed in several ways. The organism can be detected in histologic preparations of infected tissues such as lymph nodes. The mainstay of diagnosis, however, is serologic testing. Antibodies may be detected by indirect immunofluorescence or ELISA. Patients with acute infection typically have positive assays for IgM antibody, and their IgG antibody test results show seroconversion. Titers for IgM may remain positive for several months after acute infection.

Clinicians should be aware that serologic testing for toxoplasmosis is not well standardized and that only a few reference laboratories consistently provide reliable test results. When primary toxoplasmosis during pregnancy is suspected, serum specimens should be forwarded to one of these recognized referral centers for confirmation. State health departments and the CDC can provide the names of qualified reference laboratories.

Several methods have been used to diagnose fetal infection with *T gondii*. A competitive PCR test for *T gondii* can be performed on amniotic fluid obtained by amniocentesis. Fetal blood can be aspirated by cordocentesis and cultured. Fetal blood also can be assayed for total IgM concentration and IgM-specific antibody after 21–23 weeks of gestation. However, although these measures may indicate that *T gondii* is present in the fetal and placental circulation, they do not precisely define the severity of fetal infection. Ultrasound examination is valuable in this regard. Ultrasound findings that are consistent with severe fetal infection include microcephaly, ventriculomegaly, growth restriction, visceromegaly, and hydrops.

If acute fetal infection is documented, patients may be offered pregnancy termination or antibiotic treatment. A multidrug regimen including spiramycin, pyrimethamine, and sulfadiazine can eradicate microorganisms in the placenta and fetus.

Herpes Simplex

Genital herpes is a recurrent, life-long viral infection. Two serotypes of the herpes simplex virus (HSV) have been identified: herpes simplex virus 1 (HSV-1) and herpes simplex virus 2 (HSV-2). Most cases of recurrent genital herpes are caused by HSV-2. Most people infected with HSV-2 have not had their infection diagnosed. Others have mild or unrecognized infections but shed virus intermittently in the genital tract. Both HSV-1 and HSV-2 genital herpes can result in vertical transmission to the neonate (10).

The clinical diagnosis of genital herpes is both insensitive and nonspecific. The typical painful multiple vesicular or ulcerative lesions are absent in many infected women. Up to 30% of first-episode cases of genital herpes are caused by HSV-1, but recurrences are much less frequent for genital HSV-1 infection than genital HSV-2 infection.

Isolation of HSV in cell culture is the preferred virologic test in patients who present with genital ulcers or other mucocutaneous lesions. The sensitivity of culture declines rapidly as lesions begin to heal, usually within a few days of onset.

Both type-specific and nonspecific antibodies to HSV develop during the first several weeks following infection and persist indefinitely. Because almost all HSV-2 infections are sexually acquired, type-specific HSV-2 antibody indicates anogenital infection, but the presence of HSV-1 antibody does not distinguish anogenital from orolabial infection. Accurate type-specific assays for HSV antibodies must be based on the HSV-specific glycoprotein G2 for the diagnosis of infection with HSV-2 and glycoprotein G1 for diagnosis of infection with HSV-1. Such assays first became commercially available in 1999, but older assays do not accurately distinguish HSV-1 from HSV-2 antibody. Therefore, the serologic type-specific glycoprotein G-based assays should be specifically requested when serology is performed (3).

Because false-negative HSV cultures are common, especially in patients with recurrent infection or with healing lesions, type-specific serologic tests are useful in confirming a clinical diagnosis of genital herpes. Additionally, such tests can be used to diagnose persons with unrecognized infection and to manage sex partners of persons with genital herpes. Although serologic assays for HSV-2 should be available for persons who request them, screening for HSV-1 or HSV-2 infection in the general population is not indicated.

Most mothers of infants who acquire herpes neonatally lack histories of clinically evident genital herpes. The risk for transmission to the neonate from an infected mother is high (30–50%) among women who acquire genital herpes near the time of delivery and is low (<1%) among women with histories of recurrent herpes at term or who acquire genital HSV during the first half of pregnancy. Prevention of neonatal herpes depends both on preventing acquisition of genital HSV infection during late pregnancy and avoiding exposure of the infant to herpetic lesions during delivery.

Women without known genital herpes should be counseled to avoid intercourse during the third trimester with partners known or suspected of having genital herpes. In addition, pregnant women without known orolabial herpes should be advised to avoid cunnilingus during the third trimester with partners known or suspected to have orolabial herpes. In the future, type-specific serologic tests may be used to identify pregnant women at risk for HSV infection and to guide counseling with regard to the risk of acquiring genital herpes during pregnancy. Such testing and counseling may be especially important when a woman's sex partner has HSV infection.

At the onset of labor, all women should be questioned carefully about symptoms of genital herpes, including prodrome, and all women should be examined carefully for herpetic lesions. Women without symptoms or signs of genital herpes or its prodrome can deliver vaginally, but use of invasive monitors should be limited. Women with recurrent genital herpetic lesions or prodromal symptoms at the onset of labor deliver by cesarean section to prevent neonatal herpes (11).

Oral antiviral therapy (acyclovir, valacyclovir, or famciclovir) should be considered for women at or beyond 36 weeks of gestation whose first episode of HSV occurred during the current pregnancy as well as for women at risk for recurrent HSV to decrease the likelihood of HSV-shedding and need for cesarean section. Investigators have monitored more than 1,100 pregnancies in which women were exposed to acyclovir or valacyclovir and have found no evidence of adverse effects on the fetus (12).

Varicella

Varicella zoster virus (VZV), like other herpes viruses, has the capacity to exist in the body after primary infection in a latent state. Primary infection results in chickenpox, whereas reactivation leads to herpes zoster (shingles). It is highly contagious, with up to 90% of susceptible household contacts becoming infected (13). The incidence of VZV infection has fallen significantly since the licensure of the varicella vaccine in 1995. If during the initial prenatal visit no history of chickenpox is obtained, serology should be submitted for varicella IgG. If serologic testing fails to confirm immunity, postpartum vaccination (2 doses 4–8 weeks apart) is recommended. Contraception should be ensured for at least 1 month following vaccination.

The onset of maternal varicella from 5 days before to 2 days after delivery may result in an overwhelming infection in the neonate, with fatality rates as high as 30% (13). This severe infection is believed to result from fetal exposure to the virus without benefit of passively acquired maternal antibody. For this reason, varicella-zoster immune globulin (VZIG) should be administered to these infants following delivery. Primary varicella infection during the first 20 weeks of pregnancy is associated with a variety of abnormalities in the newborn, including low birth weight, hypoplasia of an extremity, skin scarring, localized muscular atrophy, encephalitis, cortical atrophy, chorioretinitis, and microcephaly. The risk of congenital varicella zoster syndrome is low (around 1%).

Varicella zoster virus infection usually is diagnosed clinically, but confirmation by culture of the vesicular fluid and ELISA testing for antibodies is available in most institutions. Primary VZV infection during pregnancy is associated with an increase risk for pneumonitis. For this reason, susceptible pregnant women with a significant exposure (live in the same house or > 5 minutes face-to-face contact, or indoor contact > 1 hour) should receive VZIG. If given within 96 hours of exposure, 80% of clinical chickenpox can be prevented, compared with a 90% rate of clinical chickenpox if no VZIG is provided. Administration of VZIG will not necessarily prevent maternal viremia and fetal infection. Pregnant women with clinical chickenpox need to be evaluated and should be monitored for symptoms and signs of varicella pneumonia. Risk factors for this serious complication include smoking, steroid use, and chronic obstructive pulmonary disease. Patients, especially in the third trimester, with an extensive rash, particularly if it is hemorrhagic in nature and involving the mucous membranes, are also at risk and hospitalization should be considered. If symptoms suggest pneumonia, a chest X-ray and arterial blood gas should be obtained. If the chest X-ray is abnormal or the pO_2 is less than 80 mm Hg, admission and parenteral therapy with acyclovir is in order. If the patient has been determined to have uncomplicated chickenpox and has presented within 24 hours of rash onset, oral acyclovir is appropriate and she can be managed as an outpatient, reassessing her status every 24–48 hours.

Parvovirus

Parvovirus B19 is the causative agent of erythema infectiosum (fifth disease). The clinical manifestations of this virus include a macular rash with a "slapped cheek" appearance that spreads to the trunk and proximal extremities and symmetrical arthralgias. The viral syndrome, which is also associated with a low-grade fever, malaise, and upper respiratory symptoms, lasts less than 3 weeks. Risk factors for infection include exposure to children and working in an elementary school; however, up to 60% of adults are seropositive, suggesting childhood disease (8). Only 3% of susceptible school employees seroconvert each year. The highest risk for infection occurs in women whose children develop the disease; nursery school teachers have the highest occupational risk.

The rate of intrauterine infection ranges from 25% to 51%, but the risk of an adverse fetal outcome is less than 5%, with the greatest risk occurring prior to 20 weeks of gestation (11). Exposed women should have serology for IgM and IgG antibodies drawn. A positive IgG and negative IgM confirms a state of immunity. Approximately 50–65% of individuals exhibit immunity as evidenced by the presence of an IgG antibody. If the period since exposure is unknown, a baseline IgG titer is obtained and repeated in 4 weeks. A 4-fold increase in IgG antibody titer indicates maternal infection; a positive IgM assay after this interval is also indicative of maternal infection, although the rate of false-positive results is high at many commercial laboratories.

The theoretic risk for the development of hydrops fetalis ranges from 0% to 8% of cases. Hydrops fetalis is believed to result from transient suppression of the erythroid cell lines of the fetal bone marrow, as well as from myocarditis. If maternal parvovirus infection is suspected, the patient should be followed by weekly ultrasound assessments for hydrops fetalis, which typically presents as fetal ascites with or without scalp edema or pleural effusion. Doppler assessment of the peak middle cerebral artery systolic velocity will detect fetal anemia before the onset of frank hydrops. Hydrops fetalis has been reported to occur as late as 10 weeks after maternal disease; therefore, assessments should be continued during this period after maternal infection. Significant hydrops can be treated with cordocentesis and intrauterine transfusion after 18 weeks of gestation. Detection of B19 DNA in fetal blood confirms the diagnosis. Follow-up in these infants has not revealed any long-term sequelae of infection.

Urinary Tract Infections

Asymptomatic Bacteriuria and Acute Cystitis

Lower urinary tract infections during pregnancy may take 2 forms: asymptomatic bacteriuria and acute cystitis. Asymptomatic bacteriuria affects 4–8% of pregnant women, and all pregnant women should be screened for asymptomatic bacteriuria by urine culture at the time of their first prenatal appointment. This is an opportunity not only to identify a uropathogen that can be treated to decrease the subsequent risk of preterm labor and pyelonephritis, but also to detect GBS bacteriuria. Acute cystitis occurs in 1–3% of obstetric patients (14).

Approximately 80% of lower urinary tract infections are caused by *Escherichia coli*; 10–15% are due to *Klebsiella pneumoniae* or *Proteus* species; 5% or fewer are caused by GBS, enterococci, or staphylococci. Anaerobic organisms are unusual pathogens except in patients who have chronic obstructions or who undergo frequent urologic examinations or procedures.

The diagnosis of asymptomatic bacteriuria is made on the basis of a positive urine culture demonstrating 105 colonies per milliliter. This urine sample should be a midstream, clean-catch specimen, preferably collected after urine has incubated in the bladder for 4–6 hours. The diagnosis of acute cystitis should be suspected when patients have dysuria, frequency, and urgency. When urine is obtained by catheterization after a short period of incubation, a colony count of 10^2 colonies per milliliter in a symptomatic patient is considered indicative of infection.

Several oral antibiotics are effective for the treatment of lower urinary tract infections: ampicillin, amoxicillin, amoxicillin–clavulanic acid, sulfisoxazole, cephalosporins, nitrofurantoin macrocrystals, trimethoprim–sulfamethoxazole, and quinolones. However, the prevalence of resistance among uropathogens is increasing to 20% or higher for ampicillin, cephalothin, and trimethoprim–sulfamethoxazole. Resistance to nitrofurantoin remains low, at 6% for all uropathogens and 1% for E coli. In addition, the quinolones are contraindicated in pregnancy because of their injurious effects on fetal cartilage in animal studies. Given equal efficacy, the agent that is least expensive and least toxic should be administered (15, 16).

The appropriate length of antibiotic treatment for uncomplicated lower urinary tract infection is controversial. Single-dose therapy appears to be less effective in obstetric patients than in nonpregnant patients. However, a 3-day course of antibiotics usually is comparable in efficacy to a 7- or 10-day course and ensures better compliance. Patients who have a poor response to this short course of therapy often have a silent upper urinary tract infection and require treatment for 2–4 weeks.

Patients should have a repeat urine culture upon completion of treatment to be certain that the infection is eradicated. The risk of recurrence later in pregnancy is 15–25%.

ACUTE PYELONEPHRITIS

Acute pyelonephritis occurs in 1–2% of pregnant women. The single most important risk factor for pyelonephritis is previously undiagnosed or inadequately treated lower urinary tract infection. In fact, approximately 40% of women with untreated asymptomatic bacteriuria develop pyelonephritis. Ascending infection is particularly likely in pregnancy because of the inhibitory effect of progesterone on ureteral peristalsis and the mechanical compression of the ureters by the enlarging uterus.

The usual clinical manifestations of acute pyelonephritis are fever, chills, flank pain and tenderness, and urinary frequency and urgency. Approximately 70–75% of cases of pyelonephritis are right sided, approximately 10–15% are left sided, and 10–15% are bilateral. Bacteremia may be present in as many as 10% of infected patients, and 1–2% of patients actually develop septic shock. A similar percentage also may manifest signs of adult respiratory distress syndrome. In patients with pyelonephritis, microscopic examination of urine typically shows leukocyte casts and bacteria. The urine culture will be positive unless the patient previously has received antibiotic treatment.

Infected patients should be hospitalized and treated with parenteral antibiotics. In some cases, outpatient management may be considered (17). Patients should be carefully selected for this approach. A third-generation cephalosporin such as ceftriaxone is an excellent empirical choice because of its uniform activity against the major uropathogens and its minimal toxicity. Patients who appear to be critically ill or who are particularly likely to have a resistant organism should be treated initially with both ampicillin and gentamicin, or with aztreonam, until sensitivity tests are completed. Parenteral antibiotics should be continued until the patient has been afebrile and asymptomatic for 24–48 hours. Once this criterion is met, the patient may be discharged from the hospital and treated with an appropriate oral antibiotic for 7–10 days. The patient's condition subsequently needs to be assessed with periodic urine cultures.

Approximately 75% of obstetric patients with pyelonephritis become afebrile within 48 hours. Almost 95% are afebrile within 72 hours. Patients who have a poor response to therapy are likely to have either a resistant organism or a urinary tract obstruction. If the latter condition is suspected, the patient should be evaluated with renal ultrasonography or intravenous pyelography. If obstruction is demonstrated, urologic consultation is indicated.

Group B Streptococcus

Group B streptococcal early-onset neonatal sepsis remains a leading infectious cause of morbidity and mortality among newborns in the United States despite the widespread acceptance of guidelines promoting the use of intrapartum antimicrobial prophylaxis. Current guidelines recommend screening all pregnant women for vaginal and rectal GBS colonization between 35 and 37 weeks of gestation. Colonized women should then be offered intrapartum antibiotics at the time of labor. All women with GBS bacteriuria during their current pregnancy or who previously gave birth to an infant with early-onset GBS disease are candidates for intrapartum antibiotic prophylaxis.

Prenatal culture-based screening for vaginal and rectal GBS colonization should be done at 35–37 weeks of gestation (18). The culture should be obtained by swabbing both the lower vagina and rectum (ie, through the anal sphincter) rather than sampling the cervix or sampling the vagina without also swabbing the rectum. Because vaginal and rectal swabs are likely to yield diverse bacteria, use of selective enrichment broth is recommended to maximize the isolation of GBS and avoid overgrowth of other organisms.

The prophylaxis regimens for women with penicillin allergy have been updated. Among penicillin-allergic women not at high risk for anaphylaxis, cefazolin, because of its narrow spectrum of activity and ability to achieve high intraamniotic concentrations, is the agent of choice for intrapartum chemoprophylaxis. For penicillin-allergic women at high risk for anaphylaxis, testing of GBS isolates from prenatal screening for susceptibility to clindamycin is recommended if feasible (19, 20). Clindamycin should be employed for intrapartum GBS prophylaxis if the screening isolate is susceptible. If the patient is at high risk for anaphylaxis and susceptibility studies are not available, vancomycin is recommended.

The presence of GBS bacteriuria in any concentration in a pregnant woman is a marker for heavy genital tract colonization. Women with GBS urinary tract infections during pregnancy should receive appropriate treatment at the time of diagnosis as well as intrapartum GBS prophylaxis.

Although a risk does exist for transmission of GBS from a colonized mother to her infant during a planned cesarean delivery performed before onset of labor in a woman with intact amniotic membranes, it is extremely low. Intrapartum antibiotic prophylaxis to prevent perinatal GBS disease is not recommended as a routine practice for women undergoing planned cesarean deliveries in the absence of labor or amniotic membrane rupture, regardless of the GBS colonization status of the mother. The new guidelines also provide an algorithm for management of patients with threatened preterm delivery (Fig. 23).

Penicillin remains the first-line agent for intrapartum antibiotic prophylaxis, with ampicillin an acceptable alternative. Women whose culture results are unknown at the time of delivery still need to be managed according to the risk-based approach, and the obstetric risk factors remain unchanged (ie, delivery at <37 weeks of gestation, duration of membrane rupture ≥18 hours, or temperature ≥100.4°F [≥38.0°C]). Women with negative vaginal and rectal GBS screening cultures within 5 weeks of delivery do not require intrapartum antimicrobial prophylaxis for GBS even if obstetric risk factors develop (ie, delivery at <37 weeks of gestation, duration of membrane rupture ≥18 hours, or temperature ≥100.4°F [≥38.0°C]). Intrapartum antimicrobial prophylaxis should be administered to women with GBS bacteriuria in any concentration during their current pregnancy or who previously gave birth to an infant with GBS disease. Finally, in the absence of GBS urinary tract infection, antimicrobial agents should not be used before the intrapartum period to treat asymptomatic GBS colonization. A complete copy of the 2002 Revised Guidelines for the Prevention of Perinatal GBS Disease is available on the CDC's web site (www.cdc.gov).

Human Immunodeficiency Virus Infection

The standard of care for the management of HIV infection continues to evolve at a rapid pace. In recognition of this fact, a web site has been created by the Public Health Service (aidsinfo.nih.gov) that provides a regularly updated guide to the management of HIV. This web site reviews recent developments in the field and should be checked frequently.

All pregnant women should have prenatal HIV testing per the recommendation of the Institute of Medicine, which recommended an informed right of refusal approach to testing. This approach requires that a prenatal patient be informed that she is going to be tested for

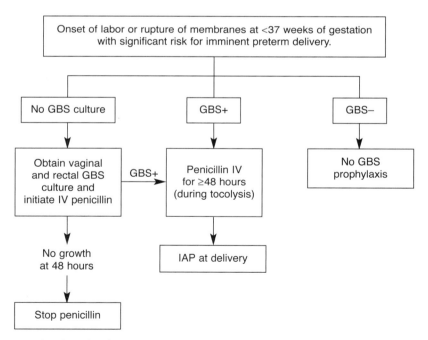

■ **FIG. 23.** Sample algorithm for group B streptococcal (GBS) prophylaxis for women with threatened preterm delivery. IV indicates intravenous; IAP, intraabdominal pressure. This algorithm is not an exclusive course of management. Variations that incorporate individual circumstances or institutional preferences may be appropriate. (Centers for Disease Control and Prevention. Prevention of perinatal group B streptococcal disease. Revised guidelines from CDC. Morb Mortal Wkly Rep MMWR 2002;51[RR-11]:1–22.)

the virus and that she has a right to refuse such testing. A written affirmative consent is not required. Up to 20% of HIV-infected women, however, do not initiate prenatal care. Given that data confirm the efficacy of intrapartum and early neonatal prophylaxis in reducing the risk of vertical transmission, efforts should be made during labor for rapidly determining the serostatus of those women using a commercially available rapid test, usually an ELISA, so that these preventive measures can be undertaken (21).

Obstetricians should ensure that highly active antiretroviral therapy (HAART) is used appropriately in the setting of pregnancy. The cornerstones of monitoring remain viral loads and CD4 counts. Monitoring in pregnancy should occur every trimester until viral load is undetectable (22). Vertical transmission is linked to viral loads, and cesarean deliveries are recommended for women whose viral loads exceed 1,000 copies/mL. For this reason, pregnant women should be informed of the advantages of initiating HAART whenever their viral loads are above 1,000 copies/mL. With appropriate therapy, viral loads should drop by more than 1 log within the first month of therapy and should eventually become undetectable. Failure to meet this goal suggests treatment failure and probable emerging resistance. For this reason, resistance testing (phenotypic and genotypic) has become a standard component of HIV care.

The combination of antepartum, intrapartum, and early neonatal therapy is optimal in preventing the vertical transmission of HIV. Initiation of therapy should occur in consultation with an expert. Adherence to therapy is crucial. It is useful to choose a regimen that spares a class of antiretroviral agents, ie, protease inhibitors or non–nucleoside reverse transcriptase inhibitors or both, in anticipation of needing to deal with failure of the initial regimen down the road. Zidovudine, which crosses the placenta well, should be used whenever possible as a component of HAART regimens. In addition, the potential risks of HAART agents, including their avidity for mitochondria, must be considered. In the mother, clinical disorders associated with mitochondrial toxicity include neuropathy, myopathy, cardiomyopathy, pancreatitis, hepatic steastosis, and lactic acidosis.

It is estimated that 70% of mother-to-child transmissions occur at delivery and about 30% in utero. About 2 of 3 in utero transmissions occur in the last 14 days before delivery. Factors other than viral load that have been linked to vertical transmission include prolonged rupture of membranes, vaginal delivery, prematurity, drug use, and breastfeeding.

External Genital Warts

Visible genital warts (formerly known as condyloma acuminata) usually are caused by human papillomavirus (HPV) type 6 or 11 (3). Depending on their size and anatomic locations, genital warts can be painful, friable, and pruritic. Because genital warts can proliferate during pregnancy, many experts advocate their removal. The primary goal of treating visible warts is the removal of symptomatic warts. Treatment can induce wart-free periods in most patients. Podophyllin, podofilox, and imiquimod should not be used in pregnancy. Topical trichloroacetic acid, judiciously placed on the warts, or cryotherapy can be recommended during pregnancy if the total wart area is small. Laser vaporization or surgical excision should be reserved for patients with a large burden of disease that could lead to pelvic outlet obstruction or excessive bleeding during vaginal delivery. Lesions commonly regress after delivery, even without specific therapy. Human papillomavirus types 6 and 11 can cause laryngeal papillomatosis in infants and children. The route of transmission is not completely understood. Because the preventive value of cesarean delivery is unknown, cesarean delivery should not be performed solely to prevent transmission of HPV infection to the newborn.

Syphilis

Syphilis is a systemic disease caused by the spirochete *Treponema pallidum*. Patients with syphilis may seek treatment for signs or symptoms of primary infection (ulcer or chancre at site of infection), secondary infection (manifestations that include rash, mucocutaneous lesions, and adenopathy), or tertiary infection (cardiac, neurologic, ophthalmic, auditory, or gummatous lesions). However, most infections are detected during the latent stage by serologic testing. All women should be screened serologically for syphilis as early as possible in pregnancy (3). In populations with high syphilis prevalence and in patients at high risk, serologic testing should be repeated at the beginning of the third trimester and again at delivery. Any woman who delivers a stillborn infant after 20 weeks of gestation should be tested for syphilis. The serologic status of an infant's mother should be determined during pregnancy before the infant is discharged from the hospital. All women with syphilis should be offered testing for HIV infection.

The specificity of serologic testing is high if both a nontreponemal screening test (VDRL or rapid plasma reagent) and a subsequent treponemal serologic test (fluorescent treponemal antibody absorption or micro-hemagglutination–*T pallidum*) are reactive. Nontreponemal test antibody titers usually correlate with disease activity, and results should be reported quantitatively. Microscopic dark-field and histologic examinations for spirochetes are most reliable when lesions are present. Seropositive pregnant women should be considered infected unless treatment history is clearly documented in a medical or health department record and sequential serologic antibody titers have declined appropriately.

Penicillin is effective for preventing transmission to the fetus and for treating established infection in the fetus. Treatment during pregnancy should be the penicillin regimen appropriate for the woman's stage of syphilis. Some experts recommend additional therapy 1 week after the initial dose, particularly for women in the third trimester of pregnancy and for those with secondary syphilis during pregnancy. Nontreponemal tests usually become nonreactive with time after treatment; however, in some women, nontreponemal antibodies can persist at a low titer for a long period of time, sometimes for the life of the patient. This response is referred to as a "sero-fast reaction." Most women with reactive treponemal tests will have reactive tests for the remainder of their lives, regardless of treatment or disease activity.

Women who are treated for syphilis during the second half of pregnancy are at risk for premature labor, fetal distress, or both if their treatment precipitates the Jarisch–Herxheimer reaction. These women should be advised to seek medical attention after treatment if they notice any change in fetal movements or if they have contractions. Stillbirth is a rare complication of treatment; however, because therapy is necessary to prevent further damage, this concern should not delay treatment.

Serologic titers should be checked monthly until the adequacy of treatment has been ensured. There are no proven alternatives to penicillin. Skin testing is helpful in most patients with a dubious history of penicillin allergy. A pregnant woman with a penicillin allergy should be treated with penicillin after desensitization. Tetracycline and doxycycline are contraindicated during pregnancy.

Bacterial Vaginosis

Bacterial vaginosis is a complex alteration of the vaginal flora characterized by a replacement of the normal H_2O_2-producing *Lactobacillus* species with high concentrations of anaerobic bacteria (eg, *Prevotella* species, *Mobiluncus* species), *Gardnerella vaginalis*, and *Mycoplasma hominis*. Women with bacterial vaginosis report an abnormal vaginal discharge associated with a fishy odor, particularly after unprotected sexual intercourse. The diagnosis of bacterial vaginosis is based on the following composite clinical criteria: homogenous white noninflammatory discharge, clue cells, pH of vaginal fluid greater than 4.5, and a fishy odor of vaginal secretions after the addition of 10% potassium hydroxide (whiff test) (3). Additional methods of diagnosis include Gram stain and a test card for the detection of elevated pH and trimethylamine.

All symptomatic pregnant women should be tested and treated. Bacterial vaginosis has been associated with PROM, preterm labor and delivery, intraamniotic fluid infection, chorioamnionitis, and postcesarean endometritis. Because treatment of bacterial vaginosis in asymptomatic pregnant women at high risk for preterm delivery

(ie, those who have previously delivered a premature infant) with a recommended regimen has reduced preterm delivery in 3 of 4 randomized controlled trials (23–26), some specialists recommend the screening and treatment of these women. However, the optimal treatment regimens have not been established.

Oral metronidazole is the treatment of choice for bacterial vaginosis. Alternative and possibly less efficacious regimens include topical metronidazole gel and oral clindamycin.

Immunizations During Pregnancy

Currently, 4 types of immunobiologic agents are available for immunization: toxoids, inactivated vaccines, live vaccines, and immune globulin preparations. As a general rule, only live viral or live bacterial vaccines are contraindicated during pregnancy (27). The most commonly used live virus vaccines in the United States are those for measles, mumps, and rubella. Varicella vaccine is also a live attenuated virus preparation.

Ideally, all women of childbearing age should be immune to measles, mumps, rubella, tetanus, pertussis, diphtheria, poliomyelitis, and varicella by virtue of either childhood vaccination or natural infection. Women who are susceptible to any of these infections may receive toxoids or inactivated vaccines (tetanus, pertussis, diphtheria, inactivated polio vaccine), if clinically indicated, during pregnancy (Table 20). Live virus vaccinations (eg, measles, mumps, rubella, varicella, or live polio vaccine) should be deferred until after delivery.

Varicella vaccine has been available since 1995 and is recommended for all susceptible persons older than 12 months. The Advisory Committee on Immunization Practices of the CDC has designated adolescents and adults living in households with children a high-risk group. Susceptible nonpregnant women of childbearing age should receive varicella vaccine and should be advised to use contraception for 1 month.

Influenza vaccine is strongly recommended for all women who are or anticipate being in the second or third trimester of pregnancy during the influenza season (see "Influenza"). Certain patients may merit special consideration for vaccination during pregnancy. Patients with risk factors for hepatitis B (see "Hepatitis B") should receive the recombinant vaccine. Patients with acute exposure to HBV also should receive hepatitis B immune globulin. Patients who live in communities where hepatitis A is endemic should receive the inactivated hepatitis A vaccine. Women who have had a splenectomy, who have sickle cell anemia, or who are immunocompromised should be vaccinated against pneumococcal infection. Finally, pregnant patients who anticipate foreign travel may require special immunizations for infections such as cholera, plague, typhoid, and viral hepatitis.

Table 20. Immunization During Pregnancy

Immunobiologic Agent	Risk From Disease to Pregnant Woman	Risk From Disease to Fetus or Neonate	Type of Immunizing Agent	Risk From Immunizing Agent to Fetus	Indications for Immunization During Pregnancy	Dose Schedule	Comments
Live Virus Vaccines							
Measles	Significant morbidity, low mortality; not altered by pregnancy	Significant increase in abortion rate; may cause malformations	Live attenuated virus vaccine	None confirmed	Contraindicated (see immune globulins)	Single dose SC, preferably as measles–mumps–rubella†	Vaccination of susceptible women should be part of postpartum care. Breastfeeding is not a contraindication.
Mumps	Low morbidity and mortality; not altered by pregnancy	Possible increased rate of abortion in first trimester	Live attenuated virus vaccine	None confirmed	Contraindicated	Single dose SC, preferably as measles–mumps–rubella	Vaccination of susceptible women should be part of postpartum care
Poliomyelitis	No increased incidence in pregnancy, but may be more severe if it does occur	Anoxic fetal damage reported; 50% mortality in neonatal disease	Live attenuated virus (oral polio vaccine) and enhanced-potency inactivated virus vaccine‡	None confirmed	Not routinely recommended for women in the United States, except women at increased risk of exposure	*Primary:* Two doses of enhanced-potency inactivated virus SC at 4–8 week intervals and a third dose 6–12 months after the second dose *Immediate protection:* One dose oral polio vaccine (in outbreak setting)	Vaccine indicated for susceptible pregnant women traveling in endemic areas or in other high-risk situations
Rubella	Low morbidity and mortality; not altered by pregnancy	High rate of abortion and congenital rubella syndrome	Live attenuated virus vaccine	None confirmed	Contraindicated, but congenital rubella syndrome has never been described after vaccine	Single dose SC, preferably as measles–mumps–rubella	Teratogenicity of vaccine is theoretic, not confirmed to date; vaccination of susceptible women should be part of postpartum care
Smallpox	High case fatality in unvaccinated populations not altered by pregnancy	Determined by maternal disease	Live vaccinia virus	—	Contraindicated	Multiple bifurcated needlesticks at single setting	Only an issue considered because of possibility of bioterrorism

TABLE 20. Immunization During Pregnancy (continued)

Immunobiologic Agent	Risk from Disease to Pregnant Woman	Risk from Disease to Fetus or Neonate	Type of Immunizing Agent	Risk from Immunizing Agent to Fetus	Indications for Immunization During Pregnancy	Dose Schedule	Comments
Live Virus Vaccines (continued)							
Varicella	Possible increase in severe pneumonia	Can cause congenital varicella in 2% of fetuses infected during the second trimester	Live attenuated virus vaccine	None confirmed	Contraindicated, but no adverse outcomes reported if given in pregnancy	Two doses needed with second dose given 4–8 weeks after first dose. Should be strongly encouraged	Teratogenicity of vaccine is theoretic, outcomes reported weeks 4–8 not confirmed to date. Vaccination of susceptible women should be considered postpartum
Yellow fever	Significant morbidity and mortality; not altered by pregnancy	Unknown	Live attenuated virus vaccine	Unknown	Contraindicated except if exposure is unavoidable	Single dose SC	Postponement of travel preferable to vaccination, if possible
Other							
Influenza	Increase in morbidity and mortality during epidemic of new antigenic strain	Possible increased abortion rate; no malformations confirmed	Inactivated virus vaccine	None confirmed	All women who are pregnant in the second and third trimester during the flu season (October–March); women at high risk for pulmonary complications regardless of trimester	One dose IM every year	—
Rabies	Near 100% fatality; not altered by pregnancy	Determined by maternal disease	Killed virus vaccine	Unknown	Indications for prophylaxis not altered by pregnancy; each case considered individually	Public health authorities to be consulted for indications, dosage, and route of administration	—

Vaccine	Effect of pregnancy on disease	Effect of disease on pregnancy	Type	Risk to fetus	Indications	Schedule	Comments
Hepatitis B	Possible increased severity during third trimester	Possible increase in abortion rate and preterm birth; neonatal hepatitis can occur; high risk of newborn carrier state	Purified surface antigen produced by recombinant technology	None reported	Preexposure and postexposure for women at risk of infection	Three-dose series IM at 0, 1, and 6 months	Used with hepatitis B immune globulin for some exposures; exposed newborn needs birth dose vaccination and immune globulin as soon as possible. All infants should receive birth dose of vaccine.
Hepatitis A	No increased risk during pregnancy	—	Inactivated virus	None reported	Preexposure and postexposure for women at risk of infection; international travelers	Two-dose schedule 6 months apart	—
Inactivated Bacterial Vaccines							
Pneumococcus	No increased risk during pregnancy; no increase in severity of disease	Unknown, but depends on maternal illness	Polyvalent polysaccharide vaccine	None reported	Recommended for women with asplenia; metabolic, renal, cardiac, pulmonary diseases; smokers; immunosuppressed. Indications not altered by pregnancy.	In adults, one SC or IM dose only; consider repeat dose in 6 years for high-risk women	—
Meningococcus	Significant morbidity and mortality; not altered by pregnancy	Unknown, but depends on maternal illness	Quadrivalent polysaccharide vaccine	None reported	Indications not altered by pregnancy; vaccination recommended in unusual outbreak situations	One SC dose; public health authorities consulted	—
Typhoid	Significant morbidity and mortality; not altered by pregnancy	Unknown	Killed or live attenuated oral bacterial vaccine	None confirmed	Not recommended routinely except for close, continued exposure or travel to endemic areas	Killed Primary: Two injections SC at least 4 weeks apart. Booster: Single dose SC or ID (depending on type of product) Booster: Schedule not yet determined	Oral vaccine preferred

(continued)

TABLE 20. Immunization During Pregnancy (continued)

Immunobiologic Agent	Risk From Disease to Pregnant Woman	Risk From Disease to Fetus or Neonate	Type of Immunizing Agent	Risk From Immunizing Agent to Fetus	Indications for Immunization During Pregnancy	Dose Schedule	Comments
Inactivated Bacterial Vaccines (continued)							
Anthrax	Significant morbidity and mortality; not altered by pregnancy	Unknown, but depends on maternal illness	Preparation from cell-free filtrate of B anthracis; no dead or live bacteria	None confirmed	Not routinely recommended unless pregnant women work directly with B anthracis, imported animal hides, potentially infected animals in high incidence areas (not United States) or military personnel deployed to high-risk exposure areas	Six-dose primary vaccination SC, then annual booster vaccination	Teratogenicity of vaccine theoretical
Toxoids							
Tetanus–diphtheria	Severe morbidity; tetanus mortality 30%; diphtheria mortality 10%; unaltered by pregnancy	Neonatal tetanus mortality 60%	Combined tetanus–diphtheria toxoids preferred: adult tetanus–diphtheria formulation	None confirmed	Lack of primary series, or no booster within past 10 years	Primary: Two doses IM at 1–2-month interval with a third dose 6–12 months after the second. Booster: Single dose IM every 10 years after completion of primary series	Updating of immune status should be part of antepartum care
Specific Immune Globulins							
Hepatitis B	Possible increased severity during third trimester	Possible increase in abortion rate and preterm birth; neonatal hepatitis can occur; high risk of carrier state in newborn	Hepatitis B immune globulin	None reported	Postexposure prophylaxis	Depends on exposure; consult Immunization Practices Advisory Committee recommendations (IM)	Usually given with hepatitis B virus vaccine; exposed newborn needs immediate postexposure prophylaxis

	Effect on Mother	Effect on Fetus or Neonate	Product	Adverse Effects	Indication	Dose	Comments
Rabies	Near 100% fatality; not altered by pregnancy	Determined by maternal disease	Rabies immune globulin	None reported	Postexposure prophylaxis	Half dose at injury site, half dose in deltoid	Used in conjunction with rabies killed virus vaccine
Tetanus	Severe morbidity; mortality 60%	Neonatal tetanus mortality 60%	Tetanus immune globulin	None reported	Postexposure prophylaxis	One dose IM	Used in conjunction with tetanus toxoid
Varicella	Possible increase in severe varicella pneumonia	Can cause congenital varicella with increased mortality in neonatal period; very rarely causes congenital defects	Varicella–zoster immune globulin (obtained from the American Red Cross)	None reported	Should be considered for healthy pregnant women exposed to varicella to protect against maternal, not congenital, infection	One dose IM within 96 hours of exposure	Indicated also for newborns of women who developed varicella within 4 days before delivery or 2 days following delivery; approximately 90–95% of adults are immune to varicella; not indicated for prevention of congenital varicella
Standard Immune Globulins							
Hepatitis A	Possible increased severity during third trimester	Probable increase in abortion rate and preterm birth; possible transmission to neonate at delivery if woman is incubating the virus or is acutely ill at that time	Standard immune globulin	None reported	Postexposure prophylaxis, but hepatitis A virus vaccine should be used with hepatitis A immune globulin	0.02 mL/kg IM in one dose of immune globulin	Immune globulin should be given as soon as possible and within 2 weeks of exposure; infants born to women who are incubating the virus or are acutely ill at delivery should receive one dose of 0.5 mL as soon as possible after birth

ID indicates intradermally; IM, intramuscularly; PO, orally; and SC, subcutaneously.

†Two doses necessary for adequate vaccination of students entering institutions of higher education, newly hired medical personnel, and international travelers.

‡Inactivated polio vaccine recommended for nonimmunized adults at increased risk.

Data from General recommendations on immunization. Recommendations of the Advisory Committee on Immunization Practices (ACIP) and the American Academy of Family Physicians (AAFP). Centers for Disease Control and Prevention. MMWR Recomm Rep; 51(RR-2):1–35. Available at http://www.cdc.gov/mmwr/preview/mmwrhtml/rr5102a1.htm. Retrieved October 11, 2002.

Adapted from Immunization during pregnancy. ACOG Committee Opinion No. 282. American College of Obstetricians and Gynecologists. Obstet Gynecol 2003;101:207–12.

References

1. Prevention of hepatitis A through active or passive immunization: Recommendations of the Advisory Committee on Immunization Practices (ACIP). MMWR Recomm Rep 1999;48(RR-12):1–37.

2. Staes CJ, Schlenker TL, Risk I, Cannon KG, Harris H, Pavia AT, et al. Sources of infection among persons with acute hepatitis A and no identified risk factors during a sustained community-wide outbreak. Pediatrics 2000;106:E54.

3. Sexually transmitted diseases treatment guidelines 2002. Centers for Disease Control and Prevention. MMWR Recomm Rep 2002;51(RR-6):1–78.

4. Hepatitis B virus: a comprehensive strategy for eliminating transmission in the United States through universal childhood vaccination. Recommendations of the Immunization Practices Advisory Committee (ACIP). MMWR Recomm Rep 1991;40(RR-13):1–25.

5. Duff P. Hepatitis in pregnancy. Semin Perinatol 1998;22:277–83.

6. Kumar RM, Uduman S, Rana S, Kochiyil JK, Usmani A, Thomas L. Sero-prevalence and mother-to-infant transmission of hepatitis E virus among pregnant women in the United Arab Emirates. Eur J Obstet Gynecol Reprod Biol 2001;100:9–15.

7. Control and prevention of rubella: evaluation and management of suspected outbreaks, rubella in pregnant women and surveillance for congenital rubella syndrome. MMWR Recomm Rep 2001;50(RR-12):1–23.

8. American College of Obstetricians and Gynecologists. Perinatal viral and parasitic infections. ACOG Practice Bulletin 20. Washington, DC: ACOG; 2000.

9. Preventing congenital toxoplasmosis. MMWR Recomm Rep 2000;49(RR-02):57–75.

10. Wald A, Zeh J, Selke S, Ashley RL, Corey L. Virologic characteristics of subclinical and symptomatic genital herpes infections. N Engl J Med 1995;333:770–5.

11. Brown ZA, Wald A, Morrow RA, Selke S, Zeh J, Corey L. Effect of serologic status and cesarean delivery on transmission rates of herpes simplex virus from mother to infant. JAMA 2003;289:203–9.

12. Sheffield JS, Hollier LM, Hill JB, Stuart GS, Wendel GD. Acyclovir prophylaxis to prevent herpes simplex virus recurrence at delivery: a systematic review. Obstet Gynecol 2003;102:1396–403.

13. Nathwani D, Maclean A, Conway S, Carrington D. Varicella infections in pregnancy and the newborn. A review prepared for the UK Advisory Group on Chickenpox on behalf of the British Society for the Study of Infection. J Infect 1998;36 (suppl 1):59–71.

14. Smaill F. Antibiotics for asymptomatic bacteriuria in pregnancy. The Cochrane Database of Systematic Reviews 2001, Issue 2. Art. No.: CD000490. DOI: 10.1002/14651858.CD000490.

15. Jamie WE, Edwards RK, Duff P. Antimicrobial susceptibility of Gram-negative uropathogens isolated from obstetric patients. Infect Dis Obstet Gynecol 2002;10:123–6.

16. Vasquez J, Villar J. Treatments for symptomatic urinary tract infections during pregnancy. The Cochrane Database of Systematic Reviews 2003;4:CD002256.

17. Wing DA, Hendershott CM, Debuque L, Millar LK. Outpatient treatment of acute pyelonephritis in pregnancy after 24 weeks. Obstet Gynecol 1999;94:683–8.

18. Schrag SJ, Zell ER, Lynfield R, Roome A, Arnold KE, Craig AS, et al. A population-based comparison of strategies to prevent early-onset group B streptococcal disease in neonates. N Engl J Med 2002;347:233–9.

19. Prevention of early-onset group B streptococcal disease in newborns. ACOG Committee Opinion No. 279. American College of Obstetricians and Gynecologists. Obstet Gynecol 2002;100:1405–12.

20. Pearlman M. Prevention of early-onset group B streptococcal disease in newborns [letter]. Obstet Gynecol 2003;102:414–5; author reply 415.

21. Minkoff H. Human immunodeficiency virus infection in pregnancy. Obstet Gynecol 2003;101:797–810.

22. Update: influenza activity—United States, 2003-2004 season, and composition of the 2004-05 influenza vaccine. Centers for Disease Control and Prevention. MMWR Morb Mortal Wkly Rep 2004;53:547l–52.

23. Hauth JC, Goldenberg RL, Andrews WW, DuBard MB, Copper RL. Reduced incidence of preterm delivery with metronidazole and erythromycin in women with bacterial vaginosis. N Engl J Med 1995;333:1732–6.

24. Morales WJ, Schorr S, Albritton J. Effect of metronidazole in patients with preterm birth in preceding pregnancy and bacterial vaginosis: a placebo-controlled, double-blind study. Am J Obstet Gynecol 1994;171:345–7; discussion 348–9.

25. McDonald HM, O'Loughlin JA, Vigneswaran R, Jolley PT, Harvey JA, Bof A, et al. Impact of metronidazole therapy on preterm birth in women with bacterial vaginosis flora (Gardnerella vaginalis): a randomized, placebo controlled trial. Br J Obstet Gynaecol 1997;104:1391–7.

26. Carey JC, Klebanoff MA, Hauth JC, Hillier SL, Thom EA, Ernest JM, et al. Metronidazole to prevent preterm delivery in pregnant women with asymptomatic bacterial vaginosis. National Institute of Child Health and Human Development Network of Maternal–Fetal Medicine Units. N Engl J Med 2000;342:534–40.

27. Immunization during pregnancy. ACOG Committee Opinion No. 282. American College of Obstetricians and Gynecologists. Obstet Gynecol 2003;101:207–12.

Pain Management in Pregnancy

ACUTE AND CHRONIC PAIN

There are 2 fundamental types of pain: nociceptive pain ("ordinary pain"), which is felt in response to a noxious stimulus, and neuropathic pain, which occurs when a pain signal originates within abnormally functioning peripheral or central neurons. Pain that lasts a month or more beyond the usual course of an acute injury or disease is defined as chronic pain. Chronic pain syndromes are just beginning to be understood and encompass multiple mechanisms operating at different sites in the nervous system and with different temporal profiles in different patients. The initial pain is initiated by the primary injury or disease, but the pain mechanism itself, not the disease or injury, leads to chronic pain (1). Chronic pelvic pain, fibromyalgia, chronic daily headaches, chronic low back pain, chronic sickle cell pain, and cancer pain are examples of chronic pain syndromes.

In most patients with chronic pain, the disease or pathology cannot be treated effectively or cured. The current approach by pain medicine specialists is to consider pain the disease and to attempt to identify and treat the mechanisms responsible for the chronic pain. This pain mechanism-based approach is very different from management based primarily on the underlying disease.

Treating pregnant women who have acute or chronic pain is complicated by the actual or potential risks to the fetus from treatment medications. Some of the following approaches can be used during pregnancy, however, to relieve pain.

Treatment of Acute Pain in Pregnancy

Most pregnant women will have pain during their pregnancy. Many will self-medicate with over-the-counter (OTC) medications such as aspirin, acetaminophen, or ibuprofen. Aspirin and NSAIDs recently have been shown to increase the risk of spontaneous abortion if taken at the time of conception or for more than 7 consecutive days during the first trimester (2). Aspirin at full dose also is associated with an increased risk of gastroschisis (3), maternal bleeding complications, and fetal bleeding complications. Because there are other, safer analgesics available, full-dose aspirin should not be used during pregnancy. Low-dose aspirin has not been associated with any fetal or maternal complications.

The appropriate treatment of acute pain is based on the cause and severity of the pain. Diagnosing and treating the underlying cause are the first considerations. Treatment for pain should start with nonpharmacologic therapies when applicable (eg, ice packs or heat). Drug therapy should be added when necessary:

- Acetaminophen is the safest pain medication for mild-to-moderate pain during pregnancy and often is effective.

- For more intense pain, especially if it has an inflammatory component, a short course (<7 days) of ibuprofen may be appropriate during the first or second trimester. After 32 weeks of gestation, ibuprofen should be used with caution and limited to 3–4 days at a time. Longer courses require monitoring of amniotic fluid for evidence of oligohydramnios.

- Acetaminophen with codeine is known to be safe throughout pregnancy and should be used for moderate to severe acute pain.

- All of the opioids are relatively safe in pregnancy. None of them is related to congenital abnormalities, and they are problematic for the fetus only if used at high doses for prolonged periods. However, if the pain treatment lasts longer than 2 weeks, referral to a pain medicine specialist should be considered.

- Cyclooxygenase (COX-2) inhibitors are used frequently for acute and chronic pain. Fetal risks are unknown but may be similar to conventional NSAIDs. Until more data are available, COX-2 inhibitors probably should be avoided during pregnancy.

Pain With Sickle Cell Disease

Women with sickle cell disease will have more frequent episodes of severe pain (known as sickle cell crisis or vasoocclusive crisis) when they become pregnant. Other precipitating factors are dehydration, exposure to cold, stress, high altitude (including flying), and infection, although there is no clear cause of pain in more than half of the cases.

Painful crises can occur in more than 50% of persons who have hemoglobin SS disease. If, for any reason, arterial oxygenation decreases, their red blood cells can become stiff and less pliable. They become deformed (sickled) and undergo membrane changes that allow an influx of calcium, leakage of potassium, and dehydration. Blood becomes even more viscous due to the body's inability to concentrate urine. The survival time of these sickled cells is shortened, and they can clump together, causing capillary venous occlusion throughout the body.

RESOURCES

Pain Management in Pregnancy

American Chronic Pain Association
www.theacpa.org

American College of Obstetricians and Gynecologists
www.acog.org

American Council for Headache Education
www.achenet.org

American Pain Foundation
www.painfoundation.org

American Society of Anesthesiologists
www.asahq.org

American Society of Regional Anesthesia and Pain Medicine
www.asra.com

National Institute of Neurological Disorders and Stroke
www.ninds.nih.gov

NIH Pain Consortium
painconsortium.nih.gov

Society for Obstetric Anesthesia and Perinatology
www.soap.org

The consequences of these vasoocclusive episodes frequently are associated with intense pain, often secondary to conditions, such as aseptic bone necrosis, painful muscle contractions, acute chest syndrome, vertebral collapse, and chronic arthritis.

Prophylactic red cell transfusion clearly decreases the frequency of pain crises, but it has not been shown to improve the outcome of the pregnancy. Because there are inherent risks of transfusion reactions, alloimmunization, and acquisition of infections, its use is controversial at present. However, prophylactic transfusion should be considered for women with a history of frequent pain crises before or during pregnancy specifically to decrease pain morbidity. Other criteria are detailed in a comprehensive guideline for management of pain crises (4).

Most therapeutic regimens include increased fluid intake, potent analgesics, and antibiotics (when necessary for infection). Less frequently, bone marrow transplantation, red cell pheresis, and hydroxyurea are administered. Magnesium compounds (such as sulfate or pidolate) have been used with success, but the exact mechanism of action is not clear. Magnesium has been shown to induce cellular hydration, inhibit calcium-mediated smooth muscle contractions, and cause vasodilation. It has also been shown to slow clotting time, which could decrease red blood cell clumping, and improve the passage of blood through smaller blood vessels. There have been reports of decreased pain during crises and shortened lengths of hospital stay among pediatric patients who have been treated with magnesium compared with placebo.

When a pregnant patient with sickle cell comes to the emergency room or labor and delivery with severe pain, it is important not to overlook the possibility of other causes, such as ectopic pregnancy, spontaneous abortion, placental abruption, appendicitis, and cholecystitis. While these conditions are being evaluated, intravenous hydration should be administered. If the patient has a viable fetus, continuous electronic monitoring should be undertaken. Once other causes are ruled out, aggressive pain management should be instituted:

- Start with IV morphine in full therapeutic doses at 2–4 hour intervals, with smaller doses for breakthrough pain. (Meperidine should be discouraged, even though many patients with sickle cell pain are accustomed to meperidine.)
- Continue treatment with patient-controlled analgesia; it prevents fluctuations in serum drug levels and reduces the time from perception of pain to administration of the analgesic.

Oxygen therapy has not been shown to be effective in decreasing the duration or intensity of the pain crisis, but should be used when there is hypoxemia or fetal distress.

When pain becomes mild to moderate, oral acetaminophen with codeine (if tolerated) or acetaminophen with oxycodone can be given. Upon discharge, the patient should be given enough oral medication to last until the next clinic visit, ideally within 5–7 days. Some patients with sickle cell disease develop chronic pain. These patients benefit from seeing a pain specialist and using combination medication for chronic pain.

Chronic Pain

Chronic pain is usually a combination of nociceptive pain and neuropathic pain. The management of chronic pain is complex and evolving rapidly as new discoveries are made. Pain medicine is a relatively new and rapidly growing specialty. The current emphasis in pain medicine is to approach chronic pain as a disease state, using pain mechanisms themselves to define the pain state and determine the best treatment regimens. Ideally, a pregnant patient with chronic pain would be managed by close cooperation between her pain physician and her obstetrician.

Prepregnancy Planning

The patient's medicines should be reviewed with the risks to the developing fetus in mind. It often takes months to find the right combination of medications to control chronic pain. The decision to change these medications is a difficult one because the benefits to the patient in terms of pain control and psychologic benefits (including treating or preventing depression) may outweigh the small risks (usually uncertain) to the fetus by remaining on the medication (Table 21). There are well-defined strategies used in chronic pain management:

- One provider should be designated to manage the pain medication. All questions and medication needs should be handled by that provider, who alone should prescribe pain medications. At the same time, there should be a plan in place for treatment of acute exacerbations of pain.

- Analgesics should be given on a fixed-dose schedule around the clock (*not* on an as-needed basis); this provides more consistent pain relief.

- The lowest dose that is effective should be used.

- Often there is synergy between 2 medications that allows effective treatment at lower doses for both, thereby minimizing side effects and fetal risks.

- Medications, especially opioids, should be administered in the way most comfortable for the patient: orally, transdermally, or by rectal suppositories.

Adjunctive Therapies in the Treatment of Chronic Pain

Psychoeducational interventions (such as detailed patient education, cognitive–behavioral therapy, relaxation techniques, and psychotherapy) and physical interventions (including physical therapy, acupuncture, and therapeutic massage) are safe and often helpful in the treatment of chronic pain in pregnancy, although rigorous studies are lacking. Involving the patient in the management of her chronic pain has been shown to increase the effectiveness of the treatment program (5, 6).

TABLE 21. Medications Frequently Used in Chronic Pain Management

Medication	Use in Pregnancy
Nonsteroidal antiinflammatory drugs (NSAIDs)	Recent evidence points to an increased risk of spontaneous miscarriage if used at the time of conception or for more than 7 consecutive days.* They should not be used chronically after 28 weeks of gestation except in rare circumstances; close ultrasound surveillance for amniotic fluid changes is mandatory.
Aspirin	Aspirin should not be used. It has the same risks as other NSAIDs and has been associated with gastroschisis.[†] Use of low-dose aspirin may be considered.
Opioids	There are no known teratogenic risks. Physical dependence of the fetus requiring withdrawal is expected if opioids are used throughout the pregnancy.
	For long-term, chronic treatment of pain, opioids can be given transdermally or by long-acting oral formulations. Fentanyl by patch has gained wide acceptance by pain physicians.
Tricyclic antidepressants	These are often used in pain management. Amitriptyline is the most studied and probably the safest during pregnancy. The others (nortriptyline, imipramine, desipramine, doxepin) are less well studied and should be avoided if possible.
Selective serotonin reuptake inhibitors (SSRIs)	These are probably safe. Their role in chronic pain management is evolving. Fluoxetine is the most studied and has been used the most in chronic pain.
Anticonvulsants	Phenytoin is associated with major and minor congenital anomalies and should be avoided. Carbamazepine and valproic acid are contraindicated because of the risk of neural tube defects.
	Gabapentin is especially helpful in treating chronic neuropathic pain. A recent study found no increased risk for congenital anomalies,[‡] but the numbers were small.

*Li DK, Liu L, Odouli R. Exposure to non-steroidal anti-inflammatory drugs during pregnancy and risk of miscarriage: population based cohort study. BMJ 2003;327:368.

[†]Werler MM, Sheehan JE, Mitchell AA. Maternal medication use and risks of gastroschisis and small intestinal atresia. Am J Epidemiol 2002; 155:26–31; Martinez-Frias ML, Rodriguez-Pinilla E, Prieto L. Prenatal exposure to salicylates and gastroschisis: a case-control study. Teratology 1997;56:241–3.

[‡]Montouris G. Gabapentin exposure in human pregnancy: results from the Gabapentin Pregnancy Registry. Epilepsy Behav 2003;4:310–4.

References

1. Ballantyne J, Fishman S, Abdi S, editors. The Massachusetts General Hospital handbook of pain management. 2nd ed. Philadelphia (PA): Lippincott Williams & Wilkins, 2002.

2. Li DK, Liu L, Odouli R. Exposure to non-steroidal anti-inflammatory drugs during pregnancy and risk of miscarriage: population based cohort study. BMJ 2003;327:368.

3. Werler MM, Sheehan JE, Mitchell AA. Maternal medication use and risks of gastroschisis and small intestinal atresia. Am J Epidemiol 2002;155:26–31.

4. Rees DC, Olujohungbe AD, Parker NE, Stephens AD, Telfer P, Wright J. Guidelines for the management of the acute painful crisis in sickle cell disease. British Committee for Standards in Haematology General Haematology Task Force by the Sickle Cell Working Party. Br J Haematol 2003;120:744–52.

5. Arnstein P, Caudill M, Mandle CL, Norris A, Beasley R. Self efficacy as a mediator of the relationship between pain intensity, disability and depression in chronic pain patients. Pain 1999;80:483–91.

6. Caudill MA. Managing pain before it manages you. Rev. ed. New York (NY): Guilford Press; 2002.

HEADACHES

Headaches are the most common recurrent pain problem among adults and are one of the most common reasons Americans visit primary care physicians, neurologists, and emergency departments. Headaches are especially common in women: lifetime incidence is 99%, with tension-type headache occurring in 88% and migraine headache in at least 18% of women. The majority of women will have headaches during their pregnancies, even those who do not have an underlying primary headache disorder.

Classifying headaches is important because management of headaches during pregnancy is influenced by the underlying headache type. The International Headache Society formalized the classification of headache in 1988, spelling out specific diagnostic criteria for primary headaches, which are migraine headaches, with and without aura, and tension-type headaches (often called muscle-contraction headaches), distinguishing them from secondary headaches, where the headaches are caused by underlying conditions, such as intracranial lesions. Symptoms of secondary headaches may include the "first and worst" headache of the patient's life. Such headaches should be evaluated in the emergency room with neurologic consultation and CT or MRI scanning.

Migraine headaches are usually unilateral, have a pulsating or throbbing quality, are moderate-to-severe in intensity (which inhibits or prohibits daily activities), and are aggravated by walking stairs or similar routine physical activity. Migraines often are accompanied by nausea or vomiting, as well as photophobia and phonophobia. Other family members often have similar headaches.

Fortunately, many women with migraines will note improvement during pregnancy (1).

Tension-type headaches are the most common and least defined of the headache syndromes. The temporal pattern is vague or inconsistent, and most patients are unable to be precise about time of onset or duration. The pain is mild to moderate, bandlike, bilateral, dull, nagging, and persistent, and often goes into the neck. Pregnancy does not have the same beneficial effect on tension-type headaches as it does on migraines.

Analgesic rebound headache (also called "transformed migraine headache") is a recently identified phenomenon that explains much about the cause of the recurrent, daily headaches which beset many patients. These patients begin with occasional migraine attacks and end up years later with chronic daily headaches due to overuse of prescription and OTC medications (2).

Prepregnancy Issues

Many women with migraine headaches are being treated with medications that should not be used during pregnancy. These include ergotamine derivatives, triptans, chronic use of NSAIDs, and certain medications used for preventive treatment: valproate and methysergide. Women planning pregnancy should discontinue these medications before conception. Aspirin should be avoided during pregnancy (with the exception of low-dose aspirin [81 mg/day] prescribed for specific medical or obstetric indications). A recent report implicates use of aspirin or NSAIDs at the time of conception or for more than 7 consecutive days during the first trimester with an increased risk of miscarriage (3). Aspirin also appears to increase the risk of fetal gastroschisis (4).

If a woman has analgesic rebound headaches, she should be referred to a headache specialist for "detoxification." This entails stopping the daily use of analgesics, sedative/tranquilizer drugs, ergotamine derivatives, and other prescription or OTC medication, with in-patient support if necessary during the withdrawal process. Successfully treated, the woman's daily headaches will abate, and medications used to treat migraine episodes will be effective once again.

Good evidence supports the use of nonpharmacologic approaches to headache treatment and prevention: relaxation training, cognitive–behavioral therapy, thermal and electromyographic biofeedback, and acupuncture (5). These could be learned before pregnancy (6). In addition, a patient can decrease migraine attacks by avoiding known triggers, adopting regular sleeping and eating patterns, exercising regularly, and avoiding cigarette smoke.

Treating Headaches During Pregnancy

Initial pharmacotherapy for migraine and tension-type headaches overlap. The goal is to stop individual attacks or to reduce the severity and duration of symptoms. As soon as the patient is aware of the onset of headache, she should rest in a dark, quiet room, avoid sensory overstimulation, and apply an ice pack to the head. The medications recommended for treatment are listed in Table 22. The patient, with input from her physician, should choose her treatment based on the intensity of the pain, selecting the medications most likely to be effective for that episode.

Prophylactic Treatment for Migraine and Tension-Type Headaches

Prophylactic treatment should be considered under the following conditions:

- The patient has at least 2 or 3 attacks per month.
- The attacks are incapacitating, or of prolonged duration or associated with focal neurologic signs.
- The patient is unable to cope with her headache.
- There are contraindications or adverse reactions to medications used for treatment.
- Attempts at nonpharmacologic prevention have failed.

The goals of preventive treatment are to decrease the frequency and intensity of the headache attacks. Table 23

TABLE 22. Medications for Treatment of Headaches During Pregnancy

Medication	Pregnancy Risk Category	Comment
Mild Intensity		
Acetaminophen ± caffeine	B	Limit dose to 1 g stat, 4 g/d; for 2–3 days
If Nausea Is Present:		
Metoclopramide	B	10 mg at onset of nausea; may repeat every 6 hours × 4
If Unable to Tolerate Oral Administration:		
Promethazine	C	At onset of nausea; may repeat in 6 hours if necessary
Mild–Moderate Intensity		
Ibuprofen	B/D*	800 mg stat, 400 mg every 4 h, up to 2,400 mg/d, 2–3 d
Or		
Naproxen sodium	B/D*	3–275 mg tablets initially, 2 tablets twice daily up to 2–3 days
Mild–Moderate Intensity, Not Responsive to Above:		
Acetaminophen/ ± caffeine/ butalbital	C/D†	Limit dose to 1–2 stat, repeat in 4 hours, 6/attack, 24/mo
Mild–Moderate Intensity, Not Responsive to Above:		
Isometheptene/acetaminophen Dichloralphenazone	B	2 capsules at onset; then 1 every 30–60 min; max 6/attack, 2 d/week
Moderate–Severe Intensity		
Acetaminophen/codeine	C/D†	Limit dose to 1–2 stat, repeat every 3-4 h, 6/attack, 16/month
Acetaminophen/hydrocodone	C/D†	limit dose to 1-2 stat, repeat q3-4 h, 6/attack, 16/month
"Rescue Medication": If Severe Intensity and Unresponsive to Above:		
Acetaminophen/oxycodone	B/D†	Limit dose to 1–2 stat, repeat every 3–4h, 6/attack, 12/mo
Or		
Hydromorphone	B/D†	Limit dose to 1–2 stat, repeat every 3–4 h, 6/attack, 12/mo

*D if used more than 2–3 days in the third trimester or at term.

†D if used for prolonged periods or in high doses at term.

TABLE 23. Preventive Medications for Migraines and Tension-type Headaches During Pregnancy

Medication	Pregnancy Risk Category	Initial Dosage	Comment
Propranolol*	C	20 mg orally 4 times daily	If well tolerated, use long-acting formulation: 80 mg daily, increasing by 80 mg every 2 weeks; ceiling 240 mg/day
Amitriptyline*	B	10 mg orally at bedtime	Drug of choice for tension-type headache; can be used together with β-antagonist; titrate slowly up to 250 mg/d
Fluoxetine†	B	20 mg/day	Works especially well if there is a component of depression present‡
Verapamil†	C	240 mg/day	Decreases the frequency of attacks, not the intensity; may take 4–6 weeks to show efficacy

*Group 1 in The U.S. Headache Consortium Guidelines: medium to high efficacy, good strength of evidence, with acceptable side effect profile.

†Group 2 in The U.S. Headache Consortium Guidelines: lower efficacy than Group 1, or limited strength of evidence, and mild to moderate side effects. (Silberstein SD. Migraine and other headache disorders. Clin Update Womens Health Care 2002;I:1–59; Silberstein SD, Freitag FG. Preventive treatment of migraine. Neurology 2003;60 suppl 2:S38–S44.)

‡d'Amato CC, Pizza V, Marmolo T, Giordano E, Alfano V, Nasta A. Fluoxetine for migraine prophylaxis: a double-blind trial. Headache 1999;39:716–9.

lists medications that can be used for prophylaxis during pregnancy. Each medication should be given an adequate trial, usually several weeks, starting low and increasing gradually until the desired effect is reached. Use of other medications should be avoided except for treatment of acute attacks.

References

1. Sances G, Granella F, Nappi RE, Fignon A, Ghiotto N, Polatti F, Nappi G. Course of migraine during pregnancy and postpartum: a prospective study. Cephalalgia 2003;23: 197–205.

2. Silberstein SD. Migraine and other headache disorders. Clin Update Womens Health Care 2002;I:1–59.

3. Li DK, Liu L, Odouli R. Exposure to non-steroidal anti-inflammatory drugs during pregnancy and risk of miscarriage: population based cohort study. BMJ 2003;327:368.

4. Werler MM, Sheehan JE, Mitchell AA. Maternal medication use and risks of gastroschisis and small intestinal atresia. Am J Epidemiol 2002;155:26–31.

5. Melchart D, Linde K, Fischer P, Berman B, White A, Vickers A, Allais G. Acupuncture for idiopathic headache. The Cochrane Database of Systematic Reviews 2001, Issue 1. Art. No.: CD001218. DOI: 10.1002/14651858.CD001218.

6. Silberstein SD. Practice parameter: evidence-based guidelines for migraine headache (an evidence-based review): report of the Quality Standards Subcommittee of the American Academy of Neurology [published erratum appears in Neurology 2000;56:142]. Neurology 2000;55: 754–62.

OBSTETRIC ANESTHESIA AND ANALGESIA

Obstetric anesthesia and analgesia comprise the multiple techniques used to alleviate pain associated with labor and delivery. *Anesthesia* refers to techniques used for surgical procedures, whereas *analgesia* means techniques for pain relief during labor or following cesarean delivery. Often, anesthesia and analgesia can be provided with the same technique (eg, spinal or epidural) by using different medications. Relief of discomfort and pain during labor and delivery is an essential part of good obstetric care (1).

Nonobstetric, or surgical, anesthesia and obstetric anesthesia differ in several significant ways (2). First and foremost, with obstetric anesthesia there are 2 patients to consider, and what may prove beneficial to one may actually be detrimental to the other. Numerous physiologic changes and an increase in certain complications during pregnancy must be taken into account. For example, pulmonary aspiration and failed tracheal intubation are more common among pregnant patients receiving general anesthesia. Desaturation occurs more quickly in pregnant women because of decreased functional residual capacity. Aortocaval compression by the enlarged uterus increases the risk of hypotension after regional anesthesia in the parturient, and total doses of local anesthetic drugs must be decreased because nerves are more sensitive to their actions during pregnancy. Two common obstetric complications are hypertension and hemorrhage, which have a significant impact on anesthetic management.

Nonpharmacologic Methods of Labor Analgesia

Nonpharmacologic methods of pain relief, either exclusively or in combination with medications, may be useful tools in helping women to cope with the pain of labor. These methods have advantages that benefit the infant by decreasing opioid use and may benefit the mother by decreasing the need for regional analgesia or by delaying placement until the active phase of labor. Methods include hydrotherapy and position changes, massage, hypnosis, psychoprophylaxis, acupuncture or acupressure, transcutaneous electrical nerve stimulation, sterile water blocks, and social and professional support (eg, doulas). Emotional support provided by doulas has been shown to decrease the use of analgesics, length of labor, and incidence of operative deliveries in healthy patients with normal labors. Other techniques do not substantially reduce the use of analgesics, but they do decrease the anxiety associated with labor.

Systemic Agents

Although the use of regional anesthesia is increasing, obstetricians still commonly use parenteral narcotics and tranquilizers for pain relief during labor. These agents are especially useful for women who have contraindications to regional anesthesia (eg, patient refusal or coagulopathy) or when an anesthesia provider is not available. All narcotics have transient effects; they cause delayed gastric emptying and nausea in the mother, respiratory depression in the mother and fetus, loss of beat-to-beat variability, and fetal neurobehavioral depression. Four narcotics are in common use today: meperidine, nalbuphine, butorphanol, and fentanyl.

Meperidine has a long history of safety in obstetrics. It produces less nausea and less newborn respiratory depression than morphine. Meperidine also is used for intravenous patient-controlled analgesia during labor. Its primary side effects are tachycardia and nausea, and its active metabolite (normeperidine) may cause mild neurobehavioral effects in the newborn for up to 3 days.

Nalbuphine is an agonist–antagonist narcotic with a protective "ceiling" that limits the amount of respiratory depression. Unfortunately, this naloxonelike activity also produces an "analgesia ceiling." Nalbuphine causes sedation but little nausea and minimal newborn effects. Its side effects include dysphoric reactions (which are common to all agonist–antagonist analgesics), withdrawal in opioid-dependent patients, and alterations in FHR tracings, described as decreased variability and loss of accelerations.

Butorphanol is also an agonist–antagonist analgesic that can be used intravenously. Its advantages and disadvantages are similar to those of nalbuphine. It can cause dysphoric reactions, withdrawal symptoms in susceptible patients, and a sinusoidal FHR pattern.

Fentanyl is a pure agonist synthetic opioid commonly used in the operating room for surgical procedures. It has a rapid onset, no active metabolites, and minimal fetal effects, and produces minimal sedation and little nausea. It also can be delivered by a patient-controlled analgesia pump during labor (3). Its drawbacks are short duration (45 minutes) of effect, accumulation with high or repeated doses, and the potential to cause respiratory depression in the mother.

The total dose of administered narcotic and the time from administration to the time of delivery govern the transfer of drug to the fetus. Thus, the smallest dose possible should be administered near delivery. The number of doses should be kept to a minimum to avoid accumulation of drug and metabolites in the fetus, especially in the case of a premature birth. Although a drug administered to the mother may be eliminated promptly and completely from her system, levels in the newborn may be elevated for a considerable length of time. Naloxone, a narcotic antagonist, is considered the drug of choice to reverse respiratory depression in the newborn associated with narcotics. It can be given intravenously, intramuscularly, subcutaneously, or via endotracheal tube.

Antiemetic agents often are used in combination with narcotics, although the commonly used opioids have a low incidence of nausea. To prevent polypharmacy, these adjuncts should not be used routinely, but only in those patients who require treatment. Promethazine is a very sedating antihistamine with weak antiemetic properties. The drug should be given intravenously, because intramuscular injection is very painful. Intravenous metoclopramide increases gastric emptying and decreases nausea. It does not cause sedation and actually may potentiate opioid analgesia. Droperidol is no longer used because of its classification. Ondansetron is a selective blocking agent of the serotonin 5-HT$_3$ receptor. It is highly effective and nonsedating, but the most expensive of these antiemetics.

The benzodiazepines, such as midazolam, are not recommended for use in laboring women because they may cause amnesia in the mother and prolonged neonatal depression with hypotonia, feeding problems, and defective temperature regulation. Barbiturates may potentiate the sedative effects of narcotics while having an antianalgesic effect. They are used primarily in the latent phase of labor to allow the mother to rest.

Regional Analgesia and Anesthesia

Regional analgesia consists of various nerve blocks that provide pain relief without loss of consciousness. Examples include local infiltration, pudendal block, paracervical block, subarachnoid or spinal block, lumbar epidural block, and combined spinal–epidural block. The latter 3 are also the most commonly used techniques for cesarean delivery.

LOCAL, PUDENDAL, AND PARACERVICAL BLOCKS

A local block is administered via infiltration of a local anesthetic, usually lidocaine, before performing an episiotomy or repairing genital lacerations. Few, if any, significant complications are associated with this technique.

Pudendal block entails infiltration of the pudendal nerve as it runs posterior to the sacrospinous ligament near the ischial spine. Lidocaine (1%) is injected on each side with careful aspiration to avoid inadvertent intravascular injection. The pudendal nerve provides sensory innervation to the perineum, anus, and vulva. This technique usually provides adequate analgesia for spontaneous delivery, assisted breech deliveries, and outlet forceps procedures. However, pudendal block may be inadequate for midpelvic delivery with forceps or vacuum extraction.

Unlike local and pudendal blocks, paracervical block provides pain relief for uterine contractions. A local anesthetic, usually lidocaine or chloroprocaine, is infiltrated at the 3-o'clock and 9-o'clock positions next to the cervix. A major complication of this technique is fetal bradycardia, which is probably secondary to uterine artery vasoconstriction induced by the local anesthetic. Thus, this is not an ideal procedure in cases of potential fetal compromise, such as a nonreassuring FHR pattern. Inadvertent intravascular injection of the local anesthetic during pudendal or paracervical block may result in maternal central nervous system stimulation and convulsions.

REGIONAL ANALGESIA

Regional analgesia can be used during the first stage of labor to block the spinal segments that transmit pain arising from the cervix and uterus (T10 to L1) and during the second stage of labor to block these segments plus those that transmit pain arising from the lower vagina, perineum, and perianal area (S2 to S4). Regional analgesia can be very adaptable in that pain relief can be provided with minimal motor block by using low concentrations of local anesthetics with narcotics, sometimes allowing ambulation during labor—the "walking epidural." For forceps delivery, extensive perineal repairs, or cesarean delivery later on, complete sensory and motor block (surgical *anesthesia*) can be provided by using higher concentrations of local anesthetics. Because the anesthetic usually is administered by continuous infusion with a catheter, the anesthetic can be administered for as long as necessary. Patient-controlled epidural analgesia allows the patient to self-administer doses from their infusion pump, providing themselves with the amount of local anesthetic solution they require for analgesia. Advantages include reduced local anesthetic use and side effects, increased patient satisfaction, and reduced clinician workload (4). After cesarean delivery, postoperative pain relief also can be provided with preservative-free narcotics such as morphine in the spinal or epidural space.

Of the various local anesthetics that can be used, 2-chloroprocaine has the fastest onset, shortest duration, and best safety profile because, as an ester, it is metabolized rapidly in plasma. It is used primarily in urgent situations. Lidocaine has an intermediate onset that can be shortened by alkalinization with bicarbonate. Often it is used for cesarean delivery. Bupivacaine has a long onset of action, which may provide better hemodynamic stability. It is highly protein bound, which minimizes placental transfer, and has the least amount of motor block for a given amount of sensory block, making it useful for labor analgesia. Ropivacaine and levo-bupivacaine are new local anesthetics with properties similar to those of bupivacaine.

A variety of opioids, such as fentanyl and sufentanil, also may be used in the subarachnoid or epidural space. Spinal opioids provide excellent analgesia without motor block (allowing ambulation) but are of limited duration (5). For this reason, an epidural catheter often is placed at the same time as the spinal dose; this is the combined spinal–epidural technique (6). Because *epidural* opioids used alone produce high blood levels and inadequate pain relief, they are used most often in combination with a dilute local anesthetic, such as 0.1% bupivacaine. The resulting synergism permits use of a much lower concentration of local anesthetic. Potential side effects of opioids include pruritus, nausea and vomiting, and respiratory depression.

Regional analgesia is contraindicated if there are no personnel present capable of dealing with complications such as total spinal block and toxic reactions to local anesthetics (Box 22). Because local anesthetics act as depressants of the central nervous system and the cardiovascular system, they can cause convulsions and cardiovascular collapse if large doses enter the cerebrospinal fluid or are injected intravascularly. The management of convulsions consists of airway protection and ventilation, placing the patient on her side to avoid aortocaval compression, and administering a small dose of thiopental or benzodiazepine if there is no hemodynamic compromise. If there are dysrhythmias, advanced cardiac life support protocols should be followed and hyperventilation used to prevent acidosis. Advanced cardiac life support protocol includes delivery within 5 minutes if an effective cardiac rhythm is not restored. Total spinal block also requires airway management and ventilation.

Another potential complication of regional anesthesia during labor is hypotension, which occurs in approximately 20% of patients. Hypotension is treated with fluids, phenylephrine or ephedrine, left uterine displacement, and elevation of the legs to prevent venous pooling (7). An anesthetic should never be given without a secure intravenous line and a blood pressure cuff in place. Some anesthesiologists may request that the obstetrician be in attendance during placement of the anesthetic because of concerns that these potential complications could cause fetal compromise.

BOX 22

Contraindications to Use of Regional Anesthesia During Labor and Delivery

Absolute Contraindications

- Patient refusal
- Hemodynamic instability from hemorrhage, sepsis, etc.
- Clinically significant coagulopathy (A specific platelet count that is predictive of regional anesthetic complications has not been determined, and isolated mild thrombocytopenia is probably not a contraindication.)
- Infection at the site where the puncture is to be made
- Absence of a physician trained in regional block or the treatment of complications
- Unavailability of monitoring equipment or necessary drugs
- Lack of adequate venous access

Relative Contraindications

- Preexisting neurologic disease
- Prior back surgery with instrumentation

The risk of postdural puncture headache is about 1% after spinal or epidural anesthesia (8). Postdural puncture headache improves when the patient is supine and worsens when the patient is upright. Treatment may be conservative (eg, analgesics for comfort and caffeine to provide cerebral vasoconstriction) or aggressive (eg, epidural blood patch). An epidural blood patch is applied by placing 15–25 mL of the patient's blood in the epidural space just below the level of the previous puncture. The choice of treatment should be based on the patient's preferences and how severely the headache restricts her activities. These headaches rarely last longer than 7 days.

The major complications of regional anesthesia include the following:

- Hypotension
- High blockade causing respiratory compromise
- Local anesthetic toxicity (epidural only)
- Postdural puncture headache (<1%)
- Infection or neurologic damage (extremely rare)

General Anesthesia

General anesthesia is used for cesarean delivery most often when rapid anesthesia is required, as with abruption, severe hemorrhage, or cord prolapse. Other common indications include patient refusal of regional anesthesia, failed or inadequate regional blocks, or medical conditions in which a fall in systemic vascular resistance would be detrimental or life threatening (eg, severe aortic stenosis or pulmonary hypertension).

General anesthesia for operative delivery is provided by using a combination of anesthetic agents to minimize the side effects and complications of each and to prevent high concentrations from reaching the fetus. A commonly used protocol might include thiopental to induce sleep and succinylcholine (a muscle relaxant) to facilitate intubation, followed by a combination of oxygen, nitrous oxide, and a volatile agent. After delivery of the fetus, narcotics are added for analgesia, and a longer-acting muscle relaxant is administered if needed.

INTRAVENOUS AGENTS

Intravenous agents are used to provide hypnosis during induction of anesthesia and before intubation. Thiopental is the most commonly used agent for this purpose; its onset is rapid and its duration of action is short because of rapid redistribution in the mother and fetus. Ketamine has sympathomimetic properties that support blood pressure and increase heart rate, making it ideal for patients with acute hemorrhage. This agent also provides intense analgesia and amnesia without respiratory depression when operative vaginal delivery or manual removal of a retained placenta is required. However, ketamine may cause troublesome hallucinations or dysphoric reactions. Also, it should be avoided in women with significant hypertension because of its sympathomimetic properties.

INHALATION AGENTS

Inhalation analgesia can be provided with nitrous oxide, but the gas must be scavenged from the environment to prevent exposure of other personnel, which is not possible outside the operating room. Other volatile anesthetic agents include isoflurane, desflurane, and sevoflurane. All of these agents provide hypnosis, amnesia, some analgesia, and some muscle relaxation. However, in high concentrations they also depress maternal cardiac output, relax uterine muscle, and increase postpartum bleeding, so they usually are combined with other agents to provide a complete anesthetic.

Complications

Complications from anesthesia are the seventh leading cause of maternal death, and failed intubation and aspiration are the leading causes of anesthesia-related death (9). Fortunately, the rate of maternal death resulting from complications of anesthesia seems to be declining, most recently to 1.8% of maternal deaths during delivery. Difficult intubation often can be predicted by the presence of medical or obstetric complications, marked obesity, short neck, receding mandible, facial edema, or anatomic anomalies of the neck and face. When providing care to a patient with these features, the clinician should consult an anesthesiologist to reduce the risk of life-threatening airway complications.

Aspiration occurs when the patient cannot protect her airway because of sedation, anesthesia, or a high regional block. Steps to prevent this serious complication consist of avoiding oral intake of solids during labor; using clear non-particulate antacids, H_2-receptor antagonists, or metoclopramide to minimize and neutralize gastric contents; and exerting cricoid pressure during induction of general anesthesia before intubation. If aspiration occurs, treatment is supportive, including ventilation and positive end expiratory pressure. Steroids and antibiotics are not indicated.

References

1. Obstetric analgesia and anesthesia. ACOG Practice Bulletin No. 36. American College of Obstetricians and Gynecologists. Obstet Gynecol 2002;100:177–91.

2. Practice guidelines for obstetrical anesthesia: a report by the American Society of Anesthesiologists Task Force on Obstetrical Anesthesia. Anesthesiology 1999;90:600–611.

3. Campbell DC. Parenteral opioids for labor analgesia. Clin Obstet Gynecol 2003;46:616–22.

4. van der Vyver M, Halpern S, Joseph G. Patient-controlled epidural analgesia versus continuous infusion for labour analgesia: a meta-analysis. Br J Anaesth 2002;89:459–65.

5. Yeh HM, Chen LK, Shyu MK, Lin CJ, Sun WZ, Wang MJ, et al. The addition of morphine prolongs fentanyl-bupivacaine spinal analgesia for the relief of labor pain. Anesth Analg 2001;92:665–8.

6. Norris MC, Fogel ST, Conway-Long C. Combined spinal-epidural versus epidural labor analgesia. Anesthesiology 2001;95:913–20.

7. Lee A, Ngan Kee WD, Gin T. A quantitative, systematic review of randomized controlled trials of ephedrine versus phenylephrine for the management of hypotension during spinal anesthesia for cesarean delivery. Anesth Analg 2002; 94:920–6.

8. Turnbull DK, Shepherd DB. Post-dural puncture headache: pathogenesis, prevention and treatment. Br J Anaesth 2003; 91:718–29.

9. Hawkins JL. Anesthesia-related maternal mortality. Clin Obstet Gynecol 2003;46:679–87.

Intrapartum Management

Management of labor may include several components, including a disciplined approach to the diagnosis of labor, monitoring of labor progress, treatment of dystocia or abnormal labor, and assessment of maternal and fetal well-being.

LABOR STIMULATION

The stimulation of uterine contractions may be characterized as labor induction or labor augmentation. Induction of labor is one of the most commonly performed obstetric procedures in the United States, with a rate approaching 20% (1). Induction of labor implies stimulation of uterine contractions previously absent with or without ruptured fetal membranes. Labor induction may be elective or indicated. Elective induction of labor is associated with an increased occurrence of cesarean delivery and operative vaginal delivery. Augmentation refers to stimulation of uterine contractions when spontaneous contractions have failed to result in progressive cervical dilation, descent of the fetus, or both. (See Box 23 for common indicators for labor stimulation.)

Techniques for induction of labor may be surgical or medical. Surgical techniques include amniotomy or stripping of membranes. Stripping of fetal membranes involves bluntly separating the chorioamnionic membrane from the wall of the cervix and the lower uterine segment. The efficacy of induction of labor by stripping of membranes is debated. Risks include potential infection, bleeding from previously undiagnosed placenta previa or low-lying placenta, and accidental rupture of membranes.

Although systemic or local administration of prostaglandin cervical gels is widely used and often successful, these gels may be associated with unwanted side effects, such as tachysystole or hyperstimulation. Variability in the definition of tachysystole and hyperstimulation exists. Tachysystole may be defined as 6 or more contractions in 10 minutes without associated abnormalities in the fetal heart rate. Although various definitions for hyperstimulation have been proposed, there is no clear definition of hyperstimulation that is applicable to all clinical settings (2).

Intracervical mechanical devices, such as the cervical balloon and laminaria, may provide cervical ripening with the advantages of low cost, less hyperstimulation, lack of systemic side effects, and easy reversibility (3). Disadvantages include risk of infection, disruption of a low-lying placenta, and mild maternal discomfort with cervical manipulation.

One technique involves extra-amniotic saline infusion whereby the cervix is visualized by sterile speculum and cleaned with povidone–iodine solution. A 22–25-gauge Foley catheter is inserted through the external os and the

---

BOX 23

Common Indications for Labor Stimulation

- Abruptio placentae
- Chorioamnionitis
- Fetal demise
- Gestational hypertension
- Premature rupture of membranes
- Postterm pregnancy
- Maternal medical conditions (eg, diabetes mellitus, renal disease, chronic pulmonary disease, chronic hypertension)
- Fetal compromise (eg, severe intrauterine growth restriction, isoimmunization)
- Preeclampsia, eclampsia
- Logistical reasons (risk of rapid labor, distance from hospital, psychosocial indications), provided term gestation is confirmed or fetal lung maturity is established.

American College of Obstetricians and Gynecologists. Induction of labor. ACOG Practice Bulletin 10. Washington, DC: ACOG; 1999.

RESOURCES

Intrapartum Management/ Surgical Complications in Pregnancy/Neonatal Resuscitation

American Academy of Pediatrics
www.aap.org

American College of Nurse Midwives
www.acnm.org

American College of Obstetricians and Gynecologists
www.acog.org

Association of Women's Health Obstetric and Neonatal Nurses
www.awhonn.org

National Institute of Child Health and Human Development
www.nichd.nih.gov

balloon is inflated above the internal os with 30–40 mL of sterile water. A normal saline solution is infused at a constant rate of 40–60 mL/h by an infusion pump. The catheter is removed by spontaneous expulsion, at rupture of membranes, or at a predetermined time limit. Oxytocin may be started concurrently or after a period of observation.

Three randomized trials comparing extraamniotic saline infusion with concomitant oxytocin infusion to vaginally administered PGE_1 (misoprostol) found the extraamniotic saline infusion technique to be associated with shorter or comparable induction to vaginal delivery times (4). In contrast, a comprehensive review of randomized studies found that use of the extraamniotic saline without concomitant oxytocin was less likely to achieve vaginal delivery within 24 hours (3) than was use of any prostaglandin for cervical ripening.

Prostaglandin

Prostaglandin (PG) E_2, $PGF_{2\alpha}$, and PGE_1 may be used for induction of labor at term and in early and middle pregnancy, when the uterus is more refractory to oxytocin. Prostaglandin E_2 can be given intravenously, orally, and intravaginally as a suppository or gel, or intraamniotically. A systematic review comprising 13 trials with more than 1,000 women enrolled compared intravenous PGE_2 and $PGF_{2\alpha}$ to intravenous oxytocin for labor induction (5). The use of intravenous prostaglandin was associated with higher rates of uterine hyperstimulation with changes in the FHR (RR 6.76, 95% CI 1.2–37.1) than was oxytocin. Intravenous prostaglandin also was associated with more maternal side effects, including gastrointestinal disorders, thrombophlebitis, and pyrexia. Use of intravenous prostaglandin was no more likely to result in vaginal delivery than was use of oxytocin.

Prostaglandin administered to the vagina or cervix is the preferred agent for preinduction cervical ripening. A comprehensive review of 57 studies involving 10,039 women found that vaginal PGE_2 compared with placebo reduced the likelihood that vaginal delivery would not be achieved within 24 hours (18% versus 99%, RR 0.19, 95% CI 0.14–0.25). There was no difference between cesarean rates, but risk of hyperstimulation with FHR changes was increased (4.6 versus 0.51, RR 4.14 95% CI 1.91–8.90) (6). In comparison to placebo, vaginal $PGF_{2\alpha}$ was associated with improved cervical scores and reduced oxytocin augmentation, but similar cesarean rates. Thus, vaginally administered prostaglandins are associated with an increase in successful vaginal delivery rates in 24 hours, no increase in operative delivery rates, and a significantly more favorable cervix within 24–48 hours. Side effects are few and include vomiting, diarrhea, and fever. In a retrospective cohort study involving 20,095 women with previous cesarean birth, the risk of uterine rupture was significantly higher with prostaglandin-induced labors than with spontaneous or non–prostaglandin-induced labor (7).

Prostaglandin formulations that have been used for cervical ripening include oral PGE_2 tablets, PGE_2 gel preparations, PGE_2 vaginal suppositories, controlled-release PGE_2 suppositories, and controlled-release PGE_2 pessaries (Table 24). Commercially available preparations are PGE_2 gel doses of 0.5 mg, oral PGE_2 tablets, and PGE_2 vaginal suppositories. The gel preparations and the vaginal suppositories are used in clinical practice to ripen the cervix. The controlled-release hydrogel pessary contains 10 mg of PGE_2 and releases about 0.8 mg of PGE_2 per hour in vitro. Both intracervical and intravaginal instillations of PGE_2 have been used to ripen the cervix. The dose of PGE_2 gel given intracervically is usually 0.5 mg (range, 0.25–1.0 mg), repeated in 6–12 hours if induction of labor is desired. The manufacturer recommends a maximum cumulative dose of 1.5 mg of dinoprostone (3 doses or 7.5 mL of gel) within a 24-hour period. The intravaginal dose is 3 mg (range 2.5–4 mg), repeated in 4–6 hours if labor is not initiated. With an unfavorable cervix (Bishop score of ≤3), 0.5 mg of PGE_2 intracervically is more effective than 4 mg of PGE_2 intravaginally. However, both routes of administration are equally effective if the cervix is favorable. With intravaginal PGE_2, multigravidas are more likely to go into labor, to have shorter labors, to require less epidural analgesia, to have more unassisted vaginal deliveries, and to have fewer cesarean deliveries than primigravidas.

Prostaglandin cervical ripeners should be administered near a labor and delivery suite, and FHR and uterine activity should be monitored continuously. An observation period of 30 minutes to 2 hours is prudent. If regular uterine activity persists, monitoring should be continued. Most physicians advocate delaying oxytocin administration for 3–12 hours after prostaglandin ripening. After use of dinoprostone in sustained-release form, delaying oxytocin induction for 30–60 minutes after removal is sufficient.

Misoprostol

Misoprostol, a synthetic PGE_1 analog, is a gastric cytoprotective agent that has been marketed in the United States since 1988 for the prevention of peptic ulcers. The advantages of misoprostol over PGE_2 derivatives include lower cost, ease of storage, and stability at room temperature, which have led to its widespread use for induction of labor in women with an unfavorable cervix. A systematic review of vaginal misoprostol for cervical ripening and induction of labor, which included 62 trials, found vaginal misoprostol to be more effective than conventional methods of cervical ripening and labor induction (8). Compared with vaginal PGE_2 and oxytocin, use of vaginal misoprostol to induce labor was associated with less epidural analgesia use and more vaginal deliveries within 24 hours but more uterine hyperstimulation. Compared with intracervical or vaginal PGE_2, oxytocin augmentation was less common with misoprostol, but meconium-stained amniotic fluid

TABLE 24. Prostaglandin Ripening Agents

Agents	Dose	Route
Dinoprostone (PGE$_2$)	0.5 mg in 2.5 mL gel	Intracervical
Dinoprostone (PGE$_2$)	10 mg (0.3 mg/h)	Intravaginal
PGE$_2$	2.5 mg gel	Intravaginal
Misoprostol (PGE$_1$)	25–50 µg*	Intravaginal

*Available as 100-µg and 200-µg tablets, which must be broken to provide 25-µg or 50-µg dose.

was more common. Lower doses of misoprostol were associated with less hyperstimulation or tachysystole than were higher doses, but there was a greater need for oxytocin augmentation. A meta-analysis raised concerns regarding the ability to evaluate the safety of higher doses of vaginal misoprostol and suggested that the 25-µg dose should be used, with redosing intervals of 3–6 hours (9). No studies indicate that intrapartum exposure to misoprostol (or other prostaglandin cervical ripening agents) has any long-term adverse health consequences to the fetus in the absence of fetal distress. These advantages have led to widespread use of misoprostol for induction of labor in women with an unfavorable cervix. Misoprostol should not be used in term pregnancies in women with previous cesarean deliveries or uterine scars because there is an increased risk of uterine rupture (10).

Although the optimal regimen to initiate and maintain effective labor without adverse fetal overtones has not been established, general guidelines for misoprostol use exist (Box 24). Maternal and fetal monitoring of women undergoing cervical ripening and induction with misoprostol should be similar to that with oxytocin induction.

Typically, misoprostol is placed intravaginally in the posterior fornix. The dose is repeated at designated intervals until an adequate contraction pattern, cervical ripening (Bishop score of >8 or dilation of >3 cm), rupture of membranes, or the maximum dose is reached. Oxytocin augmentation is permitted as necessary no less than 4 hours after the last misoprostol dose.

Recent studies have assessed the effects of oral misoprostol for labor induction. In 7 trials, which included 1,278 women randomly assigned to oral or vaginal misoprostol, oral misoprostol appeared to be less effective. More women in the oral groups failed to achieve vaginal delivery within 24 hours (11). This systematic review of oral misoprostol for induction of labor concluded it is effective; however, data on the optimal regimen and safety are lacking. Thus, its use remains investigational.

Oxytocin

Oxytocin remains the mainstay of medical therapy for labor augmentation and induction of labor in women with a favorable cervix. Factors affecting the dose response to oxytocin include cervical dilation, parity, and gestational age. Higher doses of oxytocin generally are required in a preterm nulliparous women with an unfavorable cervix. However, the prediction of an individual's oxytocin requirement before the initial infusion is impossible. The goal of oxytocin administration is to effect uterine activity that is sufficient to produce cervical change and fetal descent while avoiding nonreassuring FHR patterns. Oxytocin should be administered in a disciplined fashion by means of an infusion pump according to established departmental protocols. When oxytocin is being administered, the FHR, resting uterine tone, and frequency and duration of contractions should be monitored appropriately by electronic fetal monitoring or palpation and auscultation every 15 minutes during the first stage of labor and every 5 minutes during the second stage of labor.

Numerous protocols varying in initial dose, incremental dose increases, and time intervals between dose increases have been studied. Low-dose regimens (start-

---

BOX 24

General Principles for Misoprostol Use for Cervical Ripening or Induction

- If misoprostol is to be used for cervical ripening or labor induction in the third trimester, one quarter of a 100-µg tablet (ie, approximately 25 µg) should be considered for the initial dose. The use of higher doses (50 µg every 6 hours) may be appropriate in some situations, although increasing the dose appears to be associated with uterine tachysystole and possibly with uterine hyperstimulation and meconium staining of amniotic fluid.

- Doses should not be administered more frequently than every 3–6 hours.

- Oxytocin should not be administered less than 4 hours after the last misoprostol dose.

- Patients undergoing cervical ripening or labor induction with misoprostol for labor induction should undergo fetal heart rate and uterine activity monitoring in a hospital setting.

- Misoprostol should not be used for cerevical ripening for the induction of labor in patients with a previous cesarean birth or prior major uterine surgery.

New U.S. Food and Drug Administration labeling on Cytotec (misoprostol) use and pregnancy. ACOG Committee Opinion No. 283. American College of Obstetricians and Gynecologists. Obstet Gynecol 2003;100:1049–50.

ing dose, 0.5–2 mU/min with incremental increases of 1–2 mU/min every 15–40 minutes) were developed based on the knowledge that it takes oxytocin 40–60 minutes to reach a steady-state concentration in maternal serum. These protocols are associated with a lower incidence of uterine hyperstimulation. In the United States, high-dose protocols (starting doses, 3–6 mU/min, incremental increases 3–6 mU/min every 15–40 minutes) have been credited with shortening the time in labor and reducing the number of cesarean deliveries resulting from labor dystocia (12). The advantages of high-dose protocols appear to be more profound when used for augmentation than for induction of labor.

The principles used in administering oxytocin for labor augmentation are the same as those for oxytocin labor induction. Because oxytocin augmentation is typically prescribed in women with complete effacement and advanced cervical dilation, it is not surprising that the maximum infusion rate required is typically lower than those needed for induction.

INTRAPARTUM FETAL HEART RATE MONITORING

The goal of intrapartum FHR monitoring is to detect signs of fetal jeopardy in time to intervene before irreversible fetal damage occurs. Despite the liberal use of continuous electronic fetal monitoring in high-risk and low-risk patients, there has been no consistent decrease in the frequency of cerebral palsy in the past 2 decades. Randomized prospective trials of continuous FHR monitoring compared with intermittent auscultation reveal no differences in their ability to detect fetal compromise. Only 1 trial noted a decrease in neonatal seizures in fetuses monitored with continuous intrapartum FHR monitoring (13). Fetuses who are severely asphyxiated during the intrapartum period will have abnormal heart rate patterns. However, most patients with nonreassuring FHR patterns give birth to healthy neonates. Abnormal electronic FHR patterns are poor predictors of subsequent development of neonatal encephalopathy. Of patients who subsequently develop cerebral palsy, 4–10% have evidence of isolated intrapartum hypoxia (13, 14). Both ACOG and the American Academy of Pediatrics suggest that the FHR should be assessed in labor. Guidelines are listed in Table 25.

The most commonly used techniques for detection of FHR are the Doppler ultrasound transducer (external technique) and the fetal scalp electrode (internal technique). The internal technique has been regarded as superior to the external technique because it can assess FHR variability more accurately and is less subject to artifacts and fetal movement. The technology of auto-correlation has resulted in significant narrowing of these differences. Uterine activity usually is measured with an externally placed tocodynamometer or an intrauterine pressure catheter. The latter generally is used when there is an abnormality of labor that requires quantitation of the force of contractions. When periodic auscultation of the fetal heart either by stethoscope or Doppler technique is used, it should be evaluated and recorded after a contraction.

Fetal heart rate patterns may be described in terms of baseline features and periodic changes. In any 10-minute window, the minimum baseline for that period must be at least 2 minutes or the baseline for that period is indeterminate. The normal baseline FHR is 120–160 beats per minute. An FHR less than 120 beats per minute is considered bradycardia. Fetal bradycardia between 100 and 120 beats per minute usually can be tolerated for long periods when it is accompanied by normal FHR variability. An FHR above 160 beats per minute is considered tachycardia. Fetal tachycardia usually results from chorioamnionitis, but may be due to a number of fetal or maternal conditions, including maternal fever, thyrotoxicosis, medication, and fetal cardiac arrhythmias. Fetal tachycardia between 160 and 200 beats per minute without any other abnormalities of the FHR is usually well tolerated.

The interval between successive heartbeats in the normal fetus in characterized by variability. Short-term variability is the beat-to-beat variability or the differences between adjacent beats or several beats. Beat-to-beat variability is best assessed by an internal FHR monitor. Long-term variability consists of irregular crude sign waves with a cycle of approximately 3–6 minutes. Normal long-term FHR variability implies variability of more than 5 beats per minute. Decreased variability includes 2–5 beats per minute, and less than 2 beats per minute (straight line) implies an absence of variability. In the presence of normal FHR variability, regardless of what other FHR patterns exist, the fetus is not suffering cerebral tissue asphyxia.

Periodic FHR changes are changes in the FHR related to uterine contractions. Uterine contractions may cause intermittent decreases in intervillous space blood flow, may influence cerebral blood flow under certain circumstances and, depending on the location of the umbilical cord, may cause intermittent umbilical cord occlusion. Periodic changes in FHR include early, variable, and late decelerations. Early decelerations appear to be mild in nature and are smooth in shape. Typically, they appear as a mirror image of the uterine contraction pattern. Variable decelerations are visually apparent abrupt decreases (defined as onset of deceleration to beginning of nadir <30 seconds) in FHR below the baseline. The dip in the FHR differs in duration, profundity, and shape from contraction to contraction. Variable decelerations typically result from umbilical cord compression. Late decelerations are characterized by a drop in the FHR after the onset of contraction and a delay in the return of the FHR to baseline until after the contraction is completed. Late decelerations result from uteroplacental insufficiency. A combination of late decelerations and loss of FHR variability are essentially pathognomonic of fetal stress.

TABLE 25. Guidelines for Intrapartum Fetal Monitoring

Stage	Auscultation		Continuous Electronic Monitoring	
	Low Risk	High Risk	Low Risk	High Risk
Active phase of first stage	Evaluate and record FHR every 30 min after a contraction	Evaluate and record FHR every 15 min, preferably after a uterine contraction	Evaluate tracing at least every 30 min	Evaluate tracing at least every 15 min
Second stage	Evaluate and record FHR every 15 min	Evaluate and record FHR at least every 5 min	Evaluate tracing at least every 15 min	Evaluate tracing at least every 5 min

FHR indicates fetal heart rate.

Fetal heart rate patterns: monitoring, interpretation, and management. ACOG Technical Bulletin 207. American College of Obstetricians and Gynecologists. Washington, DC: ACOG; 1995.

In 1997 the National Institute of Child Health and Human Development Research Planning Workshop published recommendations to standardize and clarify definitions for FHR tracings (15). Those recommendations stated that a full description of an FHR tracing requires a qualitative and quantitative description of the following characteristics:

- Baseline rate
- Baseline FHR variability
- Presence of accelerations
- Periodic or episodic deceleration
- Changes or trends of FHR patterns over time

No distinction was made between short-term and long-term variability. Baseline FHR is the mean FHR rounded to increments of 5 beats per minute during a 10-minute segment. Bradycardia and tachycardia are defined as visually apparent, abrupt increases of 15 beats per minute or more above baseline for more than 15 seconds. Acceleration of 10 minutes or more is a baseline change. Late deceleration of the FHR is a visually apparent, gradual (defined as onset of deceleration of nadir ≥30 seconds) decrease and return to baseline FHR associated with a uterine contraction. Variable deceleration of the FHR is again defined as a visually apparent, abrupt decrease (defined as onset of deceleration to beginning of nadir <30 seconds) in FHR below the baseline. Baseline variability was deemed fluctuations in baseline FHR of 2 cycles per minute or greater. Variability in FHR is either absent (amplitude range, undetectable), minimal (≤5 beats per minute), moderate (6–25 beats per minute), or marked (> 25 beats per minute).

There was no consensus regarding guidelines for clinical management using FHR patterns. However, there was consensus that normal FHR tracing may include a normal baseline rate, moderate FHR variability, presence of accelerations, and absence of decelerations. Furthermore, there were several patterns believed to be predictive of current or impending fetal asphyxia. These ominous patterns include recurrent late decelerations, recurrent severe variable decelerations, or sustained bradycardia with absent FHR variability. It was recognized that many FHR tracings are intermediate between the 2 extremes. These tracings are often referred to as nonreassuring.

In the presence of nonreassuring FHR patterns, several modes of evaluation should be considered. If fetal membranes are intact, amniotomy and placement of internal electronic fetal monitors may be considered. The etiology of the FHR pattern should be determined if possible and an attempt made to correct the pattern by specifically correcting the primary problem. If nonreassuring FHR patterns persist, initial conservative measures may include changing the maternal position to the left lateral position, administering oxygen, correcting maternal hypotension, and discontinuing oxytocin, if appropriate.

If a nonreassuring FHR pattern continues, the obstetrician may consider amnioinfusion, tocolytic agents, or fetal scalp or vibroacoustic stimulation. Two meta-analyses of randomized trials of amnioinfusion in fetuses at risk for cord compression showed the procedure was associated with a 50–75% reduction in FHR abnormalities (8, 16). If the nonreassuring pattern is thought to be secondary to hyperstimulation, a tocolytic agent such as terbutaline may aid in the assessment. A Swedish trial suggested that FHR monitoring plus ST analysis of the fetal electrocardiography (ECG) may reduce both the operative delivery rate for fetal distress and the cord artery metabolic acidosis rate (17). The role of fetal ECG remains investigational. Current research suggests infection may be an important contributor to the development of cerebral palsy in distressed fetuses. At this time FHR patterns associated with fetal infection and subsequent cerebral damage have not been identified. It is important to reemphasize that the most significant prognosticator of fetal well-being is FHR variability. In the presence of FHR variability, irreversible fetal hyperoxia has not occurred.

References

1. Zhang J, Yancey MK, Henderson CE. U.S. national trends in labor induction, 1989-1998. J Reprod Med 2002;47:120–4.

2. American College of Obstetricians and Gynecologists. Induction of labor. ACOG Practice Bulletin 10. Washington, DC: ACOG; 1999.

3. Boulvain M, Kelly A, Lohse C, Stan C, Irion O. Mechanical methods for induction of labour. The Cochrane Database of Systematic Reviews 2001, Issue 4. Art. No.: CD001233. DOI: 10.1002/14651858.CD001233.

4. Wing D. Induction of labor: indications, techniques and complications. In: Rose BD, editor. UpToDate. Wellesley (MA): UpToDate; 2004.

5. Luckas M, Bricker L. Intravenous prostaglandin for induction of labour. The Cochrane Database of Systematic Reviews 2000, Issue 3. Art. No.: CD002864. DOI: 10.1002/14651858.CD002864.

6. Kelly AJ, Tan B. Intravenous oxytocin alone for cervical ripening and induction of labour. The Cochrane Database of Systematic Reviews 2001, Issue 3. Art. No.: CD003246. DOI: 10.1002/14651858.CD003246.

7. Lydon-Rochelle M, Holt VL, Easterling TR, Martin DP. Risk of uterine rupture during labor among women with a prior cesarean delivery. N Engl J Med 2001;345:3–8.

8. Hofmeyr GJ. Amnioinfusion for umbilical cord compression in labour. The Cochrane Database of Systematic Reviews 1998, Issue 1. Art. No.: CD000013. DOI: 10.1002/14651858.CD003246.

9. Sanchez-Ramos L, Kaunitz AM, Delke I. Labor induction with 25 microg versus 50 microg intravaginal misoprostol: a systematic review. Obstet Gynecol 2002;99:145–51.

10. American College of Obstetricians and Gynecologists. Response to Searle's drug warning on misoprostol. ACOG Committee Opinion 248. Washington, DC: ACOG; 2000.

11. Alfirevic Z. Oral misoprostol for induction of labor. The Cochrane Database of Systematic Reviews 2001, Issue 2. Art. No.: CD001338. DOI: 10.1002/14651858.CD001338.

12. Dystocia and augmentation of labor. ACOG Practice Bulletin No. 49. American College of Obstetricians and Gynecologists. Obstet Gynecol 2003;102:1445–54.

13. American Academy of Pediatrics; American College of Obstetricians and Gynecologists. Antepartum and intrapartum considerations and assessments. In: Neonatal encephalopathy and cerebral palsy: defining the pathogenesis and pathophysiology. Washington, DC: ACOG; 2003. p. 25–38.

14. Freeman RK. Problems with intrapartum fetal heart rate monitoring interpretation and patient management. Obstet Gynecol 2002;100:813–26.

15. Electronic fetal heart rate monitoring: research guidelines for interpretation. National Institute of Child Health and Human Development Research Planning Workshop. Am J Obstet Gynecol 1997;177:1385–90.

16. Pitt C, Sanchez-Ramos L, Kaunitz AM, Gaudier F. Prophylactic amnioinfusion for intrapartum oligohydramnios: a meta-analysis of randomized controlled trials. Obstet Gynecol 2000;96:861–6.

17. Noren H, Amer-Wahlin I, Hagberg H, Herbst A, Kjellmer I, Marsal K, et al. Fetal electrocardiography in labor and neonatal outcome: data from the Swedish randomized controlled trial on intrapartum fetal monitoring. Am J Obstet Gynecol 2003;188:183–92.

FETAL ACIDEMIA

Acidosis in the fetus often results from acute or chronic hypoperfusion and, subsequently, from hypoxia. Uteroplacental blood flow, umbilical blood flow, or both may be compromised, which first leads to CO_2 retention and then, if not corrected, to hypoxia and severe fetal acidosis. Umbilical cord blood acid–base analysis may be a useful adjunct to the Apgar score to assess retrospectively various aspects of intrapartum management. Moreover, newborn metabolic acidemia is an important criterion in defining intrapartum hypoxia sufficient to cause neonatal encephalopathy. In this context, normal umbilical cord blood gas and pH values virtually eliminate the diagnosis of severe birth asphyxia, at least to the degree associated with subsequent neurologic damage.

Collection of Umbilical Cord Blood Samples

It is of paramount importance to clamp the umbilical cord as soon after delivery as possible because the arterial pH may change significantly within 60 seconds after birth. After the cord has been clamped, blood is drawn into a 1–2-mL plastic or glass syringe that has been flushed with heparin (1,000 U/mL) or into syringes with lyophilized heparin. Too much heparin or greater concentrations may affect the accuracy of the results (1).

Blood from the umbilical artery best reflects the fetal condition, whereas venous blood reflects uteroplacental circulation. Moreover, it is possible for the pH of blood from the umbilical artery to be very low in a severely acidotic fetus secondary to cord prolapse while the pH of blood from the umbilical vein is relatively normal (2). In cases where it is difficult to obtain arterial blood from the umbilical cord (ie, in a very premature infant), it is relatively easy to obtain an arterial blood sample from the chorionic surface of the placenta (the chorionic arteries always cross over the chorionic veins) that will provide accurate results.

Umbilical Cord Values

Determinations of umbilical artery blood pH and gases are especially useful in a premature infant who may have low Apgar scores solely because of immaturity. The normal mean pH and blood gas values in umbilical cord blood for premature infants are similar to those for term infants (Table 26) (2–4).

■ TABLE 26. Normal Mean Umbilical Cord Blood pH and Blood Gas Values in Term Newborns

| | Measurement | | | | | | | |
| | Arterial | | | | Venous | | | |
Study	pH	P_{CO_2} (mm Hg)	HCO_3 (meq/L)	Base Excess (mmol/L)	pH	P_{CO_2} (mm Hg)	HCO_3 (meq/L)	Base Excess (mmol/L)
Study 1 (N = 146)*	7.28	49.2	22.3	—	7.35	38.2	20.4	—
Study 2 (N = 1,292)†	7.28	49.9	23.1	-3.6	—	—	—	—
Study 3 (N = 3,522)‡	7.27	50.3	22.0	-2.7	7.34	40.7	21.4	-2.4

*Yeomans ER, Hauth JC, Gilstrap LC III, Strickland DM. Umbilical cord pH, P_{CO_2}, and bicarbonate following uncomplicated term vaginal deliveries. Am J Obstet Gynecol 1985;151:798–800.

†Ramin SM, Gilstrap LC III, Leveno KJ, Burris J, Little BB. Umbilical artery acid-base status in the preterm infant. Obstet Gynecol 1989;74:256–8.

‡Riley RJ, Johnson JW. Collecting and analyzing cord blood gases. Clin Obstet Gynecol 1993;36:13–23.

The umbilical artery blood pH threshold for significant pathologic acidemia (below which major neurologic morbidity may occur) is most likely less than 7.00 and may be less than 6.90 (5–7). However, as many as two thirds of term infants with an umbilical artery pH of less than 7.00 are admitted to the regular nursery with no apparent morbidity.

According to the ACOG Task Force on Neonatal Encephalopathy and Cerebral Palsy (8), a newborn with an acute intrapartum hypoxic event that is severe enough to cause cerebral palsy must meet all 4 of the following criteria:

- Metabolic acidosis (ie, umbilical artery blood pH of <7.00 and base deficit >12 mmol/L) (9)
- Early onset of moderate to severe neonatal encephalopathy in term or near-term infants
- Spastic quadriplegic or dyskinetic cerebral palsy
- Exclusion of other etiologies, including trauma, infection, coagulation disorders, or genetic conditions.

The task force identified additional nonspecific criteria that collectively suggest that the event occurred during labor and delivery (≤48 hours) (8). These criteria include the following:

- Sentinel hypoxic event immediately before or during labor
- Sudden and persistent fetal bradycardia or absent FHR variability in the presence of persistent, late, or variable decelerations following an event when the FHR tracing had been reassuring
- Apgar of 0–3 for more than 5 minutes
- Multiorgan system involvement within 72 hours

- Acute nonfocal cerebral abnormality on early imaging studies

References

1. Kirshon B, Moise KJ Jr. Effect of heparin on umbilical arterial blood gases. J Reprod Med 1989;34:267–9.

2. Riley RJ, Johnson JW. Collecting and analyzing cord blood gases. Clin Obstet Gynecol 1993;36:13–23.

3. Ramin SM, Gilstrap LC 3rd, Leveno KJ, Burris J, Little BB. Umbilical artery acid-base status in the preterm infant. Obstet Gynecol 1989;74:256–8.

4. Yeomans ER, Hauth JC, Gilstrap LC 3rd, Strickland DM. Umbilical cord pH, PCO2, and bicarbonate following uncomplicated term vaginal deliveries. Am J Obstet Gynecol 1985;151:798–800.

5. Goldaber KG, Gilstrap LC 3rd, Leveno KJ, Dax JS, McIntire DD. Pathologic fetal acidemia. Obstet Gynecol 1991;78:1103–7.

6. Van den Berg PP, Nelen WL, Jongsma HW, Nijland R, Kollee LA, Nijhuis JG, et al. Neonatal complications in newborns with an umbilical artery pH <7.00. Am J Obstet Gynecol 1996;175:1152–7.

7. Andres RL, Saade G, Gilstrap LC, Wilkins I, Witlin A, Zlatnik F, et al. Association between umbilical blood gas parameters and neonatal morbidity and death in neonates with pathologic fetal acidemia. Am J Obstet Gynecol 1999; 181:867–71.

8. American Academy of Pediatrics, American College of Obstetricians and Gynecologists. Neonatal encephalopathy and cerebral palsy: defining the pathogenesis and pathophysiology. Washington, DC: ACOG; 2003.

9. Low JA, Lindsay BG, Derrick EJ. Threshold of metabolic acidosis associated with newborn complications. Am J Obstet Gynecol 1997;177:1391–4.

OPERATIVE OBSTETRICS

The cesarean delivery rate in the United States has risen steadily since 1997, and in 2002 it reached an all-time high of 26.1% (1). Several factors contributed to this dramatic reversal, as evidenced by across-the-board increases in primary, repeat, and overall cesarean delivery rates. First, heightened awareness of the potential for uterine rupture and its consequences has diminished the enthusiasm for and the frequency of vaginal birth after cesarean (VBAC). The VBAC rate has fallen to 12.6 per 100 women with a prior cesarean delivery. Second, publication of the findings of the term breech trial (2) has increased the cesarean rate for term infants in breech presentation. Third, a number of articles have been published on the subject of primary elective cesarean delivery.

Concern for pelvic floor damage associated with vaginal delivery has provided some of the impetus toward primary elective procedures. Reports highlighting maternal and perinatal morbidity have led to a marked reduction in operative vaginal delivery. In 1994 the combined incidence of forceps and vacuum deliveries was 9.5%, and in 2002 it was 5.9%, representing a 61% reduction (1). Accompanying the overall decline in operative vaginal delivery frequency is a significant change in case mix: the ratio of forceps to vacuum was 18:1 in 1980, 3:2 in 1990, and 1:2 in 2000 (3). These alterations in incidence of route (abdominal or vaginal) and method (forceps or vacuum) of delivery have implications for the acquisition and maintenance of skills for residents and specialists, respectively.

The steady decline in the frequency of forceps delivery has been accompanied by a corresponding decline in the technical skills required to perform the procedure. Such skills are acquired through training during residency; the value of technical teaching in a laboratory setting is limited. Obstetricians taking their oral board examinations report a median of 5 forceps deliveries in 1 year of case collecting (4). Such minimal use may not suffice to maintain skill in practice.

Thorough documentation in the medical record is required for all operative vaginal deliveries. A recent report partially attributed a reduction in birth trauma to a policy of preoperative documentation of the operator's findings relating to clinical pelvimetry (5). Such practice is recommended.

Forceps Delivery

Forceps may be used to benefit mother, fetus, or both. Forceps deliveries can be either indicated or elective. When forceps are used electively, the criteria for outlet forceps (Box 25) should be met. Some investigators have extended the definition of elective forceps to include "low" (as high as +2 station). Due to the inherent uncertainty in the determination of station, it is advisable to limit elective use to outlet forceps only. The main advantage to elective forceps for women and infants is shorten-

---

BOX 25

Criteria for Types of Forceps Deliveries

Outlet forceps

Scalp is visible at the introitus without separating labia

Fetal skull has reached pelvic floor

Sagittal suture is in anteroposterior diameter or right or left occiput anterior or posterior position

Fetal head is at or on perineum

Rotation does not exceed 45 degrees

Low forceps

Leading point of fetal skull is at station ≥+2 cm and not on the pelvic floor

Rotation is ≤45 degrees (left or right occiput anterior to occiput anterior, or left or right occiput posterior to occiput posterior)

Rotation is >45 degrees

Midforceps

Station is above +2 cm but head is engaged

High forceps

Not included in classification.

American College of Obstetricians and Gynecologists. Operative vaginal delivery. ACOG Practice Bulletin 17. Washington, DC: ACOG; 2000.

---

ing the second stage of labor. Morbidity for either patient is not increased when forceps are used electively. Most women in labor have epidural anesthesia, which is ideal for instrumental delivery. For the practicing obstetrician, elective forceps use helps to maintain proficiency, whereas for residents it affords necessary training for situations where delivery by forceps is indicated.

Surveys confirm that operative vaginal delivery continues to be taught in U.S. residency programs. However, high cesarean rates, preference for the vacuum extractor (see "Vacuum Extraction"), and fear of litigation have diminished the absolute number of forceps cases performed by residents.

Indications (excluding elective) for forceps delivery are all relative, not absolute. They require a skilled operator who can employ sound clinical judgment based on experience. Indications may be grouped as either maternal or fetal (Box 26).

Once an appropriate indication has been identified, prerequisites for the planned forceps delivery (Box 27) must be satisfied. Careful assessment of fetopelvic relationships to ensure success and minimize morbidity is most important. Fetal evaluation includes estimate of weight and vaginal examination to ascertain position, station, attitude, asynclitism, presence of caput (see

"Vacuum Extraction"), and molding. Also on vaginal examination the operator should evaluate the bones and soft tissue of the maternal pelvis and confirm that the cervix is fully dilated and completely retracted. This information is then synthesized along with the woman's parity, course of labor (especially the second stage), and fetal status as determined by FHR monitoring.

The optimal location to conduct an instrumental delivery may be an operating room equipped with table with a firm surface and adjustable leg holders and readily available anesthesia equipment and personnel. As a practical matter, most operative vaginal deliveries take place in a labor room. Attention should be directed to positioning the patient, especially avoiding excessive abduction and flexing of the legs. The operator must then choose an instrument best suited for the particular case. In contemporary practice the initial choice is either vacuum or forceps, usually based on the training and experience of the obstetrician. If the operator is skilled with both, patient preference may be taken into account. Many reports in the literature compare vacuum to forceps as if those were the only options. However, within each category there are additional choices (type of forceps, type of cup), again based on the clinical scenario and obstetrician's experience. The culmination of the preoperative evaluation is the actual delivery. Potential pitfalls leading to maternal or neonatal morbidity can be traced to either the preoperative assessment or the performance of the operation. Therefore, as the minimum consideration of technique, the operator should check the application of any instrument prior to initiating traction. Checks for forceps include evaluating the symmetry and depth of applica-

tion. Traction in the proper direction will eliminate wasted force and decrease the risk of injury.

As with many aspects of obstetric practice, the concept of a trial of forceps is undergoing review. A cautious approach would be to regard any operative vaginal delivery as a trial, the probability of success depending on both patient characteristics and operator skill and judgment. Currently, a trial of operative vaginal delivery should not be attempted unless success is deemed highly likely (6).

One additional consideration is whether rotational forceps delivery can be justified in contemporary obstetric practice. A solid rationale has been established for continuing to perform rotational forceps (6). One study (7) confirmed no difference in maternal outcome with only limited fetal risk when rotational forceps use was compared with that of nonrotational forceps.

Vacuum Extraction

The vacuum extractor, long preeminent in Europe, continues to grow in popularity in the United States. A device warning by the FDA (which focused on a small number of adverse outcomes instead of the frequency of those outcomes) has not curbed the enthusiasm for this method of delivery. Despite its advantages of ease of application, reduced maternal morbidity, and decreased anesthesia requirement, vacuum extraction is associated with 2 significant disadvantages: a higher failure rate and increased trauma to the neonate. More frequent retinal hemorrhages and scalp trauma may be insignificant; however, cephalohematoma formation occurs 7 times more often with vacuum than forceps. Reabsorption of loculated blood can lead to jaundice severe enough to require readmission to the hospital after the infant has been discharged. By far the most worrisome complication of vacuum extraction is subaponeurotic (subgaleal) hemorrhage, which occurs with a frequency of about 1–7/1,000 (8, 9).

The same caveat applies to morbidity from vacuum extraction as to that from forceps: the instrument is likely not to be the sole culprit. The skill and judgment of the

---

BOX 26

Indications for Operative Vaginal Delivery

No indication for operative vaginal delivery is absolute. The following indications apply when the fetal head is engaged and the cervix is fully dilated:

- Prolonged second stage:
  —Nulliparous women: lack of continuing progress for 3 hours with regional anesthesia, or 2 hours without regional anesthesia
  —Multiparous women: lack of continuing progress for 2 hours with regional anesthesia, or 1 hour without regional anesthesia
- Suspicion of immediate or potential fetal compromise
- Shortening of the second stage for maternal benefit

American College of Obstetricians and Gynecologists. Operative vaginal delivery. ACOG Practice Bulletin 17. Washington, DC: ACOG; 2000.

BOX 27

Prerequisites for Forceps Delivery

- Complete cervical dilation
- Ruptured membranes
- Head engaged
- Position known
- No fetopelvic disproportion
- Adequate anesthesia
- Experienced operator with willingness to abandon the procedure if necessary

operator contribute significantly to outcomes. The same indications and prerequisites should apply to forceps and vacuum extraction.

Guidelines for the technical aspects of vacuum extraction continue to evolve as the frequency of the operation, at least relative to forceps (3), increases. Duration of the procedure should be limited to 20 minutes. Progress in descent should accompany the first 1 or 2 traction attempts. The relationship of number of detachments ("pop-offs") of the vacuum cup to morbidity is not clear and certainly differs with station and observed descent; that is, detachment in the mid-pelvis without descent is likely to be more morbid than detachment at outlet level. The most important aspect of technique is proper placement of the cup. The presence of significant caput succedaneum adversely affects cup placement and increases failure rate for vacuum extraction. The material of the cup, metal or rigid plastic or soft plastic, also may contribute to the incidence of complications. For example, soft cups appear to be associated with a lower incidence of superficial scalp injuries than metal cups. However, the trade-off is that soft cups are associated with a higher failure rate.

Although some consider the vacuum extractor to be the instrument of first choice for operative vaginal delivery, this has not been established. A 5-year follow-up of patients enrolled in a randomized controlled study of forceps versus vacuum extraction revealed no specific maternal or child benefits or side effects for either method of delivery (10). Moreover, the frequency of neonatal intracranial hemorrhage is comparable whether delivery is accomplished by cesarean birth after labor, vacuum extraction, or forceps (11). Therefore the choice of instrument should be left to the experience and preference of the operator. If current usage trends continue unabated, forceps delivery may be severely limited by the availability of adequate training.

References

1. Martin JA, Hamilton BE, Sutton PD, Ventura SJ, Menacker F, Munson ML. Births: final data for 2002. Natl Vital Stat Rep 2003;52(10):1–113.

2. Hannah ME, Hannah WJ, Hewson SA, Hodnett ED, Saigal S, Willan AR. Planned caesarean section versus planned vaginal birth for breech presentation at term: a randomised multicentre trial. Term Breech Trial Collaborative Group. Lancet 2000;356:1375–83.

3. Kozak LJ, Weeks JD. U.S. trends in obstetric procedures, 1990-2000. Birth 2002;29:157–61.

4. Chez RA, Droegemueller W, Grant NF Jr, O'Sullivan MJ. Clinical experience reported by candidates for the American Board of Obstetrics and Gynecology 1995 and 1997 oral examinations. Am J Obstet Gynecol 2001;185:1429–32.

5. Leung WC, Lam HS, Lam KW, To M, Lee CP. Unexpected reduction in the incidence of birth trauma and birth asphyxia related to instrumental deliveries during the study period: was this the Hawthorne effect? BJOG 2003;110:319–22.

6. American College of Obstetricians and Gynecologists. Operative vaginal delivery. ACOG Practice Bulletin 17. Washington, DC: ACOG; 2000.

7. Hankins GD, Leicht T, Van Hook J, Uckan EM. The role of forceps rotation in maternal and neonatal injury. Am J Obstet Gynecol 1999;180:231–4.

8. Miksovsky P, Watson WJ. Obstetric vacuum extraction: state of the art in the new millennium. Obstet Gynecol Surv 2001;56:736–51.

9. Uchil D, Arulkumaran S. Neonatal subgaleal hemorrhage and its relationship to delivery by vacuum extraction. Obstet Gynecol Surv 2003;58:687–93.

10. Johanson RB, Heycock E, Carter J, Sultan AH, Walklate K, Jones PW. Maternal and child health after assisted vaginal delivery: five-year follow up of a randomised controlled study comparing forceps and ventouse. Br J Obstet Gynaecol 1999;106:544–9.

11. Towner D, Castro MA, Eby-Wilkens E, Gilbert WM. Effect of mode of delivery in nulliparous women on neonatal intracranial injury. N Engl J Med 1999;341:1709–14.

Cesarean Birth

Perhaps the most interesting change in obstetric practice over the past 30 years has been the increasing rate of cesarean delivery. Before 1970, the total U.S. cesarean delivery rate remained consistently under 5%. The rate began to increase in 1970, reaching 15% by 1980 and 22% by 1990 (1). During the 1990s, the national cesarean rate leveled off and remained fairly constant at about 21–22%; however, by the second year of the new millennium it had increased to more than 25%. Birth certificate data indicate that the cesarean rate plateau during the 1990s was mainly due to increasing rates of VBAC and that the recent increase in cesarean rates is predominantly due to falling VBAC rates (2). In 2002 for the first time, 1 million cesarean operations were performed in the United States. Although the "ideal" cesarean rate remains controversial, increasing cesarean rates prompted 2 health care improvement organizations to release comprehensive guidelines aimed at safely reducing cesarean rates (3, 4).

The Healthy People 2010 Work Group of the Department of Health and Human Services (DHHS), which included ACOG representatives, developed evidence-based goals for the cesarean birth rate for 2010. Data from 1996 birth certificates have been used to establish target rates for 2 patient groups that are relatively homogeneous but vary widely in cesarean delivery rates:

- Reduce the primary cesarean delivery rate among low-risk women having a first birth, defined as nulliparous patients at 37 weeks of gestation or greater with singleton vertex presentation. To set the goal, the work group used the 25th percentile of rates by state ranked in ascending order, which yields a target of 15.5% for this specific population, compared with an overall rate of 17.9% in 1996.

- Increase the rate of VBAC among low-risk women with prior cesarean delivery, defined as multiparous women with 1 prior low-transverse cesarean delivery at 37 weeks of gestation or greater with singleton fetus in vertex presentation. The national 1996 VBAC rate for this group was 30.3%; the goal set at the 75th percentile is 37%.

Characteristics of patients, including payer type, socioeconomic status, ethnicity, and education, are associated with significant variations in cesarean birth rates. Aspects of physician practice, including sole versus group practice, employment status, in-house coverage, and teaching status also affect cesarean birth rates. Hospitals that provide 24-hour, in-house, dedicated obstetric physician coverage have lower cesarean rates than do group or solo practices. Data suggest that the presence of individual obstetric nurses also affects cesarean birth rates.

When variations in primary cesarean delivery rates were examined on the basis of patient characteristics, however, the most dramatic variation in primary cesarean delivery rates was found in patients with a normal term, singleton, vertex fetus. Cesarean birth rates for high-risk patients were found to be quite similar at different hospitals. Although differences in patient characteristics do account for some variations in cesarean birth rates and explain some differences between practitioner and hospital rates, it is not apparent that higher cesarean delivery rates in lower-risk patients have improved outcomes. Therefore, for both the individual practitioner as well as hospital departments of obstetrics and gynecology, it would seem appropriate to focus on low-risk, term patients when evaluating strategies for lowering the cesarean birth rate. This group of patients represents the most likely opportunity for improvement.

The ACOG Task Force on Cesarean Delivery Rates has developed specific strategies and recommendations designed to achieve optimal cesarean delivery rates (5). Examples of these approaches include the following:

1. Hospitals should evaluate variations in cesarean delivery rates among practitioners at their institutions.

2. Hospitals or physician groups with high cesarean delivery rates can consider establishing separate 24-hour, in-house, obstetric coverage by physicians who are solely responsible for the care of the intrapartum patient.

3. Institutions with high cesarean delivery rates should review individual cesarean delivery rates for each nurse, similarly to physician-specific rates.

4. The obstetric community should educate physicians, nurses, attorneys, legislators, and the public regarding the actual relationship between brain damage and perinatal events and seek reform of the medical liability claims process.

5. Obstetric practitioners should not perform cesarean delivery for the sole indication of maternal age.

6. Obstetric practitioners should educate women about the direct association between prepregnancy weight and weight gain during pregnancy and the risk of cesarean delivery.

7. Institutions with high rates of cesarean delivery performed for dystocia when cervical dilatation was less than 3–4 cm should review their cesarean delivery rates for appropriateness.

8. Practitioners should recommend using other forms of analgesia instead of an epidural prior to cervical dilatation of 4–5 cm.

9. Induction of labor for suspected macrosomia does not improve outcome, expends considerable resources, and may increase the cesarean delivery rate.

10. Obstetric practitioners should not induce labor in patients with unfavorable cervixes before 41 completed weeks of gestation unless maternal or fetal complications constitute an indication for induction.

Several trends have recently emerged that may render achievement of DHHS Healthy People 2010 goals and ACOG Task Force goals unattainable. For example, efforts to reduce the primary cesarean delivery rate among low-risk women with term pregnancies may be hampered by increasing concerns about pelvic floor damage caused by vaginal birth. Widespread media coverage of this topic is undoubtedly responsible for at least some of the recent trend of increasing elective cesarean deliveries. However, a recent paper showing high rates of incontinence in nuns with no history of childbirth casts some doubt on the validity of claims of maternal risks of vaginal birth (6). Informed choice cesarean delivery and pelvic floor issues remain controversial.

Vaginal Birth After Cesarean Delivery

The incidence of VBAC in the United States over the past 15 years is roughly a bell-shaped curve rising from 71,000 in 1989, peaking at 116,000 in 1996, and falling to 74,000 in 2002 (2). The most serious risk associated with VBAC is the potential for uterine rupture, which can result in fetal brain injury or death. The occurrence of uterine rupture during a trial of labor in women with a prior low-transverse cesarean delivery is approximately 1%. The proportion of uterine ruptures that result in significant maternal or neonatal morbidity is difficult to determine. This reflects the fact that large multicenter studies on VBAC generally have been conducted at medical centers with 24-hour in-house obstetricians and anesthesiologists. Additionally, reports of catastrophic rupture often appear as case reports or small case series without sufficient power necessary to calculate risk.

When uterine rupture does occur, prompt intervention often results in good outcomes for both mother and infant. This is not always the case, however, and fetal death or permanent neurologic sequelae may occur in spite of optimal management. Nevertheless, the immediate availability of a physician throughout active labor who is capable of monitoring labor and performing an emergency cesarean delivery, as well as available anesthesia and personnel for an emergency cesarean delivery, can be lifesaving. Furthermore, the inability to perform emergency cesarean delivery because of unavailable surgeon or anesthesia or insufficient staff or facility can be considered a contraindication to attempting VBAC. Although studies have indicated that attempted VBAC is a reasonable option in patients with more than 1 prior cesarean delivery, multifetal gestation, and suspected fetal macrosomia, the risk of uterine rupture may be slightly increased. Following are selection criteria useful in identifying candidates for VBAC (7):

- One previous low-transverse cesarean delivery
- Clinically adequate pelvis
- No other uterine scars or previous rupture
- Physicians immediately available throughout active labor and capable of performing an emergency cesarean delivery
- Availability of anesthesia and personnel for emergency cesarean delivery

Factors that influence a decision about whether to attempt a trial of labor after a previous cesarean birth are poorly understood. Given an option, patient's choice should be allowed, and many women choose elective repeat cesarean delivery. Studies have found that VBAC rates are higher among younger physicians, in more specialized hospitals, and among patients with a lower level of education. For eligible women, it is reasonable to discuss VBAC early in pregnancy. A balanced and reasoned written informed consent is prudent, recognizing that the ultimate decision as to whether to attempt a trial of labor or undergo an elective repeat cesarean delivery resides with the patient. Sample VBAC consent forms are available for reproduction or modification (8).

The most common signs of uterine rupture are either a prolonged deceleration of the fetal heart rate lasting for several minutes, formerly termed bradycardia, or repetitive severe variable decelerations during the first stage of labor. If either of these patterns occur during a trial of labor, an emergency cesarean should be initiated as quickly as it can be safely performed (8). Because pain is the hallmark of normal labor, abdominal pain is not a reliable sign of uterine rupture. Induction of labor may increase the risk of uterine rupture in VBAC patients.

The use of prostaglandin agents for cervical ripening or induction of labor in most women with a previous cesarean delivery should be discouraged (7).

Cesarean and Puerperal Hysterectomy

Indications for both emergent and nonemergent puerperal hysterectomy have changed in recent years. Emergency hysterectomy is required in approximately 1 per 1,000 births. Historically, uterine atony unresponsive to medical management and uterine rupture were the most common indications for emergency puerperal hysterectomy. However, indications are that placenta accreta is now the most common indication for emergency hysterectomy, accounting for 50–60% of all cases. This change is related to the increasing number of cesarean deliveries over the past 2 decades and the association between prior cesarean delivery and placenta accreta in subsequent pregnancies. In a recent study, 49% of emergency hysterectomies resulted from placenta accreta, and 96% of these patients had a history of previous cesarean or curettage (9).

Indications for nonemergent puerperal hysterectomy also have changed. Debate continues about the role of scheduled cesarean hysterectomy in cases of high-grade or early invasive cervical disease, ovarian malignancies, uterine leiomyomata, or abnormal uterine bleeding. However, the use of peripartum hysterectomy solely as an elective means of permanent sterilization is no longer recommended.

Puerperal hysterectomy is associated with increased intraoperative and postoperative maternal morbidity as high as 65%, mainly related to genitourinary tract injury, longer operative times, increased blood loss, and higher rates of infection. During surgery, care should be taken to gain control of the vascular blood supply quickly and to mobilize the bladder to prevent ureteral injury.

Perimortem Cesarean Delivery

Cardiac arrest during pregnancy is a rare event. When it does occur, there is no time to consult textbooks or journal articles. Hence, it is prudent to have a general plan in mind. In the first half of gestation, emergent cesarean delivery is not recommended because it will probably not aid maternal resuscitation efforts but will cause fetal death. However, after approximately 24 weeks of gestation, perimortem cesarean delivery may aid maternal cardiopulmonary resuscitation efforts and also increase fetal survival (10). While continuing cardiopulmonary resuscitation efforts, teams responsible for the management of both mother and neonate must be rapidly assembled. Perimortem cesarean is performed without concern for a sterile operative field. Optimally, delivery of a viable fetus should occur within 5 minutes of cardiac arrest to reduce the likelihood of fetal or neonatal death or brain injury. Conversely, if cardiopulmonary resuscitation efforts have very quickly restored a spontaneous maternal pulse, it is preferable to allow intrauterine resuscitation of the fetus before delivery under sterile conditions (if the indication for cesarean delivery persists). When signs of fetal life are present (even outside this window of optimal timing), perimortem cesarean delivery should be attempted. Reports have documented intact fetal survival more than 15 minutes after cardiac arrest (11).

References

1. Martin JA, Hamilton BE, Sutton PD, Ventura SJ, Menacker F, et al. Births: final data for 2002. Natl Vital Stat Rep 2003;52(10):1–113.

2. Martin JA, Hamilton BE, Ventura SJ, Menacker F, Park MM, Sutton PD. Births: final data for 2001. Natl Vital Stat Rep 2002:51(2);1–102.

3. Flamm B, Kabcenell A, Berwick D, Roessner J. Reducing cesarean section rates while maintaining maternal and infant outcomes. Boston (MA): Institute for Healthcare Improvement; 1997.

4. The Advisory Board Company. Coming to term: innovations in safely reducing cesarean rates. Washington, DC: The Advisory Board Company; 1996.

5. American College of Obstetricians and Gynecologists. Evaluation of cesarean delivery. Washington, DC: ACOG; 2000.

6. Buchsbaum GM, Chin M, Glantz C, Guzick D. Prevalence of urinary incontinence and associated risk factors in a cohort of nuns. Obstet Gynecol 2002;100:226–9.

7. Vaginal birth after previous cesarean. ACOG Practice Bulletin No. 54. American College of Obstetricians and Gynecologists. Obstet Gynecol 2004;104:203–12.

8. Flamm BL. Vaginal birth after cesarean: reducing medical and legal risks. Clin Obstet Gynecol 2001;44:622–9.

9. Kastner ES, Figueroa R, Garry D, Maulik D. Emergency peripartum hysterectomy: experience at a community teaching hospital. Obstet Gynecol 2002;99:971–5.

10. Whitty JE. Maternal cardiac arrest in pregnancy. Clin Obstet Gynecol 2002;45:377–92.

11. Katz VL, Dotters DJ, Droegemueller W. Perimortem cesarean delivery. Obstet Gynecol 1986;68:571–6.

Vaginal Breech Delivery

Breech is the most common malpresentation at delivery. About 25–30% of all fetuses are in the breech position prior to 28 weeks of gestation. Most convert spontaneously into cephalic presentation after 34 weeks of gestation. Only 3–4% of all pregnancies reach term with a fetus in breech presentation (1). In most cases no cause is found, but factors such as prematurity, multiple gestation, polyhydramnios, placenta previa, and uterine abnormality might contribute to the breech malpresentation.

Experts have argued for decades about appropriate management of fetuses in breech presentation. Studies in the 1970s estimated perinatal morbidity and mortality of breech vaginal delivery to be 3–5 times that of infants with vertex presentation (2). Trauma and hypoxia were the 2 principal contributing factors for increased perinatal morbidity and mortality with vaginal breech delivery (Table 27). Even with introduction of pelvimetry, whether clinical or radiologic to determine the best route for breech delivery, neonatal outcomes did not improve (3).

In the 1980s, retrospective studies suggested a better perinatal outcome with cesarean delivery than with vaginal breech delivery. Meta-analysis and critical review of these reports concluded that a trial of labor produced a higher risk of fetal injury and death in term breech infants and lower risk of perinatal and neonatal morbidity with planned cesarean birth (4, 5). This led to: 1) a marked decline in vaginal deliveries of breech infants at term; and 2) a lower threshold for cesarean delivery. According to the National Center for Health Statistics, in 2002, 86.9% of fetuses with a diagnosed breech presentation were delivered by cesarean and accounted for 13% of all cesarean deliveries performed (6).

Nonrandomized studies in the 1990s to assess the relative safety of cesarean and vaginal breech deliveries for both the fetus and mother yielded contradictory results. Some studies reported no difference in neonatal outcomes between planned vaginal delivery and elective cesarean delivery but increased maternal morbidity with cesarean birth (7, 8). Others reported vaginal breech birth to be associated with higher rates of infant mortality and birth injuries than with planned cesarean births, with no significant difference in maternal morbidity. However, maternal morbidity remained higher when cesarean delivery was performed under emergent situations (9).

To address this contradiction, a large international multicenter randomized term breech trial compared a policy of planned cesarean birth with planned vaginal breech

TABLE 27. Incidence of Complications Noted With Vaginal Breech Delivery

Complication	Incidence
Intrapartum fetal death	Increased 16-fold
Intrapartum asphyxia	Increased 3.8-fold
Cord prolapse	Increased 5–20-fold
Birth trauma	Increased 13-fold
Arrest of the after-coming head	8.8%
Spinal cord injury with extended fetal head	21%
Major anomalies	16–18%
Prematurity	16–33%
Hyperextension of fetal head	5%

Reprinted from Obstetrics: normal and problem pregnancies, 4th ed. Lanni SM, Seeds JW. Malpresentations. Gabbe SG, Niebyl JR, Simpson JL, editors. p. 473–501. Copyright 2002, with permission from Elsevier.

delivery (10). In this study, perinatal mortality and serious neonatal morbidity were significantly lower with planned cesarean birth than with planned vaginal birth (17/1,039 [1.6%] versus 52/1,039 [5.0%]), and there was no difference in maternal morbidity and mortality. The benefits of planned cesarean delivery remained even after correcting for potential confounding factors such as birth weight, gestational age at delivery, maternal parity, and experience of the attending physician. The reduction in the overall perinatal morbidity was greatest among centers in countries with a low perinatal mortality rate (2/514 [0.4%] versus 29/511 [5.7%]). This study recommended the policy of planned cesarean birth for breech presentation, especially in countries with a low perinatal mortality rate. Because of the inherent strength of a large randomized study as an appropriate method to quantify the benefit from a new policy, ACOG recommends that patients with a persistent breech presentation at term in a singleton gestation should undergo a planned cesarean delivery (11).

Critical review of the term breech trial revealed major concerns (12). The trial was conducted in 121 centers in 26 countries with a marked heterogeneity of patient characteristics, obstetric providers, technical sophistication, and background perinatal mortality rates. Many of the aspects of clinical care were not adequately defined, which resulted in unbalanced groups. Pelvic adequacy was predominantly assessed clinically; only 10% of cases were assessed using X-ray pelvimetry. The attitude of the fetal head and estimated fetal weight were determined by clinical examination in only 30% and 40% of women, respectively. There were more infants larger than 4,000 g in the group of planned vaginal deliveries than in the cesarean delivery group (5.8% versus 3.1%, $P = .002$). The frequency and use of oxytocin for labor augmentation were not controlled for in the regression analyses. For perinatal outcomes, although randomization was stratified by parity and not by center or country, secondary regression analyses were based on national rather than center-specific perinatal mortality rates. Furthermore, the concept of planned cesarean delivery has circumvented external cephalic version as an effective and safe management option for breech presentation at term (13). This would make it difficult to apply the results of the term breech trial to all patients and at centers where more defined criteria are contemplated to allow vaginal breech delivery.

In addition, the long-term maternal complications of planned cesarean delivery for breech presentation, including the increased risks for repeat cesarean deliveries, are not yet adequately explored. Therefore, the clinical decision for the best route of breech delivery at term may depend on the individual patient's risk and benefit after careful assessment of maternal pelvic adequacy, estimated fetal weight, type of the breech, and position of the fetal cervical spine.

The shift toward cesarean delivery for breech presentation has led to a decrease in the number of practitioners with the skills and experience to perform vaginal breech delivery (11). Still, there are situations in which vaginal delivery of fetuses presenting as breech will be unavoidable or when an informed patient opts for vaginal breech delivery. Obstetricians should maintain and train obstetric residents in the valuable skills of vaginal breech delivery (14). The principles of atraumatic techniques used for delivery of breech infants through uterine incision are the same as for vaginal breech delivery. Faculties in academic medical centers and residency programs should stress teaching obstetric residents the skills of breech delivery during cesarean section to maintain proficiency with vaginal breech delivery.

References

1. Gregory KD, Curtin SC, Taffel SM, Notzon FC. Changes in indications for cesarean delivery: United States, 1985 and 1994. Am J Public Health 1998;88:1384–7.

2. Kauppila O. The perinatal mortality in breech deliveries and observations on affecting factors. A retrospective study of 2227 cases. Acta Obstet Gynecol Scand Suppl 1975;39:1–79.

3. van Loon AJ, Mantingh A, Serlier EK, Kroon G, Mooyaart EL, Huisjes HJ. Randomised controlled trial of magnetic resonance pelvimetry in breech presentation at term. Lancet 1997;350:1799–804.

4. Gifford DS, Morton SC, Fiske M, Kahn K. A meta-analysis of infant outcomes after breech delivery. Obstet Gynecol 1995;85:1047–54.

5. Cheng M, Hannah M. Breech delivery at term: a critical review of the literature. Obstet Gynecol 1993;82:605–18.

6. Martin JA, Hamilton BE, Sutton PD, Ventura SJ, Munson ML. Births: final data for 2002. Natl Vital Stat Rep 2003;52 (10):1–113.

7. Irion O, Hirsbrunner Almagbaly P, Morabia A. Planned vaginal delivery versus elective caesarean section; a study of 705 singleton term breech presentation. Br J Obstet Gynaecol 1998;105:710–7.

8. Sanchez-Ramos L, Wells TL, Adair CD, Arcelin G, Kaunitz AM, Wells DS. Route of breech delivery and maternal and neonatal outcomes. Int J Gynaecol Obstet 2001;73:7–14.

9. Roman J, Bakos O, Cnattingius S. Pregnancy outcomes by mode of delivery among term breech births: Swedish experience 1987-1993. Obstet Gynecol 1998;92:945–50.

10. Hannah ME, Hannah WJ, Hewson SA, Hodnett ED, Saigal S, Willan AR. Planned caesarean section versus planned vaginal birth for breech presentation at term: a randomised multicentre trial. Term Breech Trial Collaborative Group. Lancet 2000;356:1375–83.

11. Mode of term singleton breech delivery. ACOG Committee Opinion No. 265. American College of Obstetricians and Gynecologists. Obstet Gynecol 2001;98:1189–90.

12. Hauth JC, Cunningham FG. Vaginal breech delivery is still justified. Obstet Gynecol 2002;99:1115–6.

13. Hofmyer GJ, Kulier R. External cephalic version for breech presentation at term (Cochrane Review). In: The Cochrane Library, Issue 3, 2004. Chichester, UK: John Wiley & Sons, Ltd.

14. Lavin JP Jr, Eaton J, Hopkins M. Teaching vaginal breech delivery and external cephalic version. A survey of faculty attitudes. J Reprod Med 2000;45:808–12.

External Cephalic Version

Although breech presentation complicates only 3–4% of all term pregnancies, it accounts for nearly 15% of cesarean deliveries. Moreover, rates of cesarean delivery for the indication of breech presentation reached 86.9% in 2002 (1). Vaginal delivery of the breech presentation at term has been associated with higher rates of perinatal morbidity and mortality than that of the vertex presentation (2). External cephalic version has become increasingly popular because of its relatively high success rates, markedly declining rates of vaginal breech delivery, and potential to decrease the overall rate of cesarean delivery. Findings of studies that have randomized patients to external cephalic version or standard management have shown significant decreases in the overall rate of cesarean delivery. Other nonrandomized studies have shown that external cephalic version is associated with significantly lower costs than strategies that do not include a version attempt (3, 4).

Due to the likelihood of spontaneous version, potential need for reversion, and concern for iatrogenic prematurity, external cephalic version is most commonly performed after 36 weeks of gestation have been completed. A recent large randomized trial performed at 25 centers in 7 countries, however, compared outcomes in women with a singleton breech fetus who underwent either early external cephalic version (34–36 weeks of gestation) or external cephalic version at 37–38 weeks of gestation (5). Statistically significant differences in the rate of noncephalic presentation at birth in the early external cephalic version group were found (56.9% versus 66.4%, P = .09, RR 0.86, 95% CI, 0.70–1.05). Although repeat external cephalic version procedures were allowed, the rate of serious fetal complications and the rate of preterm birth at less than 37 weeks of gestation were not significantly increased in the early external cephalic version group (5).

External cephalic version can be chosen for patients who present with either a breech or transverse fetal lie. If the diagnosis is in doubt after performing either Leopold's maneuvers or pelvic examination, ultrasonography may be used to confirm the fetal presentation. Suggested criteria for performing external cephalic version include the following:

- Singleton gestation
- Reactive nonstress test prior to the procedure and before discharge
- Absence of contraindications:
  —Evidence of uteroplacental insufficiency
  —Significant third-trimester vaginal bleeding
  —Uterine malformations
  —Maternal cardiac disease
  —Uncontrolled hypertension
  —Placenta previa
  —Prior classical cesarean delivery

Limited data with regard to success rates or complications exist for the following clinical scenarios; therefore, these may be considered relative contraindications for external cephalic version:

- Suspected IUGR or fetal macrosomia
- Major fetal anomaly
- Oligohydramnios (amniotic fluid index <5 cm)
- Prior cesarean delivery or other uterine scar
- Rupture of membranes
- Early or active labor

External cephalic version involves elevating the fetus out of the maternal bony pelvis and gently guiding the fetus in a forward roll or a backward flip into a cephalic presentation. Informed consent, involving explanation of the potential benefits, risks, and alternatives, should be obtained from all patients before performing external cephalic version. The average success rate associated with external cephalic version is nearly 60%, but ranges from 35% to 86% (3). Although studies have noted increased success rates among multiparous patients, nulliparity should not be considered a contraindication (6). Other factors that have been clearly shown to be correlated with successful external cephalic version success rates have included transverse or oblique lie and advanced cervical dilatation. Conflicting information exists in the literature with regard to whether other factors may influence external cephalic version, such as amniotic fluid volume, the location of the placenta, maternal weight, fetal weight, unengaged presenting part, and the ease with which the fetal head can be palpated.

During the procedure, evaluation of the FHR should be intermittently performed either by ultrasonographic visualization or external Doppler assessment. Persistent fetal bradycardia, significant patient discomfort, and inability to alter fetal presentation despite several attempts should be considered as endpoints for discontinuing external cephalic version attempts.

No data exist to support the concept that immediate labor induction after successful external cephalic version will decrease the rate of reversion. If spontaneous rupture of membranes or labor ensue after external cephalic version, oxytocin augmentation can be considered.

After the procedure has been completed, whether successful or not, maternal and fetal monitoring should continue until fetal well-being has been established and labor has been ruled out. Anti-D immune globulin may be ordered for patients who are Rh D negative. After successful version, if the fetus has been subsequently found to be in a noncephalic presentation, repeated attempts at external cephalic version may be considered.

External cephalic version has been associated with a low incidence of immediate or delayed complications, such as placental abruption, uterine rupture, fetal or maternal hemorrhage, compound presentation, isoimmunization, transient fetal bradycardias, nonreassuring FHR patterns, and even fetal death (7). Because of the small risk of complications, it is recommended that external cephalic version be attempted in settings in which cesarean delivery services (including anesthesia and operating rooms) are readily available.

Clinicians may administer tocolytics before performing external cephalic version. Examples of tocolytics that have been employed include subcutaneous terbutaline, ritodrine, and sublingual nitroglycerin (3). There is, however, conflicting information in the literature about whether such practice actually improves the rate of successful external cephalic version. The main value of prophylactic tocolysis may be for the nulliparous patient undergoing external cephalic version. In a similar fashion, randomized trials evaluating the effect of regional anesthesia (either spinal or epidural) have reported inconsistent findings (8, 9). There is, therefore, no clear evidence to recommend the routine administration of regional anesthesia before external cephalic version; its use may be considered for patients who are unable to tolerate the discomfort of external cephalic version or in whom cesarean delivery is likely if external cephalic version is unsuccessful.

References

1. Martin JA, Hamilton BE, Sutton PD, Ventura SJ, Menacker F, Munson ML. Births: final data for 2002. Natl Vital Stat Rep 2003;52(10):1–113.

2. Hannah ME, Hannah WJ, Hewson SA, Hodnett ED, Saigal S, Willan AR. Planned caesarean section versus planned vaginal birth for breech presentation at term: a randomised multicentre trial. Term Breech Trial Collaborative Group. Lancet 2000;356:1375–83.

3. American College of Obstetricians and Gynecologists. External cephalic version. ACOG Practice Bulletin 13. Washington, DC: ACOG; 2000.

4. Mauldin JG, Mauldin PD, Feng TI, Adams EK, Durkalski VL. Determining the clinical efficacy and cost savings of successful external cephalic version. Am J Obstet Gynecol 1996;175:1639–44.

5. Hutton EK, Kaufman K, Hodnett E, Amankwah K, Hewson SA, McKay D, et al. External cephalic version beginning at 34 weeks' gestation versus 37 weeks' gestation: a randomized multicenter trial. Am J Obstet Gynecol 2003;189: 245–54.

6. Aisenbrey GA, Catanzarite VA, Nelson C. External cephalic version: predictors of success. Obstet Gynecol 1999;94: 783–6.

7. Ghidini A, Korker V. Fetal complication after external cephalic version at term: case report and literature review. J Matern Fetal Med 1999;8:190–2.

8. Dugoff L, Stamm CA, Jones OW 3rd, Mohling SI, Hawkins JL. The effect of spinal anesthesia on the success rate of external cephalic version: a randomized trial. Obstet Gynecol 1999;93:345–9.

9. Mancuso KM, Yancey MK, Murphy JA, Markenson GR. Epidural analgesia for cephalic version: a randomized trial. Obstet Gynecol 2000;95:648–51.

Shoulder Dystocia

Shoulder dystocia is an infrequent but potentially catastrophic obstetric emergency that complicates 0.2–3% of all vaginal deliveries (1). Shoulder dystocia represents the failure of delivery of the fetal shoulder(s), whether it be the anterior or posterior shoulder. Shoulder dystocia results from a size discrepancy between the fetal shoulders and the pelvic inlet. A persistent anterior–posterior orientation of the fetal shoulders at the pelvic brim occurs when there is increased resistance between the fetal skin and vaginal walls, with a large fetal chest relative to the biparietal diameter, and when normal truncal rotation does not occur (as occurs in precipitous labor). Shoulder dystocia also can result from impaction of the posterior fetal shoulder on the maternal sacral promontory.

Most practicing obstetricians have employed a clinical definition for shoulder dystocia to include those deliveries that require ancillary obstetric maneuvers (in addition to gentle downward traction on the fetal head) to effect delivery of the fetal shoulders. Several studies have added the component of time in an attempt to establish an objective definition for shoulder dystocia. Although investigators in these studies have defined shoulder dystocia as a lapse of more than 60 seconds between delivery of the fetal head and delivery of the body, these criteria have had limited application in the clinical setting (2).

It has been shown that the percentages of births complicated by shoulder dystocia increase as birth weight increases. For example, 5.2% of infants weighing 4,000–4,250 g who had unassisted births not complicated by diabetes mellitus experienced shoulder dystocia, compared with 21.1% for those infants weighing 4,750–5,000 g (3). It must be remembered, however, that approximately 40–60% of shoulder dystocias occur in infants weighing less than 4,000 g (4). From a prospective point of view, most prepregnancy and antepartum risk factors, such as previous delivery of a macrosomic infant, multiparity, excessive maternal weight gain, postterm gestation, and maternal obesity, have exceedingly poor predictive value for shoulder dystocia (4). Several risk factors, however, appear to merit special attention:

- Prior history of shoulder dystocia
- Pregestational or gestational diabetes mellitus

- Macrosomia in the current pregnancy
- Prolonged second stage
- Mid-pelvic operative vaginal delivery

Before the routine availability of ultrasonography, the term *fetal macrosomia* was applied to neonates whose birth weight exceeded either 4,000 or 4,500 g. Ultrasonographic estimation of fetal weight, performed either during the late third trimester or the intrapartum period, has been advocated to estimate the risk of shoulder dystocia via birth weight prediction. Late-pregnancy ultrasonography has been shown to display low sensitivity, exceedingly poor predictive value, decreasing accuracy with increasing birth weight, and an overall tendency to overestimate the birth weight. Studies have found that this technology's accuracy is no better than clinical palpation (Leopold maneuvers) or simply determining the parous woman's assessment of what she believes the infant will weigh (5). Induction of labor due to suspected or impending fetal macrosomia is common in the obstetric community. A prospective randomized study, involving patients who were not diabetic and with ultrasonographic fetal weight estimation of 4,000–4,500 g, has shown that this policy does not alter the incidence of shoulder dystocia (6). Retrospective case–control studies have likewise revealed an increased risk of cesarean delivery among patients undergoing such inductions. The concept of prophylactic cesarean delivery, in which an estimated fetal weight threshold of 4,500 g was employed, has likewise not been supported by either clinical data or decision analysis. Despite such evidence, it is reasonable to consider offering prophylactic cesarean delivery for suspected fetal macrosomia with estimated fetal weights greater than 5,000 g in women without diabetes and greater than 4,500 g in women with diabetes (5).

Shoulder dystocia usually is heralded by the classic "turtle sign"; after the fetal head is delivered, it retracts back tightly against the maternal perineum. Under these circumstances, some clinicians have empirically advocated immediately proceeding to delivery of the fetal shoulders to maintain the forward momentum of the fetus. Others support a short delay in delivery of the shoulders, arguing that the endogenous rotational mechanics of the second stage may spontaneously alleviate the obstruction. Patients should be instructed to stop pushing after initial recognition of the shoulder dystocia; maternal expulsive efforts will be subsequently reinstituted after maneuver(s) have converted the fetal shoulders to the oblique diameter. Additional assistance may be provided by summoning other obstetricians, an anesthetist or anesthesiologist, additional nursing support, and a pediatrician.

When faced with shoulder dystocia, most providers will employ the McRoberts maneuver, or suprapubic pressure, or both because of ease of implementation, relatively high success rate (approximately 40%), and involvement of only maternal manipulation (4). Consisting of exaggerated hyperflexion of maternal thighs upon the abdomen, the McRoberts maneuver does not change the actual dimensions of the maternal pelvis. Rather, it relieves shoulder dystocia via marked cephalad rotation of the symphysis pubis and by flattening the sacrum (7). Because McRoberts maneuver has many potential benefits, its prophylactic administration when faced with suspected fetal macrosomia or among patients deemed to be at increased risk for shoulder dystocia has been suggested. The prophylactic administration of McRoberts maneuver and suprapubic pressure, however, has not been shown to significantly shorten head-to-body delivery times (8).

Many cases of shoulder dystocia require the performance of several maneuvers to alleviate the impaction. There have been no randomized controlled trials or laboratory experiments that have directly compared these techniques. Therefore, not only is there no generally accepted standard sequence of maneuvers, but there is no evidence that any one maneuver for shoulder dystocia is superior to another with regard to rates of successful alleviation. Direct fetal manipulation techniques used to alleviate shoulder dystocia are not associated with an increased rate of bone fracture or brachial plexus injury (9). As shoulder dystocia is considered to be a "bony dystocia," episiotomy alone will not release the impacted shoulder. The need for cutting a generous episiotomy or proctoepisiotomy must therefore be based on clinical circumstances and operator judgment, such as allowing the fetal rotational maneuvers to be performed with ease or creating more room for attempted delivery of the posterior arm (10).

Other reported techniques employed in shoulder dystocia management are listed in Box 28. In the Woods

---

BOX 28

Maneuvers for the Alleviation of Shoulder Dystocia

- Maternal hip hyperflexion (McRoberts maneuver)
- Suprapubic pressure
- Rotational maneuvers
  - Woods maneuver
  - Rubin maneuver
- Delivery of the posterior arm (Barnum maneuver)
- "All fours" (Gaskin maneuver)
- Cephalic replacement
  - Zavanelli maneuver
  - Modified Zavanelli maneuver
- Symphysiotomy
- Abdominal rescue through hysterotomy

corkscrew maneuver, the practitioner attempts to abduct the posterior shoulder and rotate the fetus through a 180 degree arc by exerting pressure onto the anterior surface of the posterior shoulder (Fig. 24). The Rubin maneuver involves application of pressure to the posterior surface of the most accessible part of the fetal shoulder (usually the anterior shoulder) thereby effecting shoulder adduction (Fig. 25). By replacing the bisacromial diameter with the axillo-acromial diameter, posterior arm delivery creates a

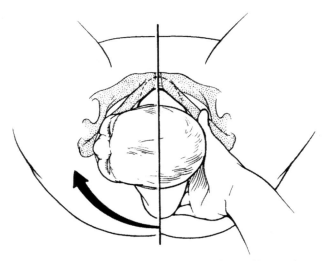

■ FIG. 24. The Woods maneuver is performed by applying pressure on the anterior surface of the posterior shoulder (shown here is a modification, in that the hand is placed on the posterior surface), with rotation of the fetus through a 180 degree arc. A reverse rotation, after the obstruction has been cleared, "corkscrews" the fetus out of the birth canal. (Cunningham FG, MacDonald PC, Gant NF, Leveno KJ, Gilstrap LC III, Hankins GD, editors. Williams obstetrics. 20th ed. Stamford [CT]: Appleton & Lange; 1997. Copyright The McGraw-Hill Companies.)

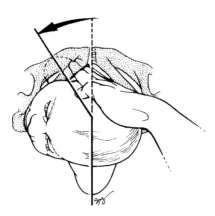

■ FIG. 25. The Rubin maneuver attempts to reduce antero-posterior shoulder dimensions by applying pressure to the posterior surface of the shoulder. (Cunningham FG, MacDonald PC, Gant NF, Leveno KJ, Gilstrap LC III, Hankins GD, editors. Williams obstetrics. 20th ed. Stamford [CT]: Appleton & Lange; 1997. Copyright The McGraw-Hill Companies.)

20% reduction in shoulder diameter (10). To perform this, pressure should be applied by the delivering provider at the antecubital fossa to flex the fetal forearm. The arm subsequently is swept out over the infant's chest and delivered over the perineum (Fig. 26).

One also may consider using the "all-fours" technique, in which the patient is rolled from her existing position onto her hands and knees. Fundal pressure as a maneuver to alleviate shoulder dystocia should be discouraged because it simply duplicates a maternal directional expulsive force that has already failed to deliver the fetal shoulders. In addition, fundal pressure has been associated with uterine rupture, Erb's palsy, and thoracic spinal cord injury in the neonate (1).

Intractable shoulder dystocias may warrant the performance of cephalic replacement, with or without subsequent cesarean delivery (Zavanelli maneuver and its modification). In the original Zavanelli maneuver, the head is rotated back to a prerestitution position, gently flexed, and then pushed back into the vagina with constant firm pressure. Tocolytic agents to relax the uterus may be useful in preparation for or during this maneuver. Other reported, but very rarely performed, techniques include symphysiotomy, intentional fetal clavicular fracture, and hysterotomy or abdominal rescue. Performance of these maneuvers will be complicated by the provider's lack of clinical experience and performance under emergent conditions.

Reported maternal complications related to shoulder dystocia have included third- or fourth-degree perineal lacerations, postpartum hemorrhage, vaginal or cervical lacerations, and symphyseal separation with lateral femoral cutaneous neuropathy. Self-limiting neonatal complications include clavicular and humeral fracture, which occur in approximately 5–10% and 7%, respectively, of shoulder dystocia cases (4). Risks to the delivery provider mainly involve litigation because shoulder dystocia accounts for a significant proportion of obstetrically related lawsuits. These medical–legal claims mainly involve Erb–Duchenne (C5 through C6) palsy or Klumpke's (C8 through T1) palsy because transient brachial plexus injury occurs in 15–20% of shoulder dystocias. Fortunately, most of these neurologic injuries resolve over time and have an estimated rate of persistence of 1–5%. Other reported neonatal complications have included a 5-minute Apgar score of less than 7 (4–12%), hypoxia/ischemia, permanent central neurologic injury, and death (0.4–1.8%) (9).

References

1. Shoulder dystocia. ACOG Practice Bulletin No. 40. American College of Obstetricians and Gynecologists. Obstet Gynecol 2002;100:1045–50.

2. Beall MH, Spong C, McKay J, Ross MG. Objective definition of shoulder dystocia: a prospective evaluation. Am J Obstet Gynecol 1998;179:934–7.

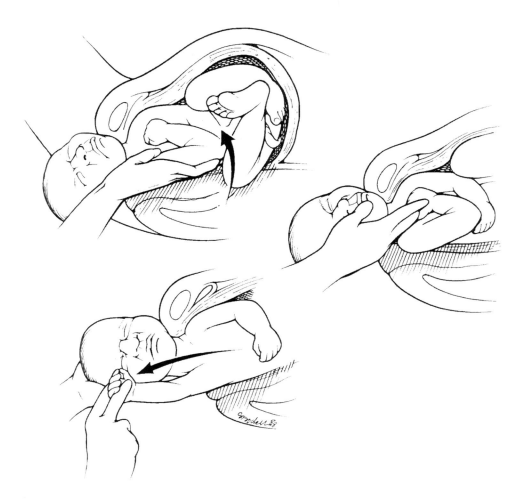

■ FIG. 26. Delivery of the posterior arm disrupts the anteroposterior alignment of the fetal shoulders. (Cunningham FG, MacDonald PC, Gant NF, Leveno KJ, Gilstrap LC III, Hankins GD, editors. Williams obstetrics. 20th ed. Stamford [CT]: Appleton & Lange; 1997. Copyright The McGraw-Hill Companies.)

3. Nesbitt TS, Gilbert WM, Herrchen B. Shoulder dystocia and associated risk factors with macrosomic infants born in California. Am J Obstet Gynecol 1998;179:476–80.

4. Gherman RB. Shoulder dystocia: an evidence-based evaluation of the obstetric nightmare. Clin Obstet Gynecol 2002; 45:345–62.

5. American College of Obstetricians and Gynecologists. Fetal macrosomia. ACOG Practice Bulletin 22. Washington, DC: ACOG; 2000.

6. Gonen O, Rosen DJ, Dolfin Z, Tepper R, Markow S, Fejgin MD. Induction of labor versus expectant management in macrosomia: a randomized study. Obstet Gynecol 1997; 89:913–7.

7. Gherman RB, Tramont J, Muffley P, Goodwin TM. Analysis of McRoberts' maneuver by X-ray pelvimetry. Obstet Gynecol 2000;95:43–7.

8. Beall MH, Spong CY, Ross MG. A randomized controlled trial of prophylactic maneuvers to reduce head-to-body delivery time in patients at risk for shoulder dystocia. Obstet Gynecol 2003;102:31–5.

9. Gherman RB, Ouzounian JG, Goodwin TM. Obstetrical maneuvers for shoulder dystocia and associated fetal morbidity. Am J Obstet Gynecol 1998;178:1126–30.

10. Poggi SH, Spong CY, Allen RH. Prioritizing posterior arm delivery during severe shoulder dystocia. Obstet Gynecol 2003;101:1068–72.

Fetal and Neonatal Injuries

Injuries that occur most often during birth include soft tissue injuries, lacerations, and fractures. Soft tissue injuries typically are identified over the presenting part and are more common with prolonged labor and the use of forceps or vacuum extraction. Early findings include localized erythema and abrasions; ecchymosis may occur later, depending on the extent of injury. Ecchymosis may be the only finding in the case of a preterm or precipitous delivery. Depending on the degree of bruising, other sequelae, such as anemia and hyperbilirubinemia, may be identified. Petechiae are common findings around the infant's head, neck, chest, and back. Although petechiae may herald a significant underlying problem, such as infection or a hemorrhagic disorder, more often they result from sudden changes in vascular pressure, such as that occurring with a tight nuchal cord or rapid expansion of the chest cavity as the neonate exits the birth canal. None of these conditions require active pediatric intervention. Affected areas should be kept clean with the expectation of spontaneous resolution within several days. Occasionally, serial hematocrits or bilirubin levels are monitored because of concerns that a significant hemorrhage has occurred.

Lacerations are sometimes identified on the cheek, forehead, jaw, occiput, shoulder, back, or buttock. These may be accidentally caused with placement of a scalp electrode, during fetal scalp pH sampling, or at the time of cesarean delivery when the lower uterine segment is sharply entered. A significant correlation between cesarean-related fetal laceration injury and nonvertex presentation has been found (1). Attempts should be made to reapproximate the wound edges with a superficial injury; deeper lacerations may require hemostasis and a layered closure.

Because the neonatal head is a common site for soft tissue injury, several specific conditions have been defined. Caput succedaneum is a finding characterized by a nondistinct area of swelling over the presenting portion of the fetal head, giving the newborn's head an oblong shape (along with molding) for the first few days of life. This entity may extend across cranial suture lines, which distinguishes it from a cephalohematoma. This latter condition occurs in 0.2–2.5% of live births and is secondary to laceration of subperiosteal vessels (2). Usually, a cephalohematoma is limited to a single cranial bone and has sharply demarcated margins at the edge of a suture line. Mechanical pressure to the fetal head is the implied etiology. An uncommon concomitant finding may be a linear, nondepressed skull fracture. No specific treatment is needed for an uncomplicated cephalohematoma. Most will spontaneously resolve in several weeks to months.

An even less common type of injury (occurring in approximately 4 of every 10,000 deliveries) is a subgaleal hemorrhage. A blood collection is identified between the galea aponeurosis and the periosteum of the skull. Because this area of loose connective tissue can accommodate a relatively large volume of blood, the neonate may present with signs of anemia or central nervous system depression. Early recognition is critical, given the very high morbidity and the mortality of approximately 25% that are associated with this condition. Since the issuance of a public health advisory by the FDA in 1998, there has been a marked increase in the reporting of this complication (3). A recent study using a large California database found that those infants delivered by vacuum extraction had a significantly higher rate of subdural or cerebral hemorrhage (odds ratio, 2.7, 95% CI, 1.9–3.9) (4).

Skull fractures are uncommon because the lack of complete mineralization of the newborn cranial bones makes them more pliable. Skull fractures should be considered with any significant soft tissue finding such as a cephalohematoma. They can sometimes be identified by palpation, although more commonly the diagnosis is established by radiography.

Two types of fractures have been characterized: linear and depressed. Both types have been described with spontaneous and instrumented deliveries, and the latter has been described with cesarean delivery. Uncomplicated linear fractures do not require treatment. However, when there is evidence of cerebrospinal fluid leakage, neurosurgical consultation should be obtained and antimicrobial therapy initiated to reduce the risk of infection. Small depressed fractures ("ping-pong" fractures) can simply be observed; larger fractures or those associated with neurologic symptoms require immediate surgical intervention. The prognosis is generally good for simple linear fractures. Depressed fractures that are identified and treated early tend to do well. Injuries that are more extensive or associated with neurologic findings carry a more guarded prognosis.

Clavicular fracture is the most common neonatal bone injury, complicating 2–3 of every 1,000 live births (5). Clavicular fracture may be associated with 3.6–9.5% of all shoulder dystocia cases; in addition, approximately one third of brachial plexus palsies are associated with a concomitant bone fracture, most commonly the clavicle (94%) (6). Many of these fractures go undetected until the newborn period, when decreased movement, deformity, or ecchymosis over the site of injury is noted. An absent Moro (startle) reflex on the affected side and crepitus with palpation also are suggestive of clavicular fracture. Most of these are greenstick fractures, although complete disruption can occur. The definitive diagnosis is established with radiography. Treatment includes pain management and immobilization of the associated arm, with an excellent prognosis for complete recovery.

The humerus is the second most common neonatal bone fracture. Typical preceding events include delivery of extended arms in a breech extraction or attempted delivery of the posterior fetal arm in an attempt to alleviate shoulder dystocia. Fractures, greenstick or complete, commonly occur in the diaphysis. Findings on physical examination of humeral injuries are similar to those of clavicular injuries: X-ray of the affected area is diagnostic. Healing is well advanced by the third week after immobilization. Fracture of the femur is much less common than the aforementioned injuries and is commonly associated with breech deliveries. The deformity is usually obvious, as is evidence of neonatal discomfort and lack of mobility. Traction–suspension casting is recommended until an adequate callus has formed.

Joint dislocations associated with birth are uncommon. Those involving the hip or knee more typically result from intrauterine positional conditions or congenital malformation. Occasionally, an extremity fracture through the epiphyseal plate is diagnosed incorrectly as a joint dislocation because it is difficult to see the poorly mineralized epiphysis on X-ray. Epiphyseal separations can occur with pulling on an extremity during an obstructed delivery. The presence of pain with motion or direct palpation should suggest this latter diagnosis. The distinction is rather important because additional diagnostic or interventional modalities may be needed to correct epiphyseal injury.

Facial nerve palsy usually results from pressure over the stylomastoid foramen, where the nerve exits the skull. Forceps-assisted delivery is associated with a higher occurrence of this injury. Facial nerve trauma also can occur during spontaneous vaginal delivery. The presumed etiology is prolonged pressure exerted by the sacral promontory. The reported incidence is approximately 0.6 per 1,000 live births and 0.7 per 1,000 liveborn cephalic singletons delivered vaginally (7). Evidence of injury may be present at birth or may be delayed until the first or second day of life. Characteristic findings on the affected side include obliteration of the nasolabial fold, inability to close the eyelid, and drooping of the corner of the mouth. Therapy should be directed toward protecting the eye from drying. Central nervous system origins for the palsy should be differentiated from peripheral nerve origins. Most traumatic facial nerve injuries resolve spontaneously over days to weeks. Other cranial nerves have the potential for injury either by direct trauma, from compression due to local tissue hemorrhage and edema, or from fracture of surrounding bony structures. These usually are identified during a routine newborn physical examination.

Injuries to the brachial plexus can result in paralysis of the muscles of the upper extremity. The overall incidence of brachial plexus palsy is 1.6 per 1,000 births. With shoulder dystocia, brachial plexus palsy is relatively common (12.7–21.4%), but the risk of permanent brachial plexus is very rare (1.6%). Several forms of nerve injury have been recognized: 1) Erb–Duchenne palsy (C5–C7) involving the upper arm; 2) Klumpke palsy (C8–T1) involving the lower arm and fingers; and 3) complete paralysis of the upper extremity (8). With involvement of the first thoracic root, disruption of sympathetic nerve fibers can lead to a concomitant ipsilateral Horner's syndrome (ptosis, miosis, and enophthalmos). Lesions at the C3 through C5 levels can result in phrenic nerve impairment. With complete paralysis, the physical examination demonstrates a flaccid arm with absent reflexes and various levels of sensory deficits. The diagnostic evaluation should rule out central nervous system lesions and local musculoskeletal abnormalities.

In the past, textbooks have stated (without evidence) that brachial plexus palsy is caused by the application of excessive lateral traction on the fetal head and neck during delivery in the presence of shoulder dystocia. Over the past several years, multiple lines of evidence have

emerged that have supported the concept that most brachial plexus palsies are not caused by the accoucheur (9, 10). This opinion is based on several findings: 1) more than 50% of cases of brachial plexus palsies are associated with uncomplicated vaginal deliveries; 2) brachial plexus palsy can occur in the posterior arm of infants whose anterior arm was impacted behind the symphysis pubis and can occur with atraumatic cesarean delivery; 3) there is no statistical correlation found between brachial plexus palsy and the experience of the obstetric provider nor the number and type of maneuvers used to alleviate shoulder dystocia; 4) rapid second-stage and disproportionate descent of the head and body of the fetus have also been implicated in the pathogenesis of the injury; and 5) mathematic and computer-simulated models have shown that maternal endogenous forces are far greater than clinician-applied exogenous delivery loads during a shoulder dystocia episode (6, 9–13).

Fortunately, spinal cord injuries are rare in the newborn and are most often associated with breech delivery. With the fetal head fixed in the uterus or pelvis, traction and hyperextension of the fetal trunk are the suggested mechanisms of injury. Spinal cord injuries have been reported with fetal version, brow and face presentations, shoulder dystocia, and in utero malpresentation. Depending on the level of injury, neonates may present as stillborns, moribund at birth with later development of profound respiratory depression, with early onset paraplegia, or with subtle late-onset neurologic spasticity.

Intraabdominal organ trauma is a very rare event but should be considered in any newborn presenting with unexplained anemia, abdominal distention, or shock. The liver is the most frequently injured organ; risk factors include breech presentation, large for gestational-age birth weights, and hepatomegaly or coagulation disorders. Rupture of the spleen, adrenal gland, and kidney also have been reported. Anomalous malformations in these organs predispose them to injury. Soft tissue injury to the external genitalia sometimes occurs, particularly in a breech delivery. These injuries are almost always self-limiting.

References

1. Smith JF, Hernandez C, Wax JR. Fetal laceration injury at cesarean delivery. Obstet Gynecol 1997;90:344–6.

2. Bofill JA, Rust OA, Devidas M, Roberts WE, Morrison JC, Martin JN Jr. Neonatal cephalohematoma from vacuum extraction. J Reprod Med 1997;42:565–9.

3. Ross MG, Fresquez M, El-Haddad MA. Effect of FDA advisory on reported vacuum-assisted delivery and morbidity. J Matern Fetal Med 2000;9:321–6.

4. Towner D, Castro MA, Eby-Wilkens E, Gilbert WM. Effect of mode of delivery in nulliparous women on neonatal intracranial injury. N Engl J Med 1999;341:1709–14.

5. Lam MH, Wong GY, Lao TT. Reappraisal of neonatal clavicular fracture: relationship between infant size and neonatal morbidity. Obstet Gynecol 2002;100:115–9.

6. Gherman RB. Shoulder dystocia: an evidence-based evaluation of the obstetric nightmare. Clin Obstet Gynecol 2002;45:345–62.

7. Perlow JH, Wigton T, Hart J, Strassner HT, Nageotte MP, Wolk BM. Birth trauma. A five year review of incidence and associated perinatal factors. J Reprod Med 1996;41: 754–60.

8. Gherman RB, Ouzounian JG, Satin AJ, Goodwin TM, Phelan JP. A comparison of shoulder dystocia-associated transient and permanent brachial plexus palsies. Obstet Gynecol 2003;102:544–8.

9. Gherman RB, Ouzounian JG, Goodwin TM. Brachial plexus palsy: an in utero injury? Am J Obstet Gynecol 1999;180:1303–7.

10. Sandmire HF, DeMott RK. Erb's palsy: concepts of causation. Obstet Gynecol 2000;95:941–2.

11. Shoulder dystocia. ACOG Practice Bulletin No. 40. American College of Obstetricians and Gynecologists. Obstet Gynecol 2002;100:1045–50.

12. Gonik B, Walker A, Grimm M. Mathematic modeling of forces associated with shoulder dystocia: a comparison of endogenous and exogenous sources. Am J Obstet Gynecol 2000;182:689–91.

13. Gonik B, Zhang N, Grimm MJ. Defining forces that are associated with shoulder dystocia: the use of a mathematic dynamic computer model. Am J Obstet Gynecol 2003; 188:1068–72.

FETAL DEATH

Fetal mortality is defined as the number of fetal deaths per 1,000 live births plus fetal deaths. (Throughout this chapter, fetal mortality is expressed by this number.) The recording of fetal death is controlled at the state level and through a collaboration, the CDC's National Vital Statistics System, has the most comprehensive source of U.S. data on fetal deaths of 20 weeks of gestation or greater. Several of the states record every pregnancy loss regardless of gestational age, but most use a lower limit of 20 weeks of gestation to define fetal death; some states also include fetal weight modifiers (1). In the United States, the incidence of fetal death has decreased for all races from 18.4 fetal deaths per 1,000 live births in 1950 to 6.5 in 2001. Although this represents a substantial decrease in fetal mortality, significant differences exist among maternal races (2).

The changing pattern of fetal death over the past 2 decades was evaluated in a nonreferred population at a tertiary center. The autopsy rate at that institution was 97% of fetal deaths, and the authors were able to explain the cause of death in almost 75% of cases. During the 20-year period studied, the number of fetal deaths due to isoimmunization and intrapartum asphyxia decreased to almost nonexistent levels, and intrauterine growth restriction decreased significantly. However, the number of unexplained fetal deaths, losses attributed to maternal

diabetes, and intrauterine infection remained relatively constant (3). Among the many possible causes of fetal loss, the most common are abruptio placentae, fetal growth restriction, lethal malformations, and intrauterine infection (see Box 29). Even though deaths attributed to growth restriction decreased by 60% at the tertiary center, SGA fetuses had a 10-fold increased risk of fetal death after correction was made for lethal anomalies. Intrauterine growth restriction was rarely noted among the SGA infants before death; this area represents a potentially preventable cause of fetal death. These findings have been confirmed by others (4). Medical risk factors associated with fetal death have been outlined by the National Center for Health Statistics. Although the figures probably represent an underestimate of the true incidence of associated maternal conditions and attributes, the data provide insights into population differences in the United States. Fig. 27 shows fetal mortality associated with various labor and delivery complications (5, 6).

Research on maternal smoking during pregnancy shows that fetal mortality is increased by 35%, from 7.2 in women who do not smoke to 9.7 in women who do smoke. Increasing the number of cigarettes smoked per day is like-

---

BOX 29

Possible Causes of Fetal Loss

- Abruptio placentae and other types of cord or placental complications
- Fetal anomaly or chromosomal anomalies
- Infection (syphilis, cytomegalovirus, parvovirus, listeria)
- Autoimmune disorder: antiphospholipid syndrome
- Fetal–maternal hemorrhage
- Isoimmunization
- Maternal medical conditions (eg, diabetes, hypertension, thyroid disorder)
- Multifetal pregnancy
  —Monoamniotic
  —Twin–twin transfusion
- Substance abuse
- Luteal phase defect
- Uterine anomalies or leiomyomas
- Incompetent cervix
- Teratogenic exposure
- Radiation
- Trauma
- Severe maternal illness
- Unexplained

wise associated with increasing fetal mortality in both black and white women. Alcohol use during pregnancy was associated with a fetal mortality of 13.3 per 1,000 live births, whereas fetal mortality was 7.5 among women who did not drink during pregnancy. Fetal mortality was 4 times higher among women who consumed 5 or more drinks weekly than among those who consumed 1 drink per week during pregnancy. The risk of fetal death was 3 times greater among black women who drank than among white women who drank (5).

The latency period (the interval between fetal death and delivery) is inversely proportional to gestational age at fetal loss. Spontaneous labor generally occurs within 2 weeks in 80–90% of cases of fetal death. A dead fetus poses little medical risk for the mother unless coagulopathy occurs (usually >4 weeks after fetal death). Weekly plasma fibrinogen levels may alert the clinician to clinically significant coagulopathy.

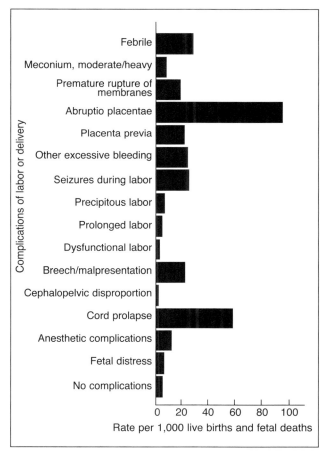

■ **FIG. 27.** Fetal mortality by selected complications of labor or delivery, 1989–1990. Data were analyzed from states with more than 80% compliance in completing the variables for prenatal care, birth weight, and method of delivery. This basic group of 29 states represented 61% of the fetal deaths during the 2 years studied. (Adapted from Hoyert DL. Medical and life-style risk factors affecting fetal mortality, 1989–90. Vital Health Stat 20. 1996;(31):1–32. Available at: http://www.cdc.gov/nchs/data/series/sr_20/sr20_031.pdf. Retrieved September 1, 2004.)

Labor may be induced with the use of oxytocin (high dose at estimated <24 weeks of gestation) and vaginal PGE$_2$ suppositories (at estimated <28 weeks of gestation). Other authors have reported success with intraamniotic PGF$_{2\alpha}$ and vaginal and oral misoprostol (7) at dosages higher than those used for induction, with fewer side effects. Although misoprostol has minimal effects and low cost, its use for induction of labor after fetal death has not been well documented in women with a uterine scar. Cesarean delivery should be avoided with late fetal death.

Every effort should be undertaken to determine the cause of fetal death. Accurate identification of an etiologic agent or process can be used to start the emotional healing process for the couple and to counsel them accurately about the risk of recurrence and the need for preconception or antenatal management in a subsequent pregnancy. Using a formal algorithm for evaluation, such as that provided in Appendix C, "Assessment of Fetal Death," will ensure that the search for the cause of death occurs in an orderly and systematic fashion. Research is under way to identify the optimal evaluation plan.

Careful review of the prenatal laboratory evaluation and record may be informative. Laboratory evaluation for all women should include a random glucose measurement, complete blood count with platelet count, maternal antibody screen, rapid plasma reagent or VDRL test, Kleihauer–Betke test, and urine toxicology sample. Selected patients may benefit from thyroid function tests, syphilis and additional serologic assessments, or lupus anticoagulant and anticardiolipin antibody screening. A carefully performed autopsy and placental examination (gross and microscopic) have been shown to significantly increase the probability of finding a cause for fetal death. Chromosomal analysis can be expensive but informative in cases of recurrent pregnancy losses, family or personal history of a fetal anomaly, malformations, growth restriction, or stigmata of aneuploidy. Chromosomal abnormalities also can be found in 6–12% of unselected stillbirths, a rate that is approximately 10 times higher than a baseline risk. Furthermore, detailed genetic studies for subtle chromosomal abnormalities may provide additional causes, such as telomere deletions. If intrauterine infection is suspected, careful culture of the maternal and fetal placental membrane surfaces may be helpful. The physician should document the status of the fetus and mother as well as other findings at delivery (Appendix C).

After careful evaluation, 25–50% of all fetal deaths remain unexplained. Couples with unexplained fetal deaths are likely to be more apprehensive during a subsequent pregnancy and require special support. Maternal assessment of fetal movement should begin at around 28 weeks of gestation. Some authors have recommended nonstress testing at 32 weeks of gestation, whereas others have suggested assessment beginning at least 1 week earlier than the gestational week at which the previous demise occurred. The timing of delivery depends on a combination of maternal anxiety, cervical ripeness, and the cause of the previous loss.

References

1. Martin JA, Hoyert DL. The national fetal death file. Semin Perinatol 2002;26:3–11.

2. DATA2010…the Healthy People 2010 Database - Jan 2004 Edition, 01/18/04, 8:08:44 pm. Focus area: 16:Maternal Infant and Child Health http://wonder.cdc.gov/scripts/broker.exe

3. Fretts RC, Boyd ME, Usher RH, Usher HA. The changing pattern of fetal death, 1961–1988. Obstet Gynecol 1992; 79:35–9.

4. Incerpi MH, Miller DA, Samadi R, Settlage RH, Goodwin TM. Stillbirth evaluation: what tests are needed? Am J Obstet Gynecol 1998;178:1121–5.

5. Hoyert DL. Medical and life-style risk factors affecting fetal mortality, 1989–90. Vital Health Stat 20 1996; (31): 1–32. Available at: http://www.cdc.gov/nchs/data/series/sr_20/sr20_031.pdf. Retrieved September 1, 2004.

6. Hoyert DL. Perinatal mortality in the United States, 1985–91. Vital Health Stat 20 1995;20(26):1–26. Available at: http://www.cdc.gov/nchs/data/series/sr-_20/sr20_026.pdf. Retrieved September 1, 2004.

7. Chittacharoen A, Herabutya Y, Punyavachira P. A randomized trial of oral and vaginal misoprostol to manage delivery in cases of fetal death. Obstet Gynecol 2003:101:70–3.

Surgical Complications in Pregnancy

From 0.5% to 2% of women require surgery during pregnancy. If diagnostic and therapeutic procedures are clearly indicated during pregnancy, they should be undertaken. The challenge is to make a prudent decision regarding the need for surgery and the appropriate approach to disease management. Adverse perinatal outcomes do not appear to be increased in the face of uncomplicated surgery or anesthesia; however, when complications arise, perinatal outcome may be affected adversely.

The largest report of anesthetic and surgical risks during pregnancy came from the Swedish Birth Registry for the years 1973–1981 (1). Nonobstetric surgery was performed on 5,405 of 720,000 pregnant women. Procedures were performed in all trimesters: 41% in the first trimester, 35% in the second trimester, and 24% in the third trimester. Abdominal surgery constituted 25% of procedures and gynecologic and urologic procedures made up another 16%. In this series, laparoscopy to rule out ectopic pregnancy was the most frequently performed procedure in the first trimester, and appendectomy was the most frequently performed procedure in the second trimester. When the authors compared the outcomes in these 5,405 pregnancies to the outcomes for the remainder of the 720,000 pregnancies in the registry, the rate of congenital malformations and stillbirths was not increased significantly. This observation is strengthened by the observation that commonly used anesthetic agents are not teratogenic (2). However, the Swedish study did document an increased occurrence of neonatal death within 7 days of surgery, low birth weight, and preterm delivery in the women who underwent surgery. These outcomes were thought to be secondary to the disease process that necessitated the surgical intervention rather than a direct effect of surgery or anesthesia.

LAPAROSCOPY

Over the past 2 decades, development of minimally invasive surgery using the laparoscope and the more widespread use of ultrasonography, CT, and MRI has revolutionized the clinical approach to patients who may require surgery, including pregnant women. The most commonly performed laparoscopic procedure in pregnant women is for diagnosis and treatment of ectopic pregnancy. In established pregnancies, cholecystectomy is the most commonly performed laparoscopic procedure (3).

Initial reassuring experience with laparoscopy in the first half of pregnancy has resulted in its use later in pregnancy for other indications, such as appendectomy, exploratory surgery, and adnexal surgery. A review of case series that included 518 women with established pregnancies who underwent laparoscopic surgery for such indications report good outcomes with regard to low birth weight, preterm labor, and low Apgar scores, but information on long-term outcomes is lacking (4).

Potential advantages to the laparoscopic approach to surgery in pregnancy include the following (5, 6):

1. Early mobilization, rapid postoperative recovery, and early return to normal activities, which can be very important because of the higher occurrence of DVT in pregnancy

2. Decreased postoperative morbidity

3. Small scars and few incisional hernias

4. Early return of gastrointestinal activity due to less manipulation of the bowel, which may result in fewer adhesions and less bowel obstruction

5. Low rate of fetal depression due to decreased pain and narcotic use

Disadvantages of the laparoscopic approach include the following:

1. Technical difficulty because of the gravid uterus

2. Possible injury to the gravid uterus

3. Potential decrease in uteroplacental blood flow because of increased intraabdominal pressure (Hypothetical risk, because maternal Valsalva, coughing, or straining maneuvers generate similar pressures.)

4. Effects of carbon dioxide or nitrous oxide pneumoperitoneum on the fetus unknown

The Society of American Gastrointestinal Endoscopic Surgeons recognizes that limited experience with surgery in pregnancy and laboratory data suggest caution when choosing the laparoscopic approach (7). They state, "Certain maneuvers must be routinely adopted in order to enhance operative safety." These include the following:

- When possible, operative intervention should be deferred until the second trimester, when fetal risk is lowest.

- Because pneumoperitoneum enhances lower extremity venous stasis already present in the pregnant patient, and because pregnancy induces a hypercoagulable state, pneumatic compression devices must be used.

- Fetal and uterine status, as well as maternal end tidal CO_2 and arterial blood gases, should be monitored.

171

- The uterus should be protected with a lead shield if intraoperative cholangiography is a possibility. Fluoroscopy should be used selectively.
- Given the enlarged uterus, abdominal access should be attained using an open technique.
- Dependent positioning should be used to shift the uterus off the inferior vena cava.
- Pneumoperitoneum pressures should be minimized (to 8–12 mm Hg) and not allowed to exceed 15 mm Hg.
- Obstetric consultation should be obtained preoperatively.

THE ACUTE ABDOMEN

Virtually all pregnant women experience abdominal pain to some degree. The pain usually results from a nonpathologic pregnancy-related cause, such as constipation or musculoskeletal pain (round ligament syndrome). However, it may be pathologic and pregnancy-related (ectopic pregnancy early in pregnancy; placental abruption late in pregnancy), or it may be pathologic and not related to the pregnancy. Fortunately, such surgical emergencies are infrequent. The most frequent cause of an acute surgical abdomen in pregnancy is appendicitis; less frequent causes include bowel obstruction and cholecystitis. The pregnant woman presents significant diagnostic dilemmas. Nausea, vomiting, and loss of appetite, common symptoms of an acute abdomen, are frequent pregnancy-related conditions. Early diagnosis of the surgical abdomen and aggressive treatment are the keys to optimal maternal and fetal outcomes.

Appendicitis

Nearly 1 in 1,000 pregnant women undergo appendectomy, and appendicitis is confirmed in two thirds of these cases (1 in nearly 1,500) (1). The physician is faced with a concern that unnecessary surgery may affect outcomes adversely and at the same time recalls Babler's admonition that "the mortality of appendicitis in pregnancy is the mortality of delay" (8). Diagnosing appendicitis in pregnancy can be a challenge. As the uterus enlarges, the appendix frequently rises with the cecum and rotates to a retrocecal position so that pain may occur in the flank, not in the right lower quadrant. Nausea, vomiting, and anorexia are common symptoms of appendicitis that also often occur in normal pregnancies. Leucocytosis is regularly encountered in normal pregnancy. Other diseases encountered in pregnancy may mimic characteristics of appendicitis, including renal colic, pyelonephritis, degeneration of a myoma, and placental abruption (Box 30) (3). Late in pregnancy, with the enlarged uterus shielding the abdominal wall and the appendix elevated and rotated toward the right flank, classic signs of peritonitis, including cervical motion, rectal tenderness, and rebound tenderness of the abdominal wall, may not be present or they may become prominent findings only late in the course of the disease when an abscess leaks or a viscus ruptures (9). As a result of these changes, and despite Babler's admonition, half of pregnant women with appendicitis have perforative appendicitis with generalized peritonitis (10), and deaths occasionally occur.

Persistent lower abdominal pain with tenderness is observed in 80% of pregnant women with appendicitis.

BOX 30

Conditions Mimicking Appendicitis

Nonobstetric

Pyelonephritis

Urinary calculi

Cholecystitis

Cholelithiasis

Bowel obstruction

Pancreatitis

Gastroenteritis

Acute mesenteric adenitis

Carcinoma of the large bowel

Rectus hematoma

External hernia

Ischemic mesenteric necrosis

Acute intermittent porphyria

Perforated duodenal ulcer

Pneumonia

Meckel's diverticulum

Tuberculous peritonitis

Obstetric/Gynecologic

Preterm labor

Abruptio placentae

Chorioamnionitis

Adnexal torsion

Ectopic/heterotopic pregnancy

Pelvic inflammatory disease

Round ligament pain

Uteroovarian vein rupture

Myomatous red degeneration

Rupture of uterine arteriovenous malformation

Uterine rupture (placenta percreta) (rudimentary uterine horn)

Sharp HT. The acute abdomen during pregnancy. Clin Obstet Gynecol 2002;45:405–13.

Most pregnant women with appendicitis are afebrile. Similar to nonpregnant patients in whom the diagnosis of appendicitis is considered, both graded compression ultrasonography and helical computed tomography have been used to assist in diagnosis during pregnancy. The ultrasonographic techniques have the limitation of being user-dependent and are unreliable in the third trimester. Helical CT shows greater promise and should be equally accurate in all 3 trimesters (3). Ultimately, in most cases the diagnosis of appendicitis in pregnancy will be made clinically.

If the diagnosis of appendicitis is seriously considered, immediate surgical exploration is warranted because rupture is so frequently encountered, and generalized peritonitis, besides putting the mother's life in danger, places the pregnancy at high risk for preterm labor and delivery with all of its attendant implications for the newborn. When surgery is undertaken early, a normal appendix may be found, but most experts agree that it is better to operate "unnecessarily" than to delay intervention until the pregnant woman has developed generalized peritonitis.

A growing body of evidence supports the safety of the laparoscopic approach to appendectomy in the first half of pregnancy (11). If laparotomy is to be performed, the incision should be made over the point of maximum tenderness on the patient's abdominal wall. If there is doubt about the diagnosis, the best approach is either through a right paramedian or vertical midline incision. In all cases, the patient should receive broad-spectrum antibiotics preoperatively, preferably a second-generation cephalosporin or semisynthetic penicillin. Antibiotics should be continued postoperatively if the appendix has ruptured or there is a periappendiceal abscess or other evidence of generalized peritonitis. In preparation for the procedure, the patient should be placed in the lateral tilt position; during the procedure, efforts should be made to maintain blood pressure in the normal range. Both of these maneuvers will optimize uterine blood flow. There is no evidence to demonstrate that continuous fetal heart rate monitoring during surgery improves outcomes, but it seems reasonable to consider its use if the patient is septic or in labor or if there is difficulty in maintaining her blood pressure.

Biliary Tract Disease

Biliary tract disease is most frequently caused by obstruction of the cystic duct, the pancreatic duct, or the common bile duct by gallstones. Symptomatic disease results in biliary colic, acute cholecystitis, jaundice, and acute pancreatitis. Biliary tract disease is the second most common surgical condition encountered in pregnancy after appendicitis. Surgery for these conditions complicates from 1 in 2,000 to 1 in 4,000 pregnancies.

By age 40 years, nearly 20% of women in the United States will have gallstones. Among these women, 1–2% per year undergo surgery for symptomatic disease. Cholecystectomy should not be performed for asymptomatic gallstones. In asymptomatic pregnant women, as many as 2.5–10% will have ultrasonographically detectable gallstones. Pregnancy is thought to increase the frequency of symptomatic gallstones because of progesterone's effect on biliary tract smooth muscle. Historically and by custom, initial episodes of biliary tract disease caused by stones had been treated medically with intravenous fluids, nasogastric suction, analgesia, and antibiotics. More recently, surgeons are beginning to advocate a more aggressive primary surgical approach, especially with the introduction of laparoscopic cholecystectomy.

This evolution in primary surgical treatment is applicable to the pregnant woman with symptomatic biliary tract disease. A consensus has developed that the pregnant patient should undergo cholecystectomy while still pregnant if conservative management fails during the initial admission, if symptoms recur upon resumption of oral intake, or if symptoms recur in the same trimester (12). Pregnant women treated medically require rehospitalization during pregnancy in more than half of cases. As many as 1 out of 3 will ultimately undergo cholecystectomy while still pregnant. Late in pregnancy, preterm labor is a significant complication in these patients, and cholecystectomy is technically more difficult to perform. Most recent reports cite better maternal and neonatal outcomes when a primary surgical approach is used (13). For all these reasons, at most major centers the pregnant woman with biliary disease caused by gallstones is treated surgically (9). In a review of 111 reported cases of laparoscopic cholecystectomy performed on pregnant women, fewer spontaneous abortions in the first trimester and a lower frequency of preterm labor in the third trimester were found with laparoscopic cholecystectomy than with the open approach. Reviewers concluded that the laparoscopic approach was safe throughout pregnancy (14).

In the nonobstetric population, approximately 45% of cases of acute pancreatitis are caused by gallstones and 35% by alcohol abuse. Less frequent causes or associated conditions include blunt abdominal trauma, abdominal surgery, connective tissue diseases, familial hypertriglyceridemia, and drugs, including diuretics, antihypertensives, and antibiotics. In marked contrast, during pregnancy gallstones are responsible for virtually all cases of acute pancreatitis.

Clinically, the presentation of acute pancreatitis is not altered by pregnancy, but when the patient presents in the third trimester, the differential diagnosis can include severe preeclampsia and fatty liver of pregnancy. Generally the patient presents with nausea, vomiting, and incapacitating epigastric pain that classically is said to radiate to the back. The patient is frequently febrile, appears ill, and is lying quietly in a fetal position. The abdomen is tender and diffusely tender with diminished to absent bowel sounds. Serum amylase can be elevated significantly (up to 3 times normal); modest elevations are seen with hepatic trauma, cholecystitis, bowel obstruction, and perforated duodenal ulcers. The patient may be hypocalcemic. The finding of elevated serum lipase may contribute to the diagnosis (Table 28). The cornerstones of management include intravenous hydration with careful electrolyte management, correction of any hypocalcemia and hyperglycemia, analgesics, and restriction of oral intake, with nasogastric suction in severe cases. Patients with fever should be treated with broad-spectrum antibiotics (15). Patients with respiratory insufficiency, shock, need for massive colloid replacement, or whose serum calcium is less than 8 mg/dL are best served by management in an intensive care setting because combinations of these findings are associated with mortality in up to 70% of cases (9).

ADNEXAL MASSES

The traditional teaching in obstetrics is that pregnant women with adnexal masses of 6 cm or greater should undergo surgery. Removal of the ovarian cyst was indicated for 3 reasons: danger of torsion, risk of malignancy, and possible obstruction of labor; these concerns continue to be applicable. The optimal time for surgery was thought to be in the second trimester, when the risk of abortion was very low and the pregnancy did not depend on a functioning corpus luteum.

Before the development of ultrasonography, adnexal masses were diagnosed by clinical examination in approximately 1 in 600 pregnancies; 3–6% of masses were malignant. In more recent studies with variable access to ultrasonography and with variation in the size of the mass included in the study, adnexal masses are diagnosed in 1 in 100 to 1 in 600 pregnancies, and from 3% to 13% are malignant or borderline tumors. Despite newer imaging technologies, in 5–10% of cases the adnexal mass is a leiomyoma. In a 12–year experience from North Carolina, adnexal masses were found in 1 in 750 pregnancies, were generally diagnosed in the second trimester, and half of the masses were benign cystic ter-

atomas. Among the 13% of masses that were malignant, two thirds were of low malignant potential (16). Earlier investigators estimated that up to 15% of adnexal masses underwent torsion in pregnancy. In contrast, another study found that when adnexal masses diagnosed using ultrasonography were followed expectantly, 2.3% (3 of 123) developed symptomatic torsion and none experienced obstruction of labor.

When masses were diagnosed in the first trimester, about 90% of mobile unilateral noncomplex cysts smaller that 5 cm and 36% of similar cysts larger than 5 cm will resolve spontaneously. Thus, it is reasonable to observe these nonsuspicious masses until the second trimester and plan surgery electively. Women who undergo emergency laparotomy for adnexal masses have poorer pregnancy outcomes than do those undergoing elective surgery (17). A straightforward protocol for the management of adnexal masses in pregnancy is shown in Figure 28 (17). Whether to approach these masses using laparoscopy or open laparotomy depends on the size of the mass, the level of suspicion for malignancy, the length of gestation, and the skills of the surgeon.

TRAUMA

Approximately two thirds of all traumas during pregnancy result from motor vehicle accidents. Other leading causes of trauma in pregnancy include falls, direct assaults to the abdomen, and gunshot wounds. In the United States, domestic violence has emerged as a major cause of trauma in pregnancy, with a prevalence of 1–7% (18). In urban inner-city environments across the United States, that prevalence is reported to range from 7% to 20%, and 60% of these women report 2 or more episodes of physical assault during their pregnancy (19).

Accidental or intentional trauma is a leading cause of mortality in reproductive-aged women. In many parts of the United States, injury-related deaths are the leading causes of nonobstetric maternal mortality (20). Fetal losses resulting from trauma can only be estimated. Extrapolations from case series suggest that 1,300 to 3,900

TABLE 28. Selected Laboratory Values in 43 Pregnant Women With Pancreatitis

Value	Pancreatitis		Normal
	Mean	Range	
Amylase (IU/L)	1,392	111–4,560	30–110
Lipase (IU/L)	6,929	36–41,842	23–208
Total bilirubin (mg/dL)	1.7	0.1–4.9	0.2–1.3
Aspartate transferase (U/L)	120	11–498	3–35
Leucocytes (per μL)	12,000	7,000–14,500	4,100–10,900

Reprinted from Am J Obstet Gynecol, Vol. 173. Ramin KD, Ramin SM, Richey SD, Cunnungham FG. Acute pancreatitis in pregnancy. p. 187–91. Copyright 1995, with permission from Elsevier.

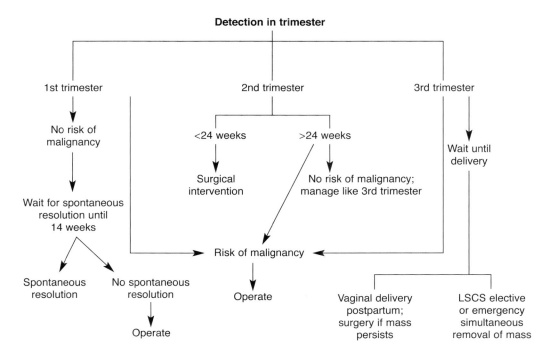

FIG. 28. Proposed protocol to manage adnexal mass during pregnancy. LSCS indicates lower segment cesarean delivery. (Archives of Gynecology and Obstetrics. Management and outcome of pregnancies complicated with adnexal masses. Agarwal N, Parul, Kriplani A, Bhatia N, Gupta A. Vol. 267, p. 151, Fig. 1, 2003. Copyright © Springer-Verlag.)

pregnancies are lost as a result of trauma. Life-threatening maternal trauma is reported to be associated with a 40–50% fetal loss rate, whereas less life-threatening trauma may be associated with a 1–5% loss rate (21). Placental abruption is the direct cause of fetal death in 50% of cases.

Pregnancy is associated with different mechanisms of injury than those found in nonpregnant women. Gestational age at the time of injury affects the pattern of maternal injury and affects the need to assess the fetal condition acutely. As pregnancy advances and the uterus rises out of the pelvis and rises in the abdomen, the uterus functions as a shield protecting the large bowel and great vessels from low abdominal trauma. At the same time, as the small bowel is displaced to the upper abdomen, trauma to the upper abdomen or trauma that displaces the gravid uterus cephalad results in a greater risk of hepatic and splenic rupture and retroperitoneal hematomas. The abdominal wall, uterine myometrium, and amniotic sac serve as buffers to afford a considerable degree of protection to the fetus from direct traumatic injury. In less than 1% of cases, blunt abdominal trauma results in fetal injury. However, indirect injury can occur from rapid compression, deceleration shearing force, or contrecoup effect, all having the potential to cause placental abruption. Although up to 40% of cases of severe maternal blunt trauma may be associated with placental abruption, even minor abdominal trauma is associated with abruption in 2–3% of cases. Uterine rupture infrequently is associated with blunt abdominal trauma. When it occurs it is usually associated with severe and direct trauma to the uterus (21).

Penetrating trauma is most commonly the consequence of gunshot or stab wounds. Depending on uterine size, the rest of the abdominal viscera are relatively protected from penetrating injury. Maternal outcomes are generally better in pregnant women than in nonpregnant individuals with similar injuries. At the same time, the likelihood of uterine injury is increased, resulting in a very high rate of fetal mortality caused by direct injury or by injury of the placenta or umbilical cord.

Management of the injured pregnant woman is directed initially at primary assessment and resuscitation of the mother followed by assessment of the fetus before conducting a secondary survey of the mother. If assessment of the fetus occurs too early in the process and before the mother is stabilized, serious or life-threatening maternal injuries may be overlooked, and clinical circumstances that can result in poor fetal oxygenation (maternal hypoxia, hypovolemia, or supine hypotension) may be ignored. The primary survey and resuscitation of the mother begins with assurance of a functioning airway, adequate ventilation, effective circulation, and an adequate circulatory volume (Fig. 29). Guidelines for airway and ventilatory management are the same as for the nonpregnant trauma patient.

A very important aspect of management is deflection of the gravid uterus from the great vessels by placing the woman in the lateral decubitus position. This simple maneuver maximizes cardiac output and ameliorates the shock state. Because maternal intravascular volume can increase by 25% through the early third trimester, the

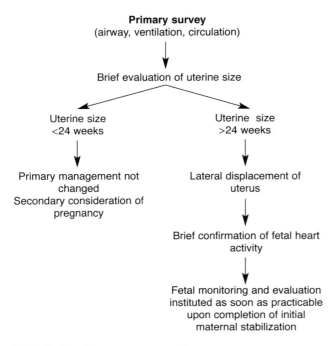

Primary survey
(airway, ventilation, circulation)

↓

Brief evaluation of uterine size

Uterine size
<24 weeks

Uterine size
>24 weeks

Primary management not
changed
Secondary consideration of
pregnancy

Lateral displacement of
uterus

↓

Brief confirmation of fetal heart
activity

↓

Fetal monitoring and evaluation
instituted as soon as practicable
upon completion of initial
maternal stabilization

■ **FIG. 29.** Obstetric aspects of primary trauma management. (Van Hook JW. Trauma in pregnancy. Clin Obstet Gynecol 2002;45[2]:414–24.)

pregnant woman can lose up to 35% of her blood volume before tachycardia or hypotension occurs. An important mechanism used by the mother to maintain a euvolemic state is to shunt one sixth of her cardiac output that perfuses the uterus into her systemic circulation. Thus, fetal bradycardia and late decelerations of the FHR can be seen on the fetal monitor. Appropriate initial maneuvers to reverse these processes include rapid infusion of colloid and type-specific blood. Pressors are to be avoided because they further decrease uterine blood flow.

Following stabilization, a more detailed secondary assessment of the mother and fetus is undertaken as is done for all trauma patients; see the Advanced Trauma Life Support Program for Doctors published by the American College of Surgeons. For the trauma patient who is more than 20 weeks pregnant, the use of electronic fetal heart rate and tocographic monitoring may be predictive in identifying the patient with placental abruption. If the frequency of uterine contractions is less than every 10 minutes during 4 hours of monitoring, placental abruption has not occurred. In contrast, among women contracting more frequently than every 10 minutes, 20% have had an abruption (21). Placental abruption usually occurs during or shortly after the traumatic event. It is therefore recommended that the pregnant trauma victim be placed on electronic fetal monitoring as soon as possible following initial stabilization. No large prospective studies have been published that validate any recommendation concerning the length of time a pregnant woman should be observed on electronic fetal monitoring. However, it seems reasonable to recommend that maternal evaluation and fetal monitoring continue so long as uterine contractions continue, a

nonreassuring fetal heart pattern persists, any vaginal bleeding continues, rupture of fetal membranes occurs, or the maternal condition remains serious (21).

Ultrasonography has not been demonstrated to be of value in making or excluding the diagnosis of placental abruption. Fetal to maternal hemorrhage can complicate maternal abdominal trauma and can result in fetal anemia, hydrops, or death. However, there is no evidence that testing for fetal to maternal hemorrhage (as with the Kleihauer–Betke test) can predict adverse immediate sequelae due to hemorrhage. It is recommended that the D-negative woman receive anti-D immune globulin in quantities sufficient to protect her from D alloimmunization. For more than 90% of women, 300 µg (1 vial) will prove sufficient.

References

1. Mazze RI, Kallen B. Appendectomy during pregnancy: a Swedish registry study of 778 cases. Obstet Gynecol 1991; 77:835–40.

2. Czeizel AE, Pataki T, Rockenbauer M. Reproductive outcome after exposure to surgery under anesthesia during pregnancy. Arch Gynecol Obstet 1998;261:193–9.

3. Sharp HT. The acute abdomen during pregnancy. Clin Obstet Gynecol 2002;45:405–13.

4. Lachman E, Schienfeld A, Voss E, Gino G, Boldes R, Levine S, et al. Pregnancy and laparoscopic surgery. J Am Assoc Gynecol Laparosc 1999;6:347–51.

5. Fatum M, Rojansky N. Laparoscopic surgery during pregnancy. Obstet Gynecol Surv 2001;56:50–9.

6. Bisharah M, Tulandi T. Laparoscopic surgery in pregnancy. Clin Obstet Gynecol 2003;46:92–7.

7. Society of American Gastrointestinal Endoscopic Surgeons. SAGES guidelines for laparoscopic surgery during pregnancy. SAGES Publication #23. Los Angeles (CA): SAGES; 2000.

8. Babler EA. Perforative appendicitis complicating pregnancy. JAMA 1908;51:1310–3.

9. Cunningham FG, Gant NF, Leveno KJ, Gilstrap LC, Hauth JC, Wenstrom KD, editors. Williams obstetrics. 21st ed. New York (NY): McGraw-Hill; 2001.

10. Tracey M, Fletcher HS. Appendicitis in pregnancy. Am Surg 2000;66:555–9; discussion 559–60.

11. Affleck DG, Handrahan DL, Egger MJ, Price RR. The laparoscopic management of appendicitis and cholelithiasis during pregnancy. Am J Surg 1999;178:523–9.

12. Barone JE, Bears S, Chen S, Tsai J, Russell JC. Outcome study of cholecystectomy during pregnancy. Am J Surg 1999;177:232–6.

13. Lee S, Bradley JP, Mele MM, Sehdev HM, Ludmir J. Cholelithiasis in pregnancy: surgical versus medical management [abstract]. Obstet Gynecol 2000;95(suppl):70s–1s.

14. Graham G, Baxi L, Tharakan T. Laparoscopic cholecystectomy during pregnancy: a case series and review of the literature. Obstet Gynecol Surv 1998;53:566–74.

15. Sainio V, Kemppainen E, Puolakkainen P, Taavitsainen M, Kivisaari L, Valtonon V, et al. Early antibiotic treatment in acute necrotizing pancreatitis. Lancet 1995;346:663–7; discussion 362–3.

16. Sherard GB 3rd, Hodson CA, Williams HJ, Semer DA, Hadi HA, Tait DL. Adnexal masses and pregnancy: a 12-year experience. Am J Obstet Gynecol 2003;189:358–62.

17. Agarwal N, Parul, Kriplani A Bhatia N, Gupta A. Management and outcome of pregnancies complicated with adnexal masses. Arch Gynecol Obstet 2003;267:148–52.

18. Gazmararian JA, Lazorick S, Spitz AM, Ballard TJ, Saltzman LE, Marks JS. Prevalence of violence against pregnant women [published erratum appears in JAMA 1997;277:1125]. JAMA 1996;275:1915–20.

19. Helton AS, McFarlane J, Anderson ET. Battered and pregnant: a prevalence study. Am J Public Health 1987;77:1337–9.

20. Fildes J, Reed L, Jones N, Martin M, Barrett J. Trauma: the leading cause of maternal death. J Trauma 1992;32:643–5.

21. American College of Obstetricians and Gynecologists. Obstetric aspects of trauma management. ACOG Educational Bulletin 251. Washington, DC: ACOG; 1998.

22. American College of Surgeons. Advanced trauma life support for doctors. 7th ed. Chicago (IL): ACS; 2003.

Neonatal Resuscitation

During birth, a cascade of physiologic events occurs in the fetus when the placenta—the primary fetal organ for gas exchange—is replaced by the lungs. Ensuring a smooth transition and optimizing outcomes requires collaborative care before, during, and after birth by obstetric and pediatric care providers, especially in complicated pregnancies.

ANTICIPATION

Ongoing risk assessment during preconceptional, prepartum, and intrapartum care can identify many of the babies who will require special attention, including resuscitation during the neonatal period. Such identification allows neonatal care providers to be fully prepared and parents counseled and involved in decision-making about neonatal care.

At least 1 person capable of initiating neonatal resuscitation and responsible for the newborn must be present for every birth (1). That person or someone else immediately available should have the skills to perform a complete resuscitation, including ventilation with bag and mask, endotracheal intubation, chest compressions, and administration of medications (1). Standards of the Joint Commission on Accreditation of Healthcare Organizations state that resuscitative services must be available throughout an organization and that qualifications must be consistent with responsibilities (2). Thus, providers of obstetric care, including physicians, nurse–midwives and nurses, should be able to initiate neonatal resuscitation and stabilization from the moment of birth as unexpected depression and complications occur. When problems are anticipated, communication and consultation with other providers who are skilled in neonatal care is advised. Certain circumstances might lead to maternal–fetal transfer to another institution in a regional system where subspecialty services, such as neonatology, pediatric surgery, neurology, and cardiology, are available.

RESUSCITATION

About 10% of babies require some help with breathing at birth, and 1% require vigorous intervention. The Neonatal Resuscitation Program (NRP) is a standardized clinical provider course sponsored by the American Heart Association and the American Academy of Pediatrics (AAP). It serves as the foundation of practically all current instruction in resuscitation in the United States and a growing portion of international teaching (3, 4).

Immediately after birth, specific steps should be taken, including drying, suctioning, and tactile stimulation of the neonate. Subsequently, continuous evaluation and judgment are employed according to specific guidelines resulting in intervention as indicated along specific pathways. Intervention is minimal if the clinician notes spontaneous respiration, a heart rate of more than 100 beats per minute, and good color. Conversely, a low heart rate (<60) with inadequate respiration or response to positive-pressure ventilation leads to additional intervention, including chest compressions and possibly medication. Effective gas exchange can be accomplished with a bag and mask in most situations. Intubation should be performed if clinically needed and a skilled provider is available.

The Apgar score is a traditional and useful tool to assess the status of a neonate in the minutes immediately after birth. It should be recorded by an independent observer at 1 and 5 minutes after delivery and at later times as needed (ie, 10 minutes and 15 minutes) until a score of 7 is obtained. Assessment and initiation of resuscitation when necessary must begin before 1 minute and should not depend on the 1-minute Apgar score. The score depicts the physiologic state of the moment; alone, it is not evidence of appropriateness of care or a predictor of neurologic sequelae (5).

STABILIZATION

Resuscitation blends into ongoing stabilization and care based on need. Many neonates that require resuscitation efforts improve rapidly, are observed for varied intervals, and transition to routine care, including being with their mothers and breastfeeding. The list of reasons why neonates require ongoing care is long, with prematurity the primary reason. Problems such as respiratory distress may need ongoing respiratory support. Problems anticipated before labor or delivery, such as congenital anomalies, may require additional assessment, such as genetic consultation and studies. Initiation of antibiotic therapy for suspected perinatally acquired infections should take place immediately. Group B streptococcal concerns should be coordinated before and after birth according to national prevention guidelines (6).

SPECIAL CONCERNS

Meconium

Resuscitation and stabilization in the presence of meconium has been the subject of study for years. Meconium as an amniotic fluid stain is present in 10–20% of deliveries, and most meconium-stained babies do not develop problems. Meconium aspiration syndrome is thought to occur in 1 in 120 liveborn babies, or about 6% of all meconium–stained babies. Serious cases have high mortality and morbidity, including pneumonitis, pneumothorax, and pulmonary artery hypertension.

When thick "pea soup" meconium is present at delivery, interventions to prevent or lessen meconium aspiration syndrome should be considered. Suctioning of the upper airway (nose, mouth, and posterior pharynx) should be performed after delivery of the head if possible. If the infant is not vigorous and thick meconium is present, NRP recommends intubation and suctioning to remove material below the glottis before positive-pressure ventilation. If the infant is active, suctioning and intubation are therapeutic options that are part of ongoing stabilization and care (3).

Resuscitation at the Threshold of Viability

Collectively, outcomes are poor for neonates born at the threshold of viability (≤25 completed weeks of gestation). Delivery room care of these so-called micropremies is the subject of ongoing concern and controversy. Parents and professionals alike have been outspoken about this issue. Most experts believe that informed parental preferences should be determined and followed concerning the degree of intervention to be undertaken. Many organizations, including ACOG and AAP, provide guidelines that address management, outcomes, and ethical concerns (7, 8).

Although some informed parents will decide that resuscitation should not be initiated, a common course is to provide individualized care that involves ongoing judgment concerning extent and duration of resuscitation on the basis of clinical course and discussions with parents when possible. Parents may be present while perinatal care is being provided to neonates, including procedures, resuscitation, and stabilization. Parents should be informed about and involved in the care of their children within the principles of family-centered care (9).

Defining Neonatal Encephalopathy and Cerebral Palsy

Understanding has emerged that factors often used to define perinatal asphyxia, such as the need for resuscitation, Apgar score, and presence of meconium, as well as nonreassuring FHR patterns, are not specific to the pathophysiologic process involved with neurologic damage. False-positive rates are significant. Approximately 70% or more of cases of neonatal encephalopathy apparently have causality that began before the onset of labor. This knowledge reinforces the need for anticipation and risk assessment well before delivery and promotes caution when discussing prognosis and outcomes after neonatal resuscitation has been necessary. Criteria that help with the definition of the relationship between acute intrapartum events and neurologic outcomes such as cerebral palsy are available (10).

OXYGEN

Long-standing recommendations for the use of supplemental oxygen during the initial acute phase of resuscitation are in place (3). However, recent research and evolving knowledge about the immediate effectiveness and the possibility of long-term sequelae of oxygen administration raise appropriate concerns. Additional studies under way may modify recommended practice (11). If in the unusual circumstance supplemental oxygen is not available, positive pressure resuscitation with room air (21% oxygen) is indicated.

References

1. American Academy of Pediatrics, American College of Obstetricians and Gynecologists. Guidelines for perinatal care. 5th ed. Elk Grove Village (IL): AAP; Washington, DC: ACOG; 2002.

2. Joint Commission on Accreditation of Healthcare Organizations. Comprehensive accreditation manual for hospitals: the official handbook: 2004 CAMH. Oakbrook Terrace (IL): JCAHO; 2004.

3. Kattwinkel J, editor. Textbook of neonatal resuscitation. 4th ed. Elk Grove Village (IL): American Academy of Pediatrics; Chicago (IL): American Heart Association; 2000.

4. Niermeyer S, Katwinkel J, Van Reempts P, Nadkarni V, Phillips B, Zideman D, et al. International Guidelines for Neonatal Resuscitation: an excerpt from the Guidelines 2000 for Cardiopulmonary Resuscitation and Emergency Cardiovascular Care: International Consensus on Science. Contributors and Reviewers for the Neonatal Resuscitation Guidelines. Pediatrics 2000;106;E29.

5. American Academy of Pediatrics, American College of Obstetricians and Gynecologists. Use and abuse of the Apgar score. ACOG Committee Opinion 174. Washington, DC: ACOG; 1996.

6. Schrag S, Gorwitz R, FultzButts K, Schuchat A. Prevention of perinatal group B streptococcal disease. Revised guidelines from CDC. MMWR Recomm Rep 2002;51 (RR-11):1–22.

7. Perinatal care at the threshold of viability. ACOG Practice Bulletin No. 38. American College of Obstetricians and Gynecologists. Obstet Gynecol 2002;100:617–24.

8. MacDonald H; American Academy of Pediatrics, Committee on Fetus and Newborn. Perinatal care at the threshold of viability. Pediatrics 2002;110:1024–7.

9. Harrison H. The principles for family-centered neonatal care. Pediatrics 1993;92:643–50.

10. American Academy of Pediatrics, American College of Obstetricians and Gynecologists. Neonatal encephalopathy and cerebral palsy: defining the pathogenesis and pathophysiology. Washington, DC: ACOG; 2003.

11. Saugstad OD, Ramji S, Irani SF, El-Meneza S, Hernanden EA, Vento M, et al. Resuscitation of newborn infants with 21% or 100% oxygen: follow-up at 18 to 24 months. Pediatrics 2003;112:296–300.

Depression During Pregnancy and the Postpartum Period

Several large-scale epidemiologic studies throughout the world have documented a prevalence of major depressive disorder in women 1.5–3 times that of men. In addition to being affected by depressive disorders at a higher rate, women are more likely than men to have chronic and recurring illness. Pregnancy, previously thought of as a time when women are at lower risk for psychiatric illness, is instead a time when 10–27% of women experience depressive symptoms or a depressive disorder (1). Not only do many women with preexisting mood symptoms continue feeling depressed during pregnancy but many women also experience the onset of a depressive disorder when pregnant. Depression has a deleterious effect on mothers and families, impeding quality of life and daily functioning. Data also suggest that the illness of depression may increase the likelihood of delivering a small-birth weight or preterm infant (2).

It remains to be determined whether rates of anxiety syndromes differ between pregnant and nonpregnant women. However, it is clear that obstetricians and gynecologists frequently encounter women with depressive and anxiety disorders.

UNIPOLAR DISORDERS

Detection of depressive disorders in obstetric and gynecology patients is low (3, 4). A recent study of 3,000 obstetrics and gynecology patients showed that 20% of patients met criteria for a psychiatric diagnosis, but of these, 77% were not recognized as depressed by their health care provider (3). One reason for low detection rates may be that the signs and symptoms characteristic of depression are difficult to distinguish from some complaints frequently brought up in normal pregnancies. For example, sleep and appetite disturbance, diminished libido, and fatigue are all common features of pregnancy. Pregnant patients with depression are more likely than those not depressed to report these problems (4). Therefore, signs to look for that may help confirm a diagnosis of depression are anhedonia (loss of interest or pleasure in previously pleasurable activities and relationships), suicidal thoughts, feelings of hopelessness and guilt, and concentration difficulties.

The hallmark symptoms of a major depressive disorder are a sustained depressed mood (usually a unipolar phenomenon) and anhedonia. The diagnostic criteria (Box 31) stipulate that the individual must have at least 5 of a possible 9 symptoms and that at least 1 symptom be depressed mood or diminished interest and pleasure.

Symptoms occur nearly every day for most of the day during the symptomatic period. Dysthymic disorder, another unipolar mood disorder, is characterized by fewer symptoms than major depressive disorder but lasts a minimum of 2 years. Depressive disorders are more likely to be episodic and recurrent rather than chronic. Depressive disorders often occur with other psychiatric disorders, resulting in greater morbidity overall. Particularly striking is the comorbidity of depressive disorders with anxiety and substance use disorders. More than 50% of patients with major depressive disorder will have a comorbid anxiety disorder, close to one fourth will have alcohol dependence, and 13% will be drug dependent (5).

A number of risk factors are associated with depression during pregnancy and the puerperium, including past history of depressive disorders, diminished partner support, marital difficulties, poor social adjustment, adverse life events, an unplanned pregnancy or uncertainty about having the child, and maternal or paternal unemployment.

Early intervention is critical to minimize the effects of maternal depression. Pregnancy constitutes an ideal time to screen for depression because a woman is likely to

RESOURCES

Depression and Other Mood Disorders in Pregnancy

The American College of Obstetricians and Gynecologists
www.acog.org

American Psychiatric Association
www.psych.org

Center for Mental Health Services (SAMHSA) National Mental Health Information Center
www.mentalhealth.org

Depression and Bipolar Support Alliance
www.dbsalliance.org

MedlinePlus: Depression
www.nlm.nih.gov/medlineplus/depression.html

National Institute of Mental Health
www.nimh.nih.gov

National Mental Health Association
www.nmha.org

have frequent contact with a health care provider. Depression screening scales are a cost-effective means for detecting depression in obstetric and gynecology settings. When implementing depression screening, providers need to consider if behavioral health care professionals are accessible on site and what type of assessment and referral will be undertaken if depression is diagnosed. See Box 32 for information on suggested screening questionnaires measuring general distress as well as depression.

The clinical course of unipolar depression varies throughout pregnancy. Most studies have found that it peaks during the first trimester, with improvement during the second trimester and an increased rate again during the third trimester. Researchers have documented that depressive symptoms during pregnancy are the strongest predictors of postpartum depression (6). Common symptoms of perinatal mood disorders (outlined in Box 33) include symptoms of major depressive disorder but also may include frequent complaints of lack of social support and misinterpretations of the infant's cues.

Postpartum Mood Disorders

Most researchers agree that postpartum mental illnesses can be divided into 3 categories: postpartum blues, postpartum depression, and postpartum psychosis.

POSTPARTUM BLUES

Postpartum blues affect 50–80% of new mothers and include symptoms of labile mood, anxiety, sleep difficulties, and irritability. Postpartum blues usually begin within the first days postpartum and should start to remit by the second week. Although postpartum blues usually do not require professional attention and subside on their own, it is important for clinicians to identify women with postpartum blues because these women are often at increased risk for developing postpartum depression. Studies have found that as many as 20% of women who experience postpartum blues ultimately develop a major

---

BOX 31

Symptoms of Major or Minor Depressive Disorder*

- Depressed, low, or blue mood most of the day, nearly every day[†]
- Markedly diminished interest or pleasure in most, if not all, activities[†]
- Decrease or increase in appetite nearly every day
- Insomnia or hypersomnia nearly every day
- Psychomotor agitation or retardation nearly every day
- Fatigue or loss of energy nearly every day
- Diminished ability to think or concentrate, or difficulty making decisions nearly every day
- Feelings of worthlessness or excessive or inappropriate guilt nearly every day
- Recurrent thoughts of death or suicidal ideation or a suicide attempt or specific plan

*Two to four symptoms for diagnosing minor depressive disorder; at least 5 for major depressive disorder.

[†]One of the starred items is required for the diagnosis.

Data from American Psychiatric Association. Diagnostic and statistical manual of mental disorders: DSM-IV-TR. 4th ed, text revision. Washington, DC: APA; 2000.

BOX 32

Depression Screening Instruments for Use in an Obstetrics and Gynecology Practice

PRIME-MD Depression Module

- 14-item self-report questionnaire
- Provides diagnosis of major and minor depressive disorders and measure of severity
- 5–20 minutes to complete

Copies and permission to use can be obtained from:

Robert L. Spitzer, MD
Chief, Biometrics Research and
Professor of Psychiatry, Columbia University
Email: RLS8@Columbia.edu

Inventory of Depressive Symptomatology (IDS)

- 28–30-item self-report form (IDS-SR) or clinician-administered (IDS-C) form
- Provides measure of illness severity
- 15–30 minutes to complete

Copies and permission to use can be obtained from:

A. John Rush, MD
University of Texas Southwestern Medical Center
5323 Harry Hines Boulevard
Dallas, TX 75235-9101

Edinburgh Postnatal Depression Scale

- 10 statements to elicit woman's feelings during the previous week
- Helps detect women with postnatal depression
- Less than 5 minutes to complete

Depression scale is available on the Internet.

Source: Cox JL, Holden JM, Sagovsky R. Detection of postnatal depression. Development of the 10-item Edinburgh Postnatal Depression Scale. Br J Psychiatry 1987;150:782–6.

BOX 33

Symptoms of Perinatal Mood Disorders

- Depressed mood
- Irritability
- Lack of interest in activities
- Insomnia
- Low energy
- Social isolation/withdrawal
- Poor memory, lack of concentration and coherent thinking
- Disorientation, bewilderment, anguish
- Frequent complaints of lack of social support
- Misinterpretations of infant's cues

---

depressive episode during the first postnatal year. Women at risk for postpartum blues are more likely to exhibit the following characteristics:

- Personal or family history of depression
- Premenstrual dysphoria
- Recent stressful life events or poor social adjustment
- Depression or anxiety during pregnancy
- Excessive fear of labor or view of the pregnancy as emotionally difficult
- Ambivalence toward the pregnancy

POSTPARTUM DEPRESSION

Postpartum depression is classified as a major depressive disorder with postpartum onset, usually in the first 4 weeks after delivery; prevalence ranges from 5% to 20%, with the highest rates in adolescents. Risk factors for postpartum depression include a history of psychiatric disorder, lack of social support, and unplanned pregnancy (Box 34).

The clinical course for women with postpartum major depressive disorder varies. Onset in most women occurs within the first month after delivery. An early study suggested that the majority of women with postpartum depression recovered within 6 months (7); however, there is a lack of clarity because another study found that 20% of women will experience chronic depression for more than 2 years (8). Longer-term follow-up indicates substantial recurrence over the next 4 years, with 50% of women continuing in treatment or again seeking treatment (7). These data on course are limited but suggest a substantial risk for chronicity and lifetime recurrence, whether the postpartum episode of depression was the first depressive event or a recurrence of an earlier illness.

A particularly dangerous consequence of a mother's postpartum depressive illness is the deleterious effect on her offspring. Postnatal depression has been shown to negatively influence infant behavior (9), cognitive development, and emotional well-being (10).

Women with mild depression generally can be managed with supportive therapy. Women with major postpartum depression generally require pharmacologic intervention with antidepressants or anxiolytic agents in addition to psychologic counseling.

POSTPARTUM PSYCHOSES

Postpartum psychoses, occurring in approximately 1–2 of 1,000 births, usually start in the first 2 weeks after delivery but occasionally begin later. Severe mental illnesses often require hospitalization. Most (75–80%) are mood disorders; 60% are depression. Risk factors include a history of mental illness, especially bipolar disorder, and current psychosocial stressors. Recurrence in subsequent pregnancies is approximately 50–80%.

Treatment consists of the use of antipsychotic and antidepressant medications and hospitalization (with the infant, if possible). Patients at high risk should be monitored carefully in the first few weeks, with special attention to obsessive thinking about harming the infant, sleep disorders, and feelings of hopelessness and anhedonia (loss of pleasure in activities previously enjoyed).

BOX 34

Risk Factors for Postpartum Depression

- Past psychiatric history
- Family history of depression or anxiety
- Personality traits (obsessive-compulsive, panic, anxiety, etc.)
- Lack of social support
- Negative life events
- Unplanned pregnancy
- Poor marital relations, or being unmarried
- Multiple births
- Occupational instability
- Poor outcomes of previous pregnancies (abortion, miscarriage, sick infant)
- Poor prenatal care
- Malnutrition
- Substance use
- Previous suicide attempts

Depression Following Pregnancy Loss

The 6-month incidence of depression in women who experienced a fetal loss (prior to 28 weeks of gestation) has been reported to be 2.5 times greater than that found in a sample of community nonpregnant women (11). In the same study, nearly three fourths of women experiencing an episode of miscarriage after depression became symptomatic for depression during the first month after their loss. Another study examining miscarriage and subsequent risk of depression found that women who experience fetal loss (at <18 weeks of gestation) and become pregnant within 1 year are at increased risk for both depression and anxiety in the third trimester of a subsequent pregnancy (12).

Parents who must cope with stillbirths, neonatal deaths, and infants born with congenital anomalies require sensitivity, compassion, and guidance from the medical care team. Clinicians need to offer counseling to these women and their partners and provide close follow-up to patients with prior depressive illnesses. Counseling should address specific issues regarding the mother's future health and pregnancies.

Pharmacotherapy

The challenge in using psychotropic medication during pregnancy (see Table 29) is to both minimize the risk to the fetus and limit the morbidity of untreated psychiatric illness of the mother. Although the focus of antidepressant treatment during pregnancy often revolves around fetal exposure to psychotropic medication, untreated depression itself may adversely affect the developing fetus (2).

Women with recurrent major depressive disorder taking antidepressant treatment medication prior to conception often are advised or choose to discontinue antidepressant medication during pregnancy or at least during the first trimester. In the general population, abrupt discontinuation of antidepressants and antipsychotics is associated with a high risk of relapse (13). Further research into relapse during pregnancy needs to be conducted, but for now, clinicians managing depression by administering maintenance medication should consider the risk of relapse, either during pregnancy or postpartum, as an important variable in treatment decisions (Fig. 30).

TRICYCLIC ANTIDEPRESSANTS

Several prospective controlled studies have been conducted on pregnant women taking tricyclic antidepressants (TCAs) and selective serotonin reuptake inhibitors (SSRIs), particularly fluoxetine. More than 450 cases of first-trimester exposure to TCAs have been examined through both prospective and retrospective studies. Overall, no significant association between fetal exposure to TCAs and risk for major congenital anomalies was found. Preferred TCAs for use during pregnancy include desipramine and nortriptyline because they are less anticholingeric and least likely to aggravate orthostatic hypotension (14). Behavioral development in children exposed in utero to TCAs is not adversely affected in terms of global intelligence, language development, or behavioral development, and timing of the antidepressant therapy (first trimester versus the entire pregnancy) does not affect behavioral outcomes (15).

Tricyclic antidepressant dosage requirements have been shown to increase across gestation, such that during the final trimester the dose required to sustain remission from depression was 1.3–2 times the nonpregnant dose. Therefore, in cases where breakthrough depressive symptoms occur, serum levels should be obtained to ensure appropriate TCA dosage. If depressive symptoms warrant, the dose of TCAs should be tapered and eventually discontinued during the 2-week period prior to the estimated delivery date to reduce the fetal drug load at birth. If a TCA is appropriate for use during pregnancy, nortriptyline is the preferable TCA because of its decade-long use and study. Other benefits of nortriptyline are its low relative anticholinergic activity and its relationship between plasma concentration and therapeutic effect (16).

SELECTIVE SEROTONIN REUPTAKE INHIBITORS

Controversy exists surrounding the relationship between SSRIs and preterm delivery and low birth weight. One study found significantly lower gestational ages and birth weights among infants exposed to an SSRI in utero but not among those exposed to a TCA (17). Other studies have hypothesized that only exposure to an SSRI in the third trimester is associated with preterm delivery. More information is needed before definitive conclusions can be reached.

Fluoxetine is the most widely studied SSRI in pregnancy. Data on more than 2,500 cases indicate no increase in risk for congenital malformations in fetuses exposed to fluoxetine. One study did demonstrate that fluoxetine was associated with premature labor and poor neonatal adaptation (18), but these findings need to be evaluated further because of the study's methodologic limitations. Data on other SSRIs such as paroxetine and sertraline are growing and appear promising, but studies are limited by sample size.

BIPOLAR DISORDERS

Because bipolar disease often occurs initially in the postpartum period, obstetrician–gynecologists frequently are involved in co-management of this disorder. Among women with known bipolar disease, up to 50% will have recurrent problems postpartum unless treatment is initiated.

TABLE 29. Pharmacotherapy for Perinatal Depression

Antidepressant	Advantages During Pregnancy	Disadvantages During Pregnancy	Recommended Dosage* (mg/day)	Percentage of Dose to Breastfeeding Infant†	Reported Side Effects to Breastfeeding Infants	Teratogenicity
Selective Serotonin Reuptake Inhibitors						
Sertraline	Expert Consensus Guidelines top choice during pregnancy (if planning to breastfeed)	No behavioral studies in human pregnancy; Increased bleeding tendency (rare)	50–200	0.4–1.0	None	Morphologic–none; Behavioral–unknown
Paroxetine	Expert Consensus Guidelines second choice during pregnancy (if planning to breastfeed)	No behavioral studies in human pregnancy; Increased bleeding tendency (rare)	20–60	0.1–4.3	None	Morphologic–none; Behavioral–unknown
Citalopram	Few interactions with other medications	No behavioral studies in human pregnancy; Increased bleeding tendency (rare)	20–40	0.7–9.0	Uneasy sleep	Morphologic–none; Behavioral–unknown
Fluoxetine	More studies in human pregnancy, including neurodevelopmental follow-up; Expert Consensus Guidelines top choice during pregnancy (if not planning to breastfeed)	Long half-life can lead to neonatal toxicity (tachypnea, respiratory distress, tremors, agitation, motor automatisms); Increased bleeding tendency (rare)	20–60	1.2–6.8	Vomiting, watery stools, excessive crying, difficulty sleeping, tremor, somnolence, hypotonia, decreased weight gain	None
Tricyclic Antidepressants						
Nortriptyline	More studies in human pregnancy, including neurodevelopmental follow-up	Maternal side effects additive to pregnancy effects (sedation, constipation, tachycardia); Orthostatic hypotension, risking decreased placental perfusion; Fetal and neonatal side effects: tachycardia, urinary retention	50–150	Not known	None	None

Desipramine	More studies in human pregnancy, including neurodevelopmental follow-up	Maternal side effects additive to pregnancy effects (sedation, constipation, tachycardia) Orthostatic hypotension, risking decreased placental perfusion Fetal and neonatal side effects: tachycardia, urinary retention	100–300	1.0	None	None
Serotonin Norepinephrine Reuptake Inhibitor						
Venlafaxine	Balanced antidepressant; may be effective when selective agents are not	No behavioral studies in human pregnancy	75–225	5.2–7.4	None	Morphologic—none Behavioral—unknown
Other						
Bupropion	No sexual side effects No excess weight gain Helps with smoking cessation	No systematic studies in human pregnancy Lowers seizure threshold Can cause insomnia	200–300	Not known	None reported to date	Unknown
Nefazodone	No sexual side effects	No systematic studies in human pregnancy Hepatotoxicity (rare)	300–600	0.45	Drowsiness, poor feeding, difficulty maintaining body temperature	Unknown
Mirtazapine	No sexual side effects Helps restore appetite in women who are not gaining weight Less likely to exacerbate nausea and vomiting	No systematic studies in human pregnancy Can cause excessive weight gain Tends to be sedating	15–45	Not known	Not known	Unknown

*Physicians may consider initiating treatment with these agents at half the lowest recommended therapeutic dose. Dosages are from Physician's Desk Reference, 56th ed.

†This is a weight adjusted estimate.

Based on Wisner KL, Parry BL, Piontek CM. Clinical practice. Postpartum depression. N Engl J Med 2002;347:194–9.

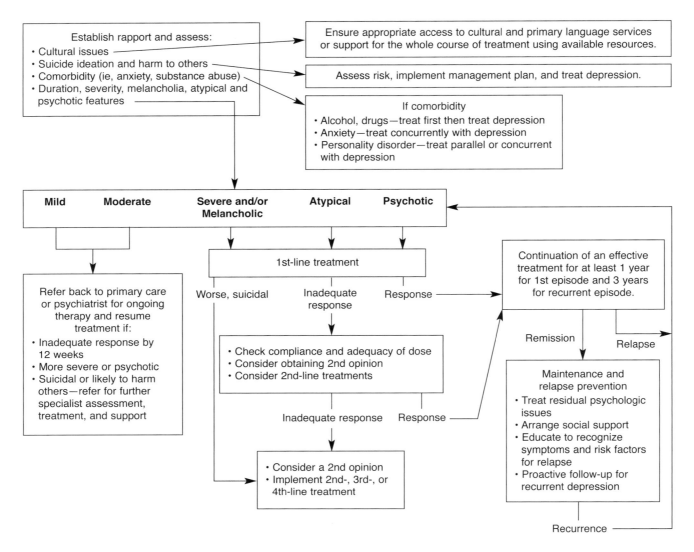

■ **FIG. 30.** Outline of treatment for depression. (Australian and New Zealand clinical practice guidelines for the treatment of depression. Aust N Z J Psychiatry 2004;38:389. Copyright Blackwell Publishing Limited.)

Diagnosis

Patients with bipolar disorders have an additional dimension: when they are ill, they may experience depression, but they also may experience mania or hypomania. Patients with mania have an expansive mood—they are elated and have increased energy and inflated self-esteem. They also have racing thoughts, poor impulse control, and extremely poor judgment.

Treatment

For women with bipolar disorder who elect to take medication during the first trimester, exposure to a psychotropic agent may be safer than exposure to multiple agents. Older agents, for which more case and cohort data have been reported, are preferable to newer agents for which data may not be available. Little data exist regarding the results of second- or third-trimester exposure to mood-stabilizing agents. Therefore, if a medication

proves effective, changing medication to avoid undocumented risk may jeopardize the woman's current stability. Notably, clinicians should use caution with women taking valproate; exposure during the first trimester carries the greatest teratogenic risk.

Lithium can be used during pregnancy to treat bipolar disorder; however, maternal serum levels, which may be affected by vomiting, sodium intake, and febrile illness, should be closely monitored. Anomalies resulting from first-trimester exposure can be identified with prenatal screening with a high-resolution ultrasound examination and fetal echocardiography at 16–18 weeks of gestation (19). As pregnancy progresses, the dose of lithium may need to be increased because renal lithium excretion increases. The use of lithium during labor requires specific precautions. Some experts advise tapering lithium a week before delivery to minimize neonatal toxic effects and to stop lithium upon the onset of labor. However, to reduce the risk of postpartum episode, treatment with lithium should be resumed immediately after birth, and plasma levels should be monitored carefully.

The most commonly prescribed benzodiazepines for individuals with bipolar disorder are lorazepam and clonazepam. The risk of physical anomalies with benzodiazepines is increased for cleft lip or palate, but these anomalies are still rare, with a risk of about 6 in 10,000 births (20). Intrauterine growth restriction has been associated with diazepam, but no association between IUGR and lorazepam or clonazepam has been described. Third-trimester exposure to benzodiazepines has resulted in acute side effects such as impaired temperature regulation, apnea, lower Apgar scores at 1 and 5 minutes, muscle hypotonia, and failure to feed. Infants born to mothers who used benzodiazepines chronically during pregnancy may evidence withdrawal symptoms; however, information is still inconclusive regarding the behavioral teratogenicity of the infant from the use of benzodiazepines during pregnancy.

Other options for the treatment of bipolar disorder among pregnant women include the use of electroconvulsive therapy (ECT) and psychosocial interventions. Electroconvulsive therapy has been shown to have a low rate of complications during pregnancy; however, fetal cardiac monitoring during ECT will allow for detection of arrhythmias and their correction. Agents routinely given in nonpregnant ECT patients to reduce bradycardia and decrease secretions should not be given during pregnancy because they increase the risk of gastric reflux.

References

1. Cooper PJ, Murray L, Hooper R, West A. The development and validation of a predictive index for postpartum depression. Psychol Med 1996;26:627–34.

2. Orr ST, James SA, Blackmore Prince C. Maternal prenatal depressive symptoms and spontaneous preterm births among African-American women in Baltimore, Maryland. Am J Epidemiol 2002;156:797–802.

3. Spitzer RL, Williams JB, Kroenke K, Hornyak R, McMurray J. Validity and utility of the PRIME-MD patient health questionnaire in assessment of 3000 obstetric-gynecology patients: the PRIME-MD Patient Health Questionnaire Obstetric Gynecology Study. Am J Obstet Gynecol 2000;183:759–69.

4. Kelly R, Zatzick D, Anders T. The detection and treatment of psychiatric disorders and substance abuse among pregnant women cared for in obstetrics. Am J Psychiatry 2001;158:213–9.

5. Kessler RC, Nelson CB, McGonagle KA, Liu J, Swartz M, Blazer DG. Comorbidity of DSM-III-R major depressive disorder in the general population: results from the US National Comorbidity Survey. Br J Psychiatry Suppl 1996;(30)17–30.

6. Kitamura T, Shima S, Sugawara M, Toda MA. Psychological and social correlates of the onset of affective disorders among pregnant women. Psychol Med 1993;23:967–75.

7. Kumar R, Robson KM. A prospective study of emotional disorders in childbearing women. Br J Psychiatry 1984;144:35–47.

8. England SJ, Ballard C, George S. Chronicity in postnatal depression. Eur J Psychiatry 1994;8:93–6.

9. Campbell SB, Cohn JF, Meyers T. Depression in first-time mothers: mother-infant interaction and depression chronicity. Dev Psychol 1995;31:349–57.

10. Murray D, Cox JL, Chapman G, Jones P. Childbirth: life event or start of a long-term difficulty? Further data from the Stoke-on-Trent controlled study of postnatal depression. Br J Psychiatry 1995;166:595–600.

11. Neugebauer R, Kline J, Shrout P, Skodol A, O'Connor P, Geller PA, et al. Major depressive disorder in the 6 months after miscarriage. JAMA 1997;277:383–8.

12. Hughes PM. Turton P. Evans CD. Stillbirth as risk factor for depression and anxiety in the subsequent pregnancy: cohort study. BMJ 1999;318:1721–4.

13. Viguera AC, Baldessarini RJ, Hegarty JD, van Kammen DP, Tohen M. Clinical risk following abrupt and gradual withdrawal of maintenance neuroleptic treatment. Arch Gen Psychiatry 1997;54:49–55.

14. Nonacs R, Cohen LS. Depression during pregnancy: diagnosis and treatment options. J Clin Psychiatry 2002;63 (suppl 7):24–30.

15. Nulman I, Rovet J, Stewart DE, Wolpin J, Gardner HA, Theis JG, et al. Neurodevelopment of children exposed in utero to antidepressant drugs. N Engl J Med 1997;336:258–62.

16. Szigethy EM, Wisner KL. Psychopharmacological treatment of mood and anxiety disorders during pregnancy. In: Steiner M, Yonkers KA, Eriksson E, editors. Mood disorders in women. London: Martin Dunitz; 2000. p. 295–311.

17. Simon GE, Cunningham ML, Davis RL. Outcomes of prenatal antidepressant exposure. Am J Psychiatry 2002;159:2055–61.

18. Chambers CD, Johnson KA, Dick LM, Felix RJ, Jones KL. Birth outcomes in pregnant women taking fluoxetine. N Engl J Med 1996;335:1010–5.

19. Altshuler LL, Cohen L, Szuba MP, Burt VK, Gitlin M, Mintz J. Pharmacologic management of psychiatric illness during pregnancy: dilemmas and guidelines. Am J Psychiatry 1996;153:592–606.

20. Dolovich LR, Addis A, Vaillancourt JM, Power JD, Koren G, Einarson TR. Benzodiazepine use in pregnancy and major malformations or oral cleft: meta-analysis of cohort and case-control studies. BMJ 1998;317:839–43.

The Puerperium

The puerperium is defined as the period following delivery and extending 6 weeks postpartum. Multiple anatomic and physiologic changes occur during this time. Tremendous adjustment is required, and certain complications (eg, infection or hemorrhage) particular to this period may occur.

INVOLUTIONAL CHANGES

At term, uterine weight is approximately 1,100 g. Within 24 hours of delivery, the fundus should be palpable at the umbilicus. By 2 weeks, the uterus is no longer palpable on abdominal examination and has decreased in weight by 50% to 500 g. By 6 weeks postpartum, the uterus has returned to almost its normal size. Ultrasound evaluation of the postpartum uterus suggests a slightly increased uterine size at 1 and 3 months postpartum in women delivered by cesarean birth compared with those undergoing vaginal delivery (1).

By day 7, most of the epithelium and stroma are similar to those of the nonpregnant state. At day 16, the proliferative endometrium is nearly restored to its nonpregnant condition except for occasional hyalinized decidual tissue and leukocytic infiltrate. Regeneration of the placental site takes longer and may not be completed until 6–7 weeks postpartum. By 1 week postpartum, the cervix should appear normal. Histologic changes remain at 6 weeks after delivery and include stromal edema and a round cell infiltrate that may last 3–4 months. The response of cervical epithelium to HPV may be altered in pregnancy and may normalize in the puerperium. In a study of 107 women with antenatal abnormal cervical cytology, 47% were found to have normalization by 6 months postpartum (2). Another investigation found only 3% of lesions had progressed following delivery (3). In addition, data suggest a decline in the percentage of patients who are positive for HPV DNA and a 48% regression of high-grade squamous intraepithelial lesions in the postpartum period (4).

Vaginal rugae reappear as vascularity and edema resolve around the third postpartum week, and the vagina resumes its typical appearance by 6–10 weeks after delivery. Vaginal atrophic changes may persist well beyond the initial 6 weeks postpartum in lactating women.

RETURN OF OVULATORY FUNCTION AND MENSTRUATION

The mean time from delivery to the return of menstruation in nonlactating women is 7–9 weeks; 70% are menstruating by 12 weeks. In lactating women, menstruation is delayed and more variable. The average time to ovulation is 45 days in nonlactating women (range, 25–72 days) and 189 days in lactating women (range, 34–256 days). Vaginal bleeding occurring within 56 days of delivery in lactating women is probably anovulatory. In lactating women, approximately 45–63% of first episodes of vaginal bleeding were anovulatory, and 41% of women who were ovulatory had luteal phase defects before 6 months postpartum. The likelihood of ovulation increases as the frequency and duration of breastfeeding decrease and supplementary feedings are used. Ovulation occurs in less than 10% of women who partially breastfeed and who experience amenorrhea in the first 6 months after delivery. In a recent study of 624 breastfeeding mothers, the median duration of amenorrhea was 8.5 months (5).

LACTATION

Because breast milk is the ideal source of nutrition for the neonate, ACOG and the AAP recommend that women

---

RESOURCES

The Puerperium

Academy of Breastfeeding Medicine
www.bfmed.org

American Academy of Pediatrics
www.aap.org

American College of Obstetricians and Gynecologists
www.acog.org

Association of Women's Health, Obstetric and Neonatal Nurses
www.awhonn.org

CDC's Breastfeeding Resources
www.cdc.gov/breastfeeding

La Leche League International
www.lalecheleague.org

March of Dimes
www.modimes.org

MEDLINEplus
medlineplus.gov

National Center for Education and Maternal Child Health
www.ncemch.org

National Institute of Child Health and Human Development
www.nichd.nih.gov

breastfeed exclusively for the first 6 months and continue breastfeeding for at least 12 months and thereafter for as long as mutually desired (6, 7). However, a 2001 national survey showed that 70% of women initiated breastfeeding but only 33% were still breastfeeding at 6 months (8). The support of the obstetrician at the postpartum follow-up visit has been correlated with an improvement in breastfeeding continuation rates.

The breast and nipples of a woman who is nursing her infant require little attention during the puerperium other than attention to cleanliness and correct positioning and latch-on of the infant to avoid nipple trauma and fissuring, which may lead to infection. Some parturients may request lactation suppression during the postpartum period. Lactation is suppressed in 60–70% of women who wear a tight brassiere and avoid stimulation of the nipples. Although breast engorgement occasionally may cause a temperature elevation of short duration, any rise in temperature during the puerperium might be a sign of infection. The FDA has recommended that no drug should be used routinely for postpartum lactation suppression. Bromocriptine, used to suppress lactation, has been associated with strokes, myocardial infarctions, seizures, and psychiatric problems in puerperal women.

Breastfeeding is contraindicated in patients with certain viral infections, such as HIV.

Benefits

The reported benefits to infants of breastfeeding include decreased risks of otitis and respiratory infections, diarrheal illness, sudden infant death, allergic and atopic disease, juvenile-onset diabetes, and childhood malignancies; fewer hospital admissions in the first year of life; and improved cognitive function. For premature infants, breast milk has been shown to reduce the risk of necrotizing enterocolitis. Maternal benefits include improved maternal–child attachment, reduced fertility due to lactational amenorrhea, and reduced incidence of some hormonally sensitive malignancies, including breast cancer. A collaborative reanalysis of 47 epidemiologic studies found a 7% reduction in breast cancer risk for each birth and a 4.3% reduction for each 12 months of breastfeeding (9). Breastfeeding also requires less preparation and is less expensive than bottle-feeding.

Risks of breastfeeding include exhaustion, atrophic vaginitis, and mastitis (see "Mastitis"). Women should drink when thirsty, eat a balanced diet, and get plenty of rest. Lubricants can be used to relieve atrophic vaginitis. Women who have infections that could be transmitted to the neonate or who take certain medications should not breastfeed (see "Teratogenic Agents").

Breast Changes

Pregnancy is accompanied by a marked increase in breast ductal sprouting, branching, and lobular formation, which are influenced by luteal and placental hormones (primarily human placental lactogen, prolactin, and hCG). Ductal sprouting is predominantly estrogen mediated, and lobular formation is primarily progesterone related. Prolactin also is essential. Colostrum secretion occurs in gestations of 16 weeks or more. Stage I of lactogenesis begins 12 weeks before delivery. High prolactin levels during pregnancy are not associated with milk production because of progesterone antagonism to the stimulatory action of prolactin.

After delivery, milk secretion begins as progesterone falls while prolactin levels remain high. Stage II of lactogenesis is marked by a peak in plasma α-lactalbumin levels; blood flow, oxygen, and glucose uptake and citrate concentration increase. On day 2 or 3 postpartum, a copious increase in milk volume occurs; this is commonly referred to as "milk coming in." The initial volume of less than 100 mL/d will increase to an average maximum of 600 mL/d at 96 hours. Delayed onset of this stage of lactation greater than 72 hours after delivery should be noted as a potential concern. A recent study found this to occur in approximately 22% of new mothers. Infants of these women were 7 times more likely to experience excessive weight loss (10). Because of concerns regarding potential dehydration and jaundice in newborn breastfeeding infants, it is recommended that the newborn have a pediatric evaluation 48–72 hours after hospital discharge.

Maintaining lactogenesis depends on suckling after the third day postpartum. Changes in milk composition then occur gradually over the next 10 days. Stage III of lactogenesis, or galactopoiesis, is the maintenance of milk secretion. Lactation at this time requires not only an intact hypothalamic–pituitary axis for milk synthesis but also removal of milk from the breasts. In most women, adequate milk supply results from adequate frequency of breastfeeding.

Hormonal Influences

Prolactin is a key hormone in lactation. Many drugs and hormones, such as estrogen, thyrotropin-releasing hormone, neuroleptics, phenothiazines, and metoclopramide, can elevate prolactin. Prolactin levels are suppressed by levodopa, ergots, clomiphene, monoamine oxidase inhibitors, PGE, and $PGF_{2\alpha}$. Suckling or nipple stimulation provides the stimulus for the release of prolactin during breastfeeding. By 14 days after delivery, prolactin returns to baseline levels if the breasts are not stimulated. In breastfeeding mothers, baseline prolactin levels decrease over the first 6 months; however, a surge in prolactin over baseline continues to be associated with suckling. The time at which prolactin levels return to normal prepregnant levels depends on the frequency of nursing. Prolactin levels peak 30–60 minutes after a nursing episode begins. Milk volume is not related directly to plasma prolactin concentrations.

Milk Ejection Reflex

The milk ejection reflex involves a neural afferent pathway and an endocrine efferent pathway. After the neural stimulus is received through the neurohypophysis, oxytocin is released from the posterior pituitary. Oxytocin induces contraction of the myoepithelial cells in the alveoli, causing ejection of milk. Although suckling is a stimulus for oxytocin release, other stimuli often result in women experiencing "let down" upon hearing, seeing, or thinking of the infant. Alcohol inhibits milk ejection in a dose-related fashion.

Milk Composition

The composition of human milk is dynamic and adapts to the needs of the infant. The rate-limiting enzyme in lactose synthesis is α-lactalbumin, which is inhibited by progesterone. Glucose is critical to milk volume. The protein composition of human milk is 60% lactalbumin and 40% casein. Lactoferrin is an important protein present in human milk because it binds iron and has been shown to inhibit the growth of certain iron-dependent bacteria in the infant gastrointestinal tract. Immunoglobulin G (IgG) and IgA are present in breast milk. Secretory IgA is the primary immunoglobulin and is highest in colostrum. It is present in the intestines of breastfed infants, remains stable at low pH, is resistant to proteolytic enzymes, and provides protection from organisms invading the mucosa. All vitamins except vitamin K are present in breast milk. Supplementation of certain other vitamins may be indicated in specific circumstances. Vitamin B_{12} supplement may be indicated for mothers who are vegans. Vitamin D supplementation may be indicated for infants who are breastfeeding and have dark pigmentation and lack of sun exposure. Iron supplementation may be indicated after 6 months of life if sufficient quantities are not obtained from the infant's diet.

Human milk is dynamic and varies in composition over time and during each feeding. The initial "foremilk" is lower in fat than the "hindmilk." Fat content is also higher in morning feedings. Colostrum is relatively higher in protein, minerals, and immunologic properties than is mature milk. Colostrum gradually converts to mature milk over 7–10 days, and fat content increases from 2% to 3.6%. Levels of lactose, calories, and water-soluble vitamins increase, while immunoglobulins, protein, and fat-soluble vitamins decrease. The average additional caloric requirement of the mother is 640 kcal per day over the first 6 months and 510 kcal per day after 6 months. Expressed breast milk from a milk bank may be used in certain situations if the mother is unable to establish an adequate milk supply; however, availability of milk from milk banks varies around the country.

POSTPARTUM CARE

Routine Care

Immediately after delivery, the healthy newborn should be given to the mother unless specific circumstances dictate otherwise. Skin-to-skin contact will assist with infant thermal regulation and maternal–infant attachment. Breastfeeding in the first hour of life is correlated with improved success with lactation. The healthy infant may be bathed and other necessary protocols performed at a later time.

A vaginal discharge of lochia rubra, composed of blood and decidua, lasts 3–4 days after delivery. This discharge then becomes watery lochia serosa, lasting 2–3 weeks, and finally changes to yellowish-white lochia alba.

Afterpains occur because of vigorous uterine contractions. These tend to be more problematic in multiparous patients and frequently are associated with nursing as a result of oxytocin release. Nonsteroidal antiinflammatory agents are useful for analgesia.

If testing for HIV was performed upon admission to the hospital, results should be reviewed and posttest counseling performed as appropriate. Rh D-negative mothers of Rh D-positive infants should be given 300 µg of anti-D immune globulin. Routine screening for syphilis also should be performed. Screening for hepatitis B virus is recommended. Hepatitis B immunization is routinely offered for infants, but nonimmunized mothers at risk also should be offered vaccination. If the mother is

---

RESOURCES

Postpartum Care/Complications

American Academy of Pediatrics
www.aap.org

American College of Obstetricians and Gynecologists
www.acog.org

Association of Women's Health, Obstetric and Neonatal Nurses
www.awhonn.org

March of Dimes
www.modimes.org

National Center for Education and Maternal Child Health
www.ncemch.org

National Institute of Child Health and Human Development
www.nichd.nih.gov

Planned Parenthood Federation of America
www.plannedparenthood.org

not immune to rubella, vaccination should be given before she is discharged from the hospital. Both hepatitis B and rubella vaccination are compatible with breastfeeding. The routine evaluation of postdelivery hemoglobin may be unwarranted in the uncomplicated, stable patient.

A relatively common complication of the early puerperium is urinary retention with bladder distention, secondary to trauma or the effects of anesthesia.

Before the patient is discharged, the normal postpartum changes to expect and signs of possible complications should be reviewed (Box 35). Topics include abnormal bleeding, restriction of activities, signs of infection, postpartum blues, contraception, basic assessment

of the newborn, and common difficulties with breastfeeding, if applicable.

The new mother needs support and reassurance during the postpartum period to instill a sense of maternal confidence and to encourage a healthy mother–infant relationship. The father should be encouraged to participate in the care of the neonate, not only to provide additional support for the mother, but also to enhance the father–infant relationship.

Changes in Sexual Function

Reports indicate that women's interest in sexual relations changes after childbirth; 47–57% of women interviewed 3 months postpartum noted decreased interest. This is commonly attributed to fatigue, pain, and concern over injury. More than 80% of women have resumed coitus by 6 weeks postpartum. An increase in vaginal atrophy and a decrease in lubrication commonly occur in exclusively breastfeeding mothers.

Contraception

Contraceptive options should be reviewed postpartum. In nonlactating women, oral contraceptives can be begun 2 weeks after delivery unless otherwise contraindicated. For lactating women, estrogen-containing oral contraceptives should be deferred for 4 weeks or more until lactation is well established. A more favorable alternative in the breastfeeding population may be progestin-only contraceptives, which do not appear to impair lactation. Alternatives include the daily progesterone-only "minipill" and depot medroxyprogesterone acetate (DMPA) injections. Use of DMPA should be initiated 6 weeks postpartum, although rarely individual circumstances may indicate initiation sooner. An intrauterine device is ideally placed 6 or more weeks after delivery to avoid an increased risk of expulsion or perforation. Diaphragm refitting is best delayed for at least 6 weeks. The lactational amenorrhea method of contraception may be used with relative confidence in motivated patients. To be most effective (approximately 98%) in the first 6 months, this technique requires amenorrhea, breastfeeding at least 8 times daily with maximum intervals of 6 hours, and essentially no supplemental feeding.

Future Pregnancy Counseling

The postpartum visit is an ideal time to discuss the planning of future pregnancies. One study found that the optimal interval between live births is 18–23 months to achieve the lowest risk for low birth weight, SGA infants, and preterm birth (11). Recently, women with an interpregnancy interval of less than 6 months were found to be more likely to experience preterm delivery and neonatal death unrelated to congenital anomalies in the second pregnancy (12).

BOX 35

In-Hospital Postpartum Care Checklist

- Review pertinent laboratory tests: blood type and screen, hepatitis B surface antigen, syphilis testing, human immunovirus test results if performed (provide posttest counseling), hemoglobin results (pre- and postdelivery where applicable). Provide treatments when indicated.

- Provide appropriate maternal vaccinations: Hepatitis B (if at risk and not previously vaccinated), rubella (if not immune), flu (if season warrants and not already given)

- Provide prescriptions for medications.

- Assure proper education regarding appropriate incisional or peri-care.

- Discuss restrictions (ie, no driving while taking narcotics, nothing per vagina, no heavy lifting).

- Discuss expected timing of follow-up visits (ie, incision check after cesarean and standard postpartum visit)

- Provide patient with education on basic breastfeeding management and appropriate resources for additional support if needed after hospital discharge.

- Review the patient's plans for contraception and prescribe as appropriate.

- Assess whether the parent's questions about care and follow-up of the newborn have been answered and whether a plan for a pediatric visit has been recommended.

- Provide education about postpartum blues and postpartum depression and notify patient (and ideally other family members as well) of reasons to seek assistance.

- Discuss warning signs of complications and how to notify appropriate health care personnel (ie: heavy bleeding, worsening abdominal pain, fever).

POSTPARTUM COMPLICATIONS

Hemorrhage

The diagnosis of postpartum hemorrhage is based primarily on the estimate and judgment of the clinician. However, it generally implies bleeding to a degree that threatens to cause, or is associated with, hemodynamic instability. Postpartum hemorrhage is classified as either early (first 24 hours after delivery) or late (after 24 hours but before 6 weeks after delivery).

EARLY HEMORRHAGE

The etiology of early postpartum hemorrhage includes uterine atony, lacerations, uterine inversion, retained placental fragments, and coagulopathy. The most common cause of postpartum hemorrhage is uterine atony, which in turn may be associated with overdistention of the uterus, protracted labor, macrosomia, high parity, intra-amniotic infection, and use of uterine-relaxing agents. The most common causes of late postpartum hemorrhage are subinvolution of the placental site, infection, and retained products of conception.

Management of postpartum hemorrhage consists of ascertaining its etiology, providing volume replacement, monitoring vital signs and urine output, and correcting the cause. Appropriate laboratory tests may include assessments of prothrombin time, partial thromboplastin time, platelet count, and fibrinogen levels to assist in the diagnosis of coagulopathy, if suspected.

Medical management consists primarily of drugs to treat or prevent uterine atony. Surgical management is necessary in women for whom medical management fails. Surgery may involve ligation of the uterine arteries, ligation of the uteroovarian arteries, ligation of the hypogastric arteries, or hysterectomy (13). Hypogastric artery ligation is technically difficult and requires special surgical skill. In the presence of life-threatening bleeding, hysterectomy is often the quickest and safest procedure.

LATE HEMORRHAGE

Treatment of late postpartum hemorrhage consists of the medical modalities listed in Table 30 and volume replacement. Antibiotics should be used if infection is suspected. Curettage may lead to increased bleeding and should be used only if medical therapy fails and retained products of conception are suspected on ultrasound examination. Unless hemorrhage is profuse, angiographic embolization also may be considered before hypogastric artery ligation or hysterectomy (14).

Postpartum Infection

UTERINE INFECTION

The most common cause of postpartum or puerperal fever is uterine infection. Such an infection may be called endometritis, endomyometritis, endoparametritis, or simply metritis. Both the frequency and severity of infection are greater after abdominal delivery than after vaginal delivery. The incidence of infection after vaginal delivery is only 1–3%, whereas the incidence after abdominal delivery is 5–30%. Women who undergo emergency or nonelective procedures (with labor, rupture of membranes, or both) are at the greatest risk for infection and are most likely to benefit from prophylactic antibiotics.

Labor and ruptured membranes are probably the 2 most common risk factors associated with infection after cesarean delivery. The number of vaginal examinations, socioeconomic status, and internal fetal monitoring also have been implicated, but their independent effects are difficult to document.

The microbiology of endometritis following cesarean delivery is polymicrobial, comprising a mixture of aerobes and anaerobes. Commonly isolated aerobes include gram-negative bacilli (eg, *Escherichia coli)* and gram-positive cocci (eg, group B streptococci). Anaerobic organisms clearly have major roles in infection (80% of specimens) after cesarean delivery. The most commonly isolated organism is often a species of Bacteroides. Anaerobic cocci also are commonly found.

The diagnosis of endometritis is based primarily on the presence of fever and the absence of other causes of fever. Uterine tenderness, especially parametrial, and purulent or foul-smelling lochia are also common findings. Laboratory studies, with the exception of blood cultures, are not particularly helpful.

The regimen commonly used as a standard for treatment is clindamycin–gentamicin, a combination that generally is curative in 85–95% of patients. Because of the potential toxicity of clindamycin–gentamicin, as well as the combined cost of these antibiotics, the possibility of using one of the newer penicillins or cephalosporins for single-drug therapy has attracted some interest. Good results have been reported with a number of these including cefoxitin, cefoperazone, cefotaxime, piperacillin, cefotetan, and clindamycin–aztreonam. Newer antibiotics containing a penicillin derivative and a β-lactamase inhibitor are also effective. Treatment generally should be continued until the patient is afebrile for 24–48 hours and then discontinued.

Causes of initial failure of antibiotic therapy include abscess, resistant organisms, wound infection, infection at other sites, or septic thrombophlebitis. Computed tomography–directed percutaneous needle drainage or surgical drainage, especially for an abscess, occasionally may be necessary. Hysterectomy may rarely be required. Treatment of a wound infection consists of drainage and débridement. Antibiotics should be used for significant induration. A puerperal infection in the pelvis may extend along the veins, resulting in septic pelvic thrombophlebitis. Treatment usually is directed at the pelvic infection, and antibiotics are indicated for therapy. The use of anticoagulants with full heparinization is controversial but is used by some clinicians.

TABLE 30. Uterotonic Agents for Postpartum Hemorrhage

Medication	Dose	Primary (Alternate) Route	Frequency of Dose	Side Effects	Comments and Contraindications
Oxytocin	10–40 U in 1,000 mL of normal saline or lactated Ringer's solution	IV (IM, IMM)	Continuous infusion	Usually none, but nausea, vomiting, and water intoxication have been reported	No contraindications
Methylergonovine	0.2 mg	IM (IMM)	Every 2–4 h	Hypertension, hypotension, nausea, vomiting	Contraindications include hypertension and preeclampsia
15-methyl-PGF$_{2\alpha}$	0.25 mg	IM (IMM)	Every 15–90 min, not to exceed 8 doses	Vomiting, diarrhea, nausea, flushing or hot flashes, chills or shivering	Contraindications include active cardiac, pulmonary renal, or hepatic disease
Dinoprostone (PGE$_2$)	20 mg	PR	Every 2 h	Vomiting, diarrhea, nausea, fever, headache, chills or shivering	Should be avoided in hypotensive patients because of vasodilation; if available, 15- methyl-PGF$_{2\alpha}$ is preferable
Misoprostol* (PGE$_1$)	400–800 µg	PR (PO)		Vomiting, diarrhea, nausea, fever, chills shivering, headache	No contraindications

IV indicates intravenous; IM, intramuscular; IMM, intramyometrial; PR, per rectum; PO, orally; PGE$_1$, prostaglandin E$_1$; PGE$_2$, prostaglandin E$_2$; PGF$_{2\alpha}$, prostaglandin F$_{2\alpha}$.

*Drug "could be useful." Mousa HA, Alfirevic Z. Treatment for primary postpartum haemorrhage. The Cochrane Database of Systematic Reviews 2003, Issue 1. Art. No.: CD003249. DOI: 10.1002/14651858.CD003249.

Adapted from American College of Obstetricians and Gynecologists. Postpartum hemorrhage. ACOG Educational Bulletin 243. Washington, DC: ACOG, 1998.

The efficacy of prophylactic antibiotics in women at risk for endometritis is now well established. A single dose of antibiotic should be used for prophylaxis and initiated after umbilical cord clamping. A "first-generation" cephalosporin is generally effective for this purpose. Although the newer, broader-spectrum antibiotics are effective for prophylaxis, there is no evidence that they are more effective than the older, less-expensive choices.

URINARY TRACT INFECTIONS

Urinary tract infections occur in approximately 5% of puerperal women. Predisposing factors include prolonged labor, urinary retention, and indwelling catheters. Acute pyelonephritis is characterized by chills, spiking fever, costovertebral angle tenderness, and frequently, nausea and vomiting.

MASTITIS

A recent study found that 9.5% of breastfeeding women experienced at least one provider diagnosed episode of mastitis in the first 12 weeks of nursing (15). Risk factors suggested for mastitis include impaired emptying of the breast, plugged ducts, nipple trauma, engorgement, low-ered maternal defenses, and missed feedings. Most often, mastitis is caused by *Staphylococcus aureus*. Other common organisms are group A or group B streptococci, *E coli*, and *Haemophilus* species.

Treatment includes continuation of breastfeeding or emptying of the breast with a pump and the use of appropriate antibiotics. The breast milk remains safe for the full term, healthy infant. Drugs of choice include penicillinase-resistant penicillins (such as dicloxacillin) or a cephalosporin. Clindamycin can be attempted in cases of severe penicillin hypersensitivity. For a hospital-acquired infection, recurrences or failure to respond after 48 hours of therapy, a mid-stream breast milk culture collected in a sterile container may be useful in guiding therapy.

Symptoms of a breast abscess may be similar to that of mastitis, but a fluctuant mass is also present. Persistent fever after initiating antibiotics also may suggest abscess. Because of the unique anatomy of the breast, destruction of breast tissue may be far more extensive than a superficial physical examination would suggest. Treatment requires adequate drainage of the abscess with continued full therapeutic doses of antibiotics for 10 days. Preferably, the incision is placed away from the nipple–areolar complex.

EPISIOTOMY INFECTION

Episiotomy infections are relatively uncommon, but when they do occur, especially in association with a third- or fourth-degree laceration, they may be associated with significant morbidity. Diagnosis generally is based on purulent discharge in association with redness and induration. Treatment consists of opening the episiotomy and removing all sutures. The episiotomy should be irrigated with copious fluid, followed by débridement of the wound. The area needs to be inspected for any dead tissue suggesting necrotizing fasciitis. Proper care requires that the wound be cleaned at least twice daily, and it is suggested that sitz baths be used liberally. Broad-spectrum antibiotics also should be used.

Urinary and Rectal Incontinence

The pelvic floor may be changed significantly from pregnancy and the birthing process. This is evidenced by the increased incidence of stress urinary incontinence and fecal incontinence after delivery. Fecal incontinence is reported in approximately 5% of vaginally delivered patients (16). Although some have attributed these changes to damage secondary to operative vaginal delivery, these pelvic floor complications have been reported with spontaneous vaginal delivery and even cesarean delivery. Some of these changes also can be attributed to aging.

Postpartum Thyroid Dysfunction

Abnormalities of thyroid function occur in approximately 5% of puerperal women. Thyroid dysfunction is transient and often goes undiagnosed because vague symptoms are attributed to the postpartum period. A thyrotoxic phase occurs in 75% of individuals 2–3 months postpartum. Symptoms include fatigue, weight loss, palpitations, and dizziness. A hypothyroid phase then ensues 4–8 months postpartum, which may be more clinically apparent with complaints of fatigue and weight gain. A goiter is present in 50% of patients. Most patients then return to euthyroidism in 3–5 months, although 10–30% becomes permanently hypothyroid. Treatment is often expectant but may be necessary if symptoms warrant. There is an increased rate of recurrence with future pregnancies (10–25%), permanent hypothyroidism, and other autoimmune diseases.

Postpartum Depression and Mood Changes

Depression to some degree is common in the postpartum period. It can range from postpartum blues, which dissipate in 2–3 weeks, to major postpartum depression, which usually requires medication and psychologic counseling (see "Depression").

References

1. Negishi H, Kishida T, Yamada H, Hirayama E, Mikuni M, Fujimoto S. Changes in uterine size after vaginal delivery and cesarean section determined by vaginal sonography in the puerperium. Arch Gynecol Obstet 1999;263:13–6.

2. Strinic T, Bukovic D, Karelovic D, Bojie L, Stipic I. The effect of delivery on regression of abnormal cervical cytologic findings. Coll Antropol 2002;26(2):577–82.

3. Siddiqui G, Kurzel RB, Lampley EC, Kang HS, Blankstein J. Cervical dysplasia in pregnancy: progression versus regression post-partum. Int J Fertil Womens Med 2001; 46:278–80.

4. Ahdoot D, Van Nostrand KM, Nguyen NJ, Tewari DS, Kurasaki T, DiSaia PJ, et al. The effect of route of delivery on regression of abnormal cervical cytologic findings in the postpartum period. Am J Obstet Gynecol 1998;178: 1116–20.

5. Gross B, Burger H; WHO Task Force on methods for the natural regulation of fertility. Breastfeeding patterns and return to fertility in Australian women. Aust N Z J Obstet Gynaecol 2002;42:148–54.

6. American College of Obstetricians and Gynecologists. Breastfeeding: maternal and infant aspects. ACOG Educational Bulletin 258. Washington, DC: ACOG; 2000.

7. Breastfeeding and the use of human milk. American Academy of Pediatrics; Work Group on Breastfeeding. Pediatrics 1997;100:1035–9.

8. Ryan AS, Wenjun Z, Acosta A. Breastfeeding continues to increase into the new millennium. Pediatrics 2002;110: 1103–9.

9. Collaborative Group on Hormonal Factors in Breast Cancer. Breast cancer and breastfeeding: collaborative reanalysis of individual data from 47 epidemiological studies in 30 countries, including 50302 women with breast cancer and 96973 women without the disease. Lancet 2002;360:187–95.

10. Dewey KG, Nommsen-Rivers LA, Heinig MJ, Cohen RJ. Risk factors for suboptimal infant breastfeeding behavior, delayed onset of lactation, and excess neonatal weight loss. Pediatrics 2003;112:607–19.

11. Zhu BP, Rolfs RT, Nangle BE, Horan JM. Effect of the interval between pregnancies on perinatal outcomes. N Engl J Med 1999;340:589–94.

12. Smith GC, Pell JP, Dobbie R. Interpregnancy interval and risk of preterm birth and neonatal death: retrospective cohort study [published erratum appears in BMJ 2003;327: 851]. BMJ 2003;327:313.

13. Papp Z. Massive obstetric hemorrhage. J Perinat Med 2003; 31:408–14.

14. Hong TM, Tseng HS, Lee RC, Wang JH, Chang CY. Uterine artery embolization: an effective treatment for intractable obstetric haemorrhage. Clin Radiol 2004;59: 96–101.

15. Foxman B, D'Arcy H, Gillespie B, Bobo JK, Schwartz K. Lactation mastitis: occurrence and medical management among 946 breastfeeding women in the United States. Am J Epidemiol 2002;155:103–14.

16. Meyer S, Schreyer A, De Grandi P, Hohlfeld P. The effects of birth on urinary continence mechanisms and other pelvic-floor characteristics. Obstet Gynecol 1998;92:613–8.

Appendix A
Information Resources

PATIENT EDUCATION MATERIALS

The following patient education pamphlets are available from ACOG. For ordering information and a complete current list, call 800-762-2264, ext 133.

Pregnancy

Alcohol and Pregnancy (2000)	AP132
Amniocentesis and Chorionic Villus Sampling (1999)	AP107
Birth Defects (2005)	AP146
Bleeding During Pregnancy (1999)	AP038
Car Safety for You and Your Baby (1999)	AP018
Childhood Illnesses and Pregnancy (2002)	AP157
Diabetes and Pregnancy (2000)	AP051
Diagnosing Birth Defects (2005)	AP164
Drugs and Pregnancy (2002)	AP104
Early Pregnancy Loss: Miscarriage and Molar Pregnancy (2002)	AP090
Easing Back Pain During Pregnancy (1997)	AP115
Ectopic Pregnancy (2002)	AP155
Especially for Fathers (1998)	AP032
Exercise During Pregnancy (2003)	AP119
Genetic Disorders in Pregnancy (2005)	AP094
Good Health Before Pregnancy: Preconceptional Care (1999)	AP056
Group B Streptococcus and Pregnancy (2003)	AP105
Having a Baby (For Adolescents) (2001)	AP103
Having Twins (2004)	AP092
Hepatitis B Virus in Pregnancy (2000)	AP093
High Blood Pressure During Pregnancy (2004)	AP034
HIV Testing and Pregnancy (2000)	AP113
How Your Baby Grows During Pregnancy (2002)	AP156
If Your Baby Is Breech (2002)	AP079
Later Childbearing (1999)	AP060
Maternal Serum Screening for Birth Defects (2005)	AP165
Morning Sickness (1999)	AP126
Nutrition During Pregnancy (2002)	AP001

Pregnancy Choices: Raising the Baby, Adoption, and Abortion (2002)	AP102
Pregnancy Options for Adolescents (2003)	FS013
Repeated Miscarriage (2000)	AP100
Routine Tests in Pregnancy (2000)	AP133
The Rh Factor: How It Can Affect Your Pregnancy (1999)	AP027
Seizure Disorders in Pregnancy (1999)	AP129
Special Tests for Monitoring Fetal Health (2002)	AP098
Toxoplasmosis and Pregnancy (2003)	AP160
Travel During Pregnancy (2001)	AP055
What to Expect After Your Due Date (2002)	AP069
Working During Your Pregnancy: Risks and Rights (2001)	AP044

Labor, Delivery, And Postpartum Care

Breastfeeding Your Baby (2001)	AP029
Cesarean Birth (2005)	AP006
Fetal Heart Rate Monitoring During Labor (2001)	AP015
Getting in Shape After Your Baby is Born (2000)	AP131
How to Tell When Labor Begins (1999)	AP004
Labor Induction (2001)	AP154
Newborn Circumcision (1999)	AP039
Pain Relief During Labor and Delivery (2004)	AP086
Postpartum Depression (1999)	AP091
Preterm Labor (2004)	AP087
Vaginal Birth After Cesarean Delivery (1999)	AP070

Other

Planning Your Pregnancy and Birth, Third Edition	AB003S
You and Your Baby: Prenatal Care, Labor and Delivery, and Postpartum Care	AB005
Healthy Mother's Food Wheel	AA005
You and Your Baby: Changes During Pregnancy (Poster)	AA438
Breastfeeding Your Baby (Poster)	AA462
Exercises During Pregnancy and After the Baby Is Born (Poster)	AA270

WOMEN'S HEALTH WEB SITES*

Consumer Resources

The American College of Obstetricians and Gynecologists
http://www.acog.org

American Self-Help Clearinghouse Self-Help Sourcebook Online
http://mentalhelp.net/selfhelp

ASHA: American Social Health Association
http://www.ashastd.org

Emory MedWeb
http://www.medweb.emory.edu/MedWeb

healthfinder
http://www.healthfinder.gov

Mayo Clinic
http://www.mayohealth.org

Medem
http://www.medem.com

MedlinePlus
http://medlineplus.gov

National Women's Health Information Center
http://www.4woman.org

NOAH: New York Online Access to Health Home Page
http://www.noah-health.org

OncoLink
http://www.oncolink.upenn.edu

Sexuality and You
http://sexualityandu.ca

Organizations

American Academy of Dermatology
www.aad.org

American Academy of Family Physicians
www.aafp.org

American Academy of Pediatrics
www.aap.org

American Autoimmune Related Disease Association
www.aarda.org

American Board of Obstetrics and Gynecology, Inc.
www.abog.org

*This list and other resource lists throughout this volume were prepared by ACOG Resource Center librarians from other sources and are provided for information only. Referral to these sites does not imply the endorsement of the American College of Obstetricians and Gynecologists. This list is not meant to be comprehensive; the exclusion of a site does not reflect the quality of that site. Please note that sites and URLs are subject to change without warning. Sites were checked November 19, 2004.

American Cancer Society
www.cancer.org

American College of Cardiology
www.acc.org

American College of Obstetricians and Gynecologists
www.acog.org

American College of Osteopathic Obstetricians and Gynecologists
www.acoog.com

American College of Physicians/American Society of Internal Medicine
www.acponline.org

American College of Radiology
www.acr.org

American College of Rheumatology
www.rheumatology.org

American Diabetes Association
www.eatright.org

American Foundation for Urologic Disease
www.afud.org

American Heart Association
www.americanheart.org

American Lung Association
www.lungusa.org

American Medical Association
www.ama-assn.org

American Psychiatric Association
www.psych.org

American Society for Reproductive Medicine
www.asrm.org

Association of Reproductive Health Professionals
www.arhp.org

Association of Women's Health, Obstetric and Neonatal Nurses
www.awhonn.org

Jacobs Institute of Women's Health
www.jiwh.org

National Association for Continence
www.nafc.org

National Association for Women's Health
www.nawh.org

National Headache Foundation
www.headaches.org

National Mental Health Association
www.nmha.org

Societies of Interest to Obstetrics & Gynecology
www.il-st-acad-sci.org/health/obsoc.html

The Thyroid Foundation of America
www.tsh.org

General Resources

Kaisernetwork.org
kaisernetwork.org

MedWeb: Biomedical Internet Resources
www.medweb.emory.edu/MedWeb

NCEMCH : National Center for Education in Maternal and Child Health
www.ncemch.org/default.html

The National Women's Health Information Center
www.4woman.gov

OBGYN.net - The Obstetrics & Gynecology Network
www.obgyn.net/home.htm

Reproductive Health Gateway
www.rhgateway.org

Quackwatch: Your Guide to Health Fraud, Quackery, and Intelligent Decisions
www.quackwatch.com

Evidence-Based Medicine

Bandolier Home Page
www.jr2.ox.ac.uk/Bandolier

Centre for Evidence-Based Medicine
cebm.net

Cochrane Collaboration
www.cochrane.org

EBM Home Page
www-hsl.mcmaster.ca/ebm

University of York NHS Centre for Reviews and Dissemination
www.york.ac.uk/inst/crd

Government

Centers for Disease Control and Prevention (CDC)
www.cdc.gov

AHRQ: Agency for Healthcare Research and Quality (a.k.a. AHCPR)
www.ahcpr.gov

Food and Drug Administration Home Page
www.fda.gov

Centers for Medicare & Medicaid Services
www.cms.hhs.gov

Department of Labor
www.dol.gov

Healthy People 2010
www.healthypeople.gov

Library of Congress Home Page
www.loc.gov

National Institutes of Health
www.nih.gov

U.S. Surgeon General
www.surgeongeneral.gov/sgoffice.htm

Guidelines

AHRQ Guidelines
www.ahrq.gov

Centers for Disease Control and Prevention (CDC)
www.cdc.gov

Joint Commission on Accreditation of Healthcare Organizations
www.jcaho.org

Guide to US Preventive Services
www.ahcpr.gov/clinic/uspstfix.htm

National Guideline Clearinghouse
www.guideline.gov

National Academy of Science
www.nas.edu

International

International Federation of Gynecology & Obstetrics (FIGO)
www.figo.org

Royal College of Obstetricians and Gynaecologists
www.rcog.org.uk

Society of Obstetricians and Gynaecologists of Canada
www.sogc.org

United Nations and Other International Organizations
http://www.un.org

World Health Organization WWW Home Page
http://www.who.int/en

MEDLINE

PUBMED
http://www.PubMed.gov

Statistics

Fedstats: One Stop Shopping for Federal Statistics
http://www.fedstats.gov

National Center for Health Statistics
http://www.cdc.gov/nchs

SEER Homepage
http://seer.cancer.gov

TERATOGEN INFORMATION

Reprotox – 301-514-3081; www.reprotox.org

Teris - 206-543-2465;
www.depts.washington.edu/~terisweb

Organization of Teratology Information Services
www.otispregnancy.org/

Appendix B
ACOG Antepartum Record

DATE _____

NAME _____
        LAST   FIRST   MIDDLE

ID # _____ HOSPITAL OF DELIVERY _____

NEWBORN'S PHYSICIAN _____ REFERRED BY _____

| FINAL EDD _____ | PRIMARY PROVIDER/GROUP _____ |

BIRTH DATE	AGE	RACE	MARITAL STATUS	ADDRESS
MONTH DAY YEAR			S M W D SEP	
OCCUPATION		EDUCATION (LAST GRADE COMPLETED)		ZIP PHONE (H) (O)
LANGUAGE				INSURANCE CARRIER/MEDICAID #
HUSBAND/DOMESTIC PARTNER		PHONE		POLICY #
FATHER OF BABY		PHONE		EMERGENCY CONTACT PHONE

TOTAL PREG	FULL TERM	PREMATURE	AB, INDUCED	AB, SPONTANEOUS	ECTOPICS	MULTIPLE BIRTHS	LIVING

MENSTRUAL HISTORY

LMP ☐ DEFINITE ☐ APPROXIMATE (MONTH KNOWN)   MENSES MONTHLY ☐ YES ☐ NO   FREQUENCY: Q _____ DAYS   MENARCHE _____ (AGE ONSET)

☐ UNKNOWN ☐ NORMAL AMOUNT/DURATION   PRIOR MENSES _____ DATE   ON BCP AT CONCEPT ☐ YES ☐ NO   hCG + ____/____/____

☐ FINAL _____

PAST PREGNANCIES (LAST SIX)

DATE MONTH/ YEAR	GA WEEKS	LENGTH OF LABOR	BIRTH WEIGHT	SEX M/F	TYPE DELIVERY	ANES.	PLACE OF DELIVERY	PRETERM LABOR YES/NO	COMMENTS/ COMPLICATIONS

MEDICAL HISTORY

	○ Neg. + Pos.	DETAIL POSITIVE REMARKS INCLUDE DATE & TREATMENT		○ Neg. + Pos.	DETAIL POSITIVE REMARKS INCLUDE DATE & TREATMENT
1. DIABETES			17. D (Rh) SENSITIZED		
2. HYPERTENSION			18. PULMONARY (TB, ASTHMA)		
3. HEART DISEASE			19. SEASONAL ALLERGIES		
4. AUTOIMMUNE DISORDER			20. DRUG/LATEX ALLERGIES/ REACTIONS		
5. KIDNEY DISEASE/UTI					
6. NEUROLOGIC/EPILEPSY			21. BREAST		
7. PSYCHIATRIC			22. GYN SURGERY		
8. DEPRESSION/POSTPARTUM DEPRESSION			23. OPERATIONS/ HOSPITALIZATIONS (YEAR & REASON)		
9. HEPATITIS/LIVER DISEASE					
10. VARICOSITIES/PHLEBITIS					
11. THYROID DYSFUNCTION			24. ANESTHETIC COMPLICATIONS		
12. TRAUMA/VIOLENCE			25. HISTORY OF ABNORMAL PAP		
13. HISTORY OF BLOOD TRANSFUS.			26. UTERINE ANOMALY/DES		

	AMT/DAY PREPREG	AMT/DAY PREG	# YEARS USE			
14. TOBACCO				27. INFERTILITY		
15. ALCOHOL				28. RELEVANT FAMILY HISTORY		
16. ILLICIT/RECREATIONAL DRUGS				29. OTHER		

COMMENTS _____

Version 5. Copyright © 2002 The American College of Obstetricians and Gynecologists, 409 12th Street, SW, PO Box 96920, Washington, DC 20090-6920   AA128   1 2 3 4 5 / 6 5 4 3 2

ACOG ANTEPARTUM RECORD (FORM A)

SYMPTOMS SINCE LMP

GENETIC SCREENING/TERATOLOGY COUNSELING
INCLUDES PATIENT, BABY'S FATHER, OR ANYONE IN EITHER FAMILY WITH:

	YES	NO		YES	NO
1. PATIENT'S AGE ≥ 35 YEARS AS OF ESTIMATED DATE OF DELIVERY			12. HUNTINGTON'S CHOREA		
2. THALASSEMIA (ITALIAN, GREEK, MEDITERRANEAN, OR ASIAN BACKGROUND): MCV <80			13. MENTAL RETARDATION/AUTISM		
			IF YES, WAS PERSON TESTED FOR FRAGILE X?		
3. NEURAL TUBE DEFECT (MENINGOMYELOCELE, SPINA BIFIDA, OR ANENCEPHALY)			14. OTHER INHERITED GENETIC OR CHROMOSOMAL DISORDER		
4. CONGENITAL HEART DEFECT			15. MATERNAL METABOLIC DISORDER (EG, TYPE 1 DIABETES, PKU)		
5. DOWN SYNDROME			16. PATIENT OR BABY'S FATHER HAD A CHILD WITH BIRTH DEFECTS NOT LISTED ABOVE		
6. TAY–SACHS (EG, JEWISH, CAJUN, FRENCH CANADIAN)			17. RECURRENT PREGNANCY LOSS, OR A STILLBIRTH		
7. CANAVAN DISEASE			18. MEDICATIONS (INCLUDING SUPPLEMENTS, VITAMINS, HERBS OR OTC DRUGS)/ILLICIT/RECREATIONAL DRUGS/ALCOHOL SINCE LAST MENSTRUAL PERIOD		
8. SICKLE CELL DISEASE OR TRAIT (AFRICAN)					
9. HEMOPHILIA OR OTHER BLOOD DISORDERS			IF YES, AGENT(S) AND STRENGTH/DOSAGE		
10. MUSCULAR DYSTROPHY					
11. CYSTIC FIBROSIS			19. ANY OTHER		

COMMENTS/COUNSELING _____

_____

INFECTION HISTORY	YES	NO		YES	NO
1. LIVE WITH SOMEONE WITH TB OR EXPOSED TO TB			4. HISTORY OF STD, GONORRHEA, CHLAMYDIA, HPV, SYPHILIS		
2. PATIENT OR PARTNER HAS HISTORY OF GENITAL HERPES			5. OTHER (See Comments)		
3. RASH OR VIRAL ILLNESS SINCE LAST MENSTRUAL PERIOD					

COMMENTS _____

_____ **INTERVIEWER'S SIGNATURE** _____

INITIAL PHYSICAL EXAMINATION

DATE _____ / _____ / _____   HEIGHT _____   BP_____

1. HEENT	☐ NORMAL	☐ ABNORMAL	12. VULVA	☐ NORMAL	☐ CONDYLOMA	☐ LESIONS
2. FUNDI	☐ NORMAL	☐ ABNORMAL	13. VAGINA	☐ NORMAL	☐ INFLAMMATION	☐ DISCHARGE
3. TEETH	☐ NORMAL	☐ ABNORMAL	14. CERVIX	☐ NORMAL	☐ INFLAMMATION	☐ LESIONS
4. THYROID	☐ NORMAL	☐ ABNORMAL	15. UTERUS SIZE	_____ WEEKS		☐ FIBROIDS
5. BREASTS	☐ NORMAL	☐ ABNORMAL	16. ADNEXA	☐ NORMAL	☐ MASS	
6. LUNGS	☐ NORMAL	☐ ABNORMAL	17. RECTUM	☐ NORMAL	☐ ABNORMAL	
7. HEART	☐ NORMAL	☐ ABNORMAL	18. DIAGONAL CONJUGATE	☐ REACHED	☐ NO	_____ CM
8. ABDOMEN	☐ NORMAL	☐ ABNORMAL	19. SPINES	☐ AVERAGE	☐ PROMINENT	☐ BLUNT
9. EXTREMITIES	☐ NORMAL	☐ ABNORMAL	20. SACRUM	☐ CONCAVE	☐ STRAIGHT	☐ ANTERIOR
10. SKIN	☐ NORMAL	☐ ABNORMAL	21. SUBPUBIC ARCH	☐ NORMAL	☐ WIDE	☐ NARROW
11. LYMPH NODES	☐ NORMAL	☐ ABNORMAL	22. GYNECOID PELVIC TYPE	☐ YES	☐ NO	

COMMENTS (Number and explain abnormals) _____

_____

_____ **EXAM BY** _____

ACOG ANTEPARTUM RECORD (FORM B)

NAME _____
        LAST   FIRST   MIDDLE

DRUG ALLERGY	LATEX ALLERGY	

IS BLOOD TRANSFUSION ACCEPTABLE IN AN EMERGENCY?   ☐ YES   ☐ NO   ANESTHESIA CONSULT PLANNED   ☐ YES   ☐ NO

PROBLEMS/PLANS

1. _____

2. _____

3. _____

4. _____

5. _____

6. _____

MEDICATION LIST   Start date   Stop date

1. _____ ____/____/____ ____/____/____

2. _____ ____/____/____ ____/____/____

3. _____ ____/____/____ ____/____/____

4. _____ ____/____/____ ____/____/____

5. _____ ____/____/____ ____/____/____

6.   ____/____/____ ____/____/____

EDD CONFIRMATION

INITIAL EDD

LMP   ____/____/____   =   EDD ____/____/____

INITIAL EXAM   ____/____/____ = ____ WKS = EDD ____/____/____

ULTRASOUND   ____/____/____ = ____ WKS = EDD ____/____/____

INITIAL EDD   ____/____/____   INITIALED BY _____

18–20-WEEK EDD UPDATE

QUICKENING   ____/____/____   +22 WKS =   ____/____/____

FUNDAL HT.
AT UMBIL.   ____/____/____   +20 WKS =   ____/____/____

ULTRASOUND   ____/____/____ = ____ WKS =   ____/____/____

FINAL EDD   ____/____/____   INITIALED BY _____

PREPREGNANCY WEIGHT
_____

	WEEKS GEST. (BEST EST.)	FUNDAL HEIGHT (CM)	PRESENTATION	FHR	FETAL MOVEMENT	PRETERM LABOR SIGNS/SYMPTOMS: +=PRESENT o=ABSENT	CERVIX EXAM (DIL./EFF./STA.) ULTRASOUND LENGTH	BLOOD PRESSURE	WEIGHT	URINE (ALBUMIN/GLUCOSE)	NEXT APPOINTMENT	PROVIDER (INITIALS)

COMMENTS

PROBLEMS _____

COMMENTS _____

ACOG ANTEPARTUM RECORD (FORM C)

LABORATORY AND EDUCATION

INITIAL LABS	DATE	RESULT	REVIEWED
BLOOD TYPE	/ /	A B AB O	
D (Rh) TYPE	/ /		
ANTIBODY SCREEN	/ /		
HCT/HGB	/ /	_____ % _____ g/dL	
PAP TEST	/ /	NORMAL/ABNORMAL/_____	
RUBELLA	/ /		
VDRL	/ /		
URINE CULTURE/SCREEN	/ /		
HBsAg	/ /		
HIV COUNSELING/TESTING*	/ /	POS. NEG. DECLINED	
OPTIONAL LABS	**DATE**	**RESULT**	
HGB ELECTROPHORESIS	/ /	AA AS SS AC SC AF $\uparrow A_2$	
PPD	/ /		
CHLAMYDIA	/ /		
GONORRHEA	/ /		
GENETIC SCREENING TESTS (SEE FORM B)	/ /		
OTHER			
8–18-WEEK LABS (WHEN INDICATED/ ELECTED)	**DATE**	**RESULT**	
ULTRASOUND	/ /		
MSAFP/MULTIPLE MARKERS	/ /		
AMNIO/CVS	/ /		
KARYOTYPE	/ /	46, XX OR 46, XY/OTHER_____	
AMNIOTIC FLUID (AFP)	/ /	NORMAL_____ ABNORMAL_____	
24–28-WEEK LABS (WHEN INDICATED)	**DATE**	**RESULT**	
HCT/HGB	/ /	_____ % _____ g/dL	
DIABETES SCREEN	/ /	1 HOUR_____	
GTT (IF SCREEN ABNORMAL)	/ /	_____FBS _____1 HOUR _____2 HOUR _____3 HOUR	
D (Rh) ANTIBODY SCREEN	/ /		
ANTI-D IMMUNE GLOBULIN (RhIG) GIVEN (28 WKS)	/ /	SIGNATURE _____	
32–36-WEEK LABS (WHEN INDICATED)	**DATE**	**RESULT**	
HCT/HGB (RECOMMENDED)	/ /	_____ % _____ g/dL	
ULTRASOUND	/ /		
VDRL	/ /		
GONORRHEA	/ /		
CHLAMYDIA	/ /		
GROUP B STREP IF USING CULTURE STRATEGY. N/A IF USING RISK STRATEGY. (35–37 WKS)	/ /		

COMMENTS/ADDITIONAL LABS

*Check state requirements before recording results.

PROVIDER SIGNATURE (AS REQUIRED)_____

ACOG ANTEPARTUM RECORD (FORM D)

NAME _____
         LAST   FIRST   MIDDLE

PLANS/EDUCATION
(COUNSELED ☐)—BY TRIMESTER. INITIAL AND DATE WHEN DISCUSSED.

	COMPLETED	NEED FOR FURTHER DISCUSSION
FIRST TRIMESTER		
☐ HIV AND OTHER ROUTINE PRENATAL TESTS		
☐ RISK FACTORS IDENTIFIED BY PRENATAL HISTORY		
☐ ANTICIPATED COURSE OF PRENATAL CARE		
☐ NUTRITION AND WEIGHT GAIN COUNSELING		
☐ TOXOPLASMOSIS PRECAUTIONS (CATS/RAW MEAT)		
☐ SEXUAL ACTIVITY		
☐ EXERCISE		
☐ ENVIRONMENTAL/WORK HAZARDS		
☐ TRAVEL		
☐ TOBACCO (ASK, ADVISE, ASSESS, ASSIST, AND ARRANGE)		
☐ ALCOHOL		
☐ ILLICIT/RECREATIONAL DRUGS		
☐ USE OF ANY MEDICATIONS (INCLUDING SUPPLEMENTS, VITAMINS, HERBS, OR OTC DRUGS)		
☐ INDICATIONS FOR ULTRASOUND		
☐ DOMESTIC VIOLENCE		
☐ SEAT BELT USE		
☐ CHILDBIRTH CLASSES/HOSPITAL FACILITIES		
SECOND TRIMESTER		
☐ SIGNS AND SYMPTOMS OF PRETERM LABOR		
☐ ABNORMAL LAB VALUES		
☐ INFLUENZA VACCINE		
☐ SELECTING A PEDIATRICIAN		
☐ POSTPARTUM FAMILY PLANNING/TUBAL STERILIZATION		
THIRD TRIMESTER		
☐ ANESTHESIA/ANALGESIA PLANS		
☐ FETAL MOVEMENT MONITORING		
☐ LABOR SIGNS		
☐ VBAC COUNSELING		
☐ SIGNS AND SYMPTOMS OF PREGNANCY-INDUCED HYPERTENSION		
☐ POSTTERM COUNSELING		
☐ CIRCUMCISION		
☐ BREAST OR BOTTLE FEEDING		
☐ POSTPARTUM DEPRESSION		
☐ NEWBORN CAR SEAT		
☐ FAMILY MEDICAL LEAVE OR DISABILITY FORMS		
REQUESTS		

TUBAL STERILIZATION CONSENT SIGNED   DATE   INITIALS
                                   ___/___/___   _____

HISTORY AND PHYSICAL HAS BEEN SENT TO HOSPITAL, IF APPLICABLE.   DATE   INITIALS
                                   ___/___/___   _____

ACOG ANTEPARTUM RECORD (FORM E)

Version 5. Copyright © 2002 The American College of Obstetricians and Gynecologists, 409 12th Street, SW, PO Box 96920, Washington, DC 20090-6920   AA128   1 2 3 4 5 / 6 5 4 3 2

Plans/Education Notes

_____
_____
_____
_____
_____
_____
_____
_____
_____
_____
_____
_____
_____
_____
_____
_____
_____
_____
_____
_____
_____
_____
_____
_____
_____
_____
_____
_____
_____
_____
_____

ACOG ANTEPARTUM RECORD (FORM E, _continued_)

Appendix C
Assessment of Fetal Death

Physician Responsibilities	Nursing Responsibilities Page i

_____ Review of prenatal records and laboratory results
 	
_____ Maternal testing
    All patients
        ☐ Random glucose
        ☐ CBC with platelet count
        ☐ Antibody screen
        ☐ VDRL
        ☐ Kleihauer-Betke
        ☐ Urine toxicology screen
    Selected patients
        ☐ Thyroid function testing
        ☐ CMV titer (IgM, acute and convalescent IgG)
        ☐ Lupus anticoagulant/anticardiolipin antibody
 	
_____ Genetic w/u indicated _____/ contacted_____
 	
_____ Confirm completion of stillbirth/fetal examination (page ii) and placement on mother's chart
 	
Consents obtained:
    _____ Autopsy
    _____ Others (eg, photographs)
    _____
    _____
 	
_____ Placenta sent to pathology
 	
_____ Fetal death/stillborn autopsy form (page iii) completed
 	
Additional studies:
    _____ Photographs
    _____ Viral cultures
    _____ X-rays
    _____ Bacterial cultures
    _____ Others _____
    _____
	Saw baby: ☐ Mother ☐ Father ☐ Other
	
	Held baby: ☐ Mother ☐ Father ☐ Other
	
	Baby's name _____
	
	    _____ Keepsakes given to family by hospital:
	        ☐ Commemorative card
	        ☐ Footprints
	        ☐ Photo
	        ☐ Blanket
	        ☐ Bracelet
	        ☐ Tape measure
	        ☐ Baptismal card/blessing card
	        ☐ Referral to support organization
	        ☐ Lock of hair
	        ☐ Booklets (specify) _____
	        _____
	        _____
	        _____
	
	Unit chosen:
	    ☐ Ob ☐ Gyn
	
	Resources:
	    ☐ Social services ☐ Chaplain
	    ☐ Community support ☐ Mental health
	    groups
	
	☐ Burial options explained
	    Option chosen _____
	
	☐ Grief process explained to:
	    ☐ Mother ☐ Father ☐ Other
	
	☐ Address/telephone number on in-patient admission record verified for follow-up call
	
	Comments _____
	_____
	_____
	_____
	_____

(Continued)

Fetal Death/Stillborn Examination   Page ii

Key: +, present; –, absent; ?, unsure

Date _____

Weight _____   Head circumference _____   Crown–heel length (stretched) _____

General _____   Macerated _____   Intact _____

Other (describe) _____

Head
___ Normal
___ Hydrocephalic
___ Scalp defects
___ Anencephalic
___ Abnormal skull shape
___ Collapsed
___ Other (describe) _____
_____

Eyes
___ Normal
___ Close together
___ Far apart
___ Straight
___ Up slanting
___ Down slanting
___ Abnormally small
___ Abnormally large
___ Epicanthus
___ Other (describe) _____
_____

Nose
___ Normal
___ Other (describe) _____

Mouth
___ Normal
___ Cleft palate
___ Cleft lip
___ Large tongue
___ Small chin
___ Other (describe) _____
_____

Ears
___ Normal
___ Lowset (top below eyes)
___ Tags
___ Pits
___ Symmetric
___ Other (describe) _____
_____

Neck
___ Normal
___ Excess skin

Neck *(continued)*
___ Cystic mass
___ Other (describe) _____
_____

Chest
___ Normal
___ Asymmetric
___ Small
___ Other (describe) _____
_____

Abdomen
___ Normal
___ Distension
___ Omphalocele
___ Gastroschisis
___ Hernia
___ 3-vessel cord
___ Other (describe) _____
_____

Back
___ Normal
___ Spina bifida (defect level___)
___ Scoliosis
___ Kyphosis
___ Other (describe) _____
_____

Limbs
Length: nl, short, long
Form: nl, symmetric missing parts
Position: nl, abnl

Arms	Length	Form	Position
Right	_____	_____	_____
Left	_____	_____	_____

Legs	Length	Form	Position
Right	_____	_____	_____
Left	_____	_____	_____

Hands
Right
___ Fingers (#)
___ Webbing/syndactyly
___ Transverse crease
___ Other (describe) _____
_____

Hands *(continued)*
Left
___ Fingers (#)
___ Webbing/syndactyly
___ Transverse crease
___ Other (describe) _____
_____

Feet
Right
___ Toes (#)
___ Webbing
___ Wide space between toes 1-2
___ Other (describe) _____
_____

Left
___ Toes (#)
___ Webbing
___ Wide space between toes 1-2
___ Other (describe) _____
_____

Nails
___ Normal
___ Small (which ones?_____)
___ Other (describe) _____
_____

Genitalia
___ Normal
___ Imperforate anus
___ Ambiguous genitalia (describe)
_____

Male
___ Hypospadias
___ Chordee
___ Undescended testes
___ Other (describe) _____

Female
___ Normal urethral opening
___ Clitoromegaly
___ Other (describe) _____
_____

(Continued)

| **Fetal Death/Stillborn Autopsy** | Page iii |

To accompany body to morgue: Fill in as completely as possible

Date _____

Medical record # _____

Mother _____

Fetus _____

Name _____

LMP _____

Estimated gestational age_____Weeks

Gravida_____ Para_____ A_____ Living children_____

Ultrasound dx _____

_____

_____

Placenta examination _____

_____

_____

Cord examination _____

_____

_____

Cytogenetics obtained:

　Blood:　☐ Yes　☐ No

　Skin:　☐ Yes　☐ No

Alpha-fetoprotein _____

Prenatal assessment _____

Labor:

　Spontaneous _____

　Induced _____

Delivery:

　Date _____　Time _____

　Vaginal _____

　Cesarean _____

Pregnancy complications _____

_____

_____

_____

_____

Delivery complications _____

_____

_____

_____

Indication(s) for pathologic examination _____

_____

_____

_____

_____

Special requests for gross and microscopic evaluation

_____

_____

_____

Attending clinician _____

Phone number _____

Courtesy of Medical College of Virginia, Richmond.

Index